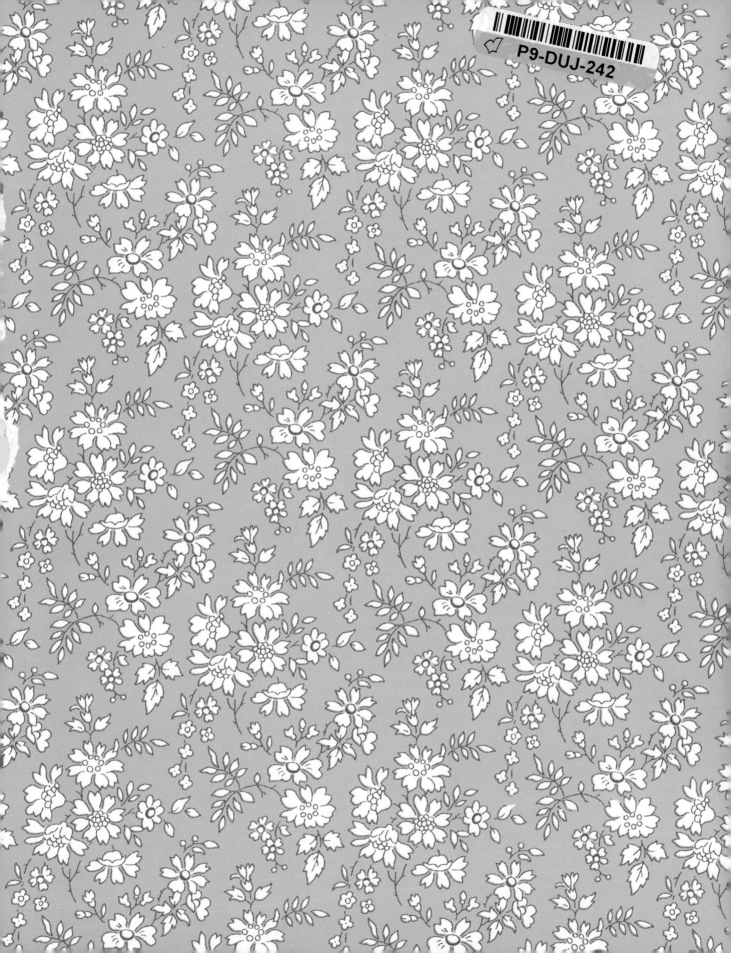

P9-DUJ-242

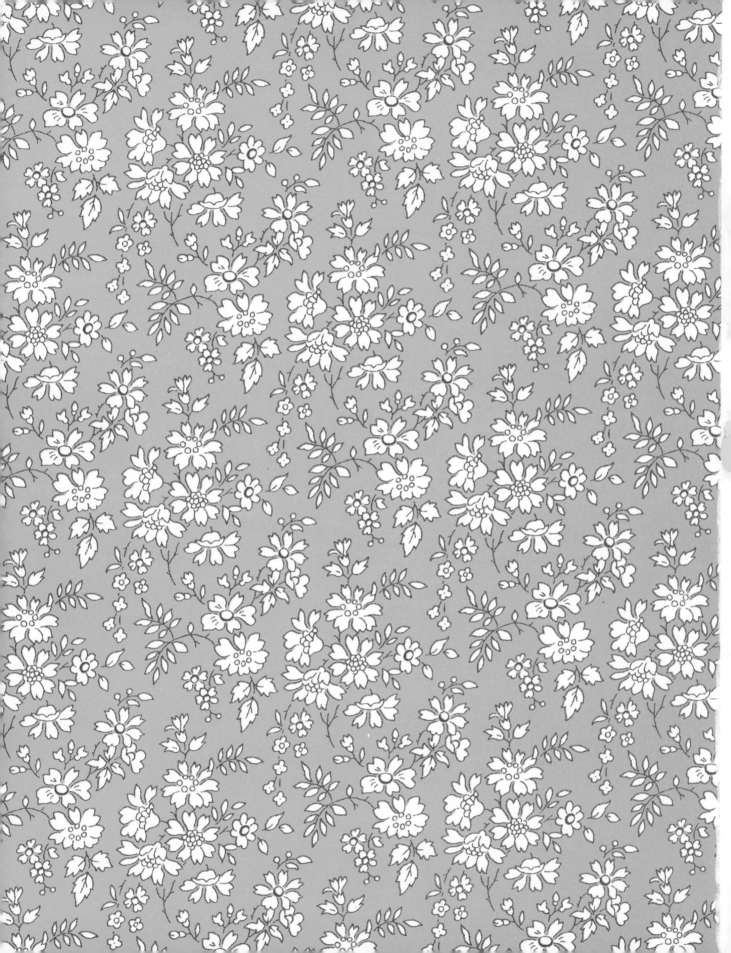

Small Plates & Sweet Treats

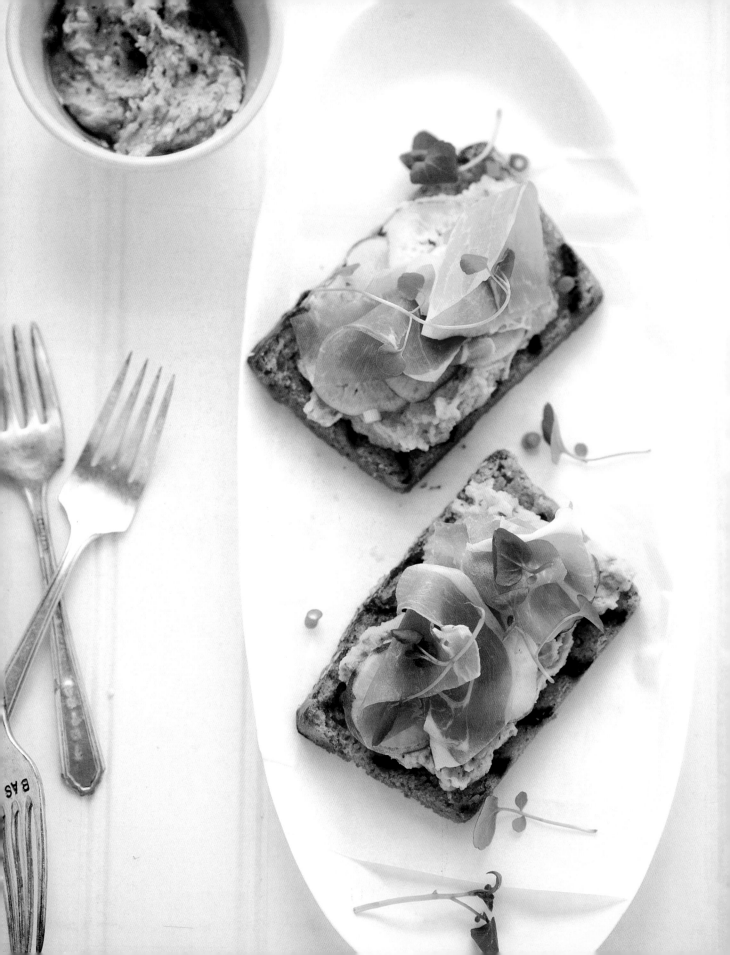

Small Plates & Sweet Treats

MY FAMILY'S JOURNEY TO
gluten-free cooking

Aran Goyoaga

CREATOR OF *cannelle et vanille*

LITTLE, BROWN AND COMPANY
NEW YORK BOSTON LONDON

This book is not intended as a substitute for the medical advice of physicians. The reader should regularly consult a physician in all matters relating to his or her health, and particularly with respect to any symptoms that may require diagnosis or medical attention.

Text and photographs copyright © 2012 by Aran Goyoaga

All rights reserved. In accordance with the US Copyright Act of 1976, the scanning, uploading, and electronic sharing of any part of this book without the permission of the publisher is unlawful piracy and theft of the author's intellectual property. If you would like to use material from the book (other than for review purposes), prior written permission must be obtained by contacting the publisher at permissions@hbgusa.com. Thank you for your support of the author's rights.

Little, Brown and Company
Hachette Book Group
237 Park Avenue, New York, NY 10017
www.littlebrown.com

First Edition: October 2012

Little, Brown and Company is a division of Hachette Book Group, Inc.
The Little, Brown name and logo are trademarks of Hachette Book Group, Inc.

The publisher is not responsible for websites (or their content) that are not owned by the publisher.

The Hachette Speakers Bureau provides a wide range of authors for speaking events. To find out more, go to www.hachettespeakersbureau.com or call (866) 376-6591.

Author photographs on pages viii and 224 copyright © 2012 by Lena Hyde
Photograph on page 90, top left, by Nadia Dole
Endpapers: Liberty fabric reproduced with permission from Liberty Ltd, London

Library of Congress Cataloging-in-Publication Data
Goyoaga, Aran.
    Small plates and sweet treats : my family's journey to gluten-free cooking / Aran Goyoaga.—1st ed.
        p. cm.
    Includes index.
    ISBN 978-0-316-18745-9
    1. Gluten-free diet—Recipes.   2. Gluten-free foods.   I. Title.
    RM237.86.G69 2012
    641.3—dc23   2011043637

10 9 8 7 6 5 4 3 2 1

Design by Laura Palese

Printed in China

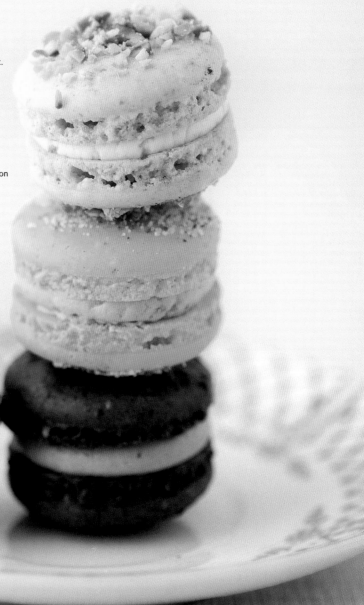

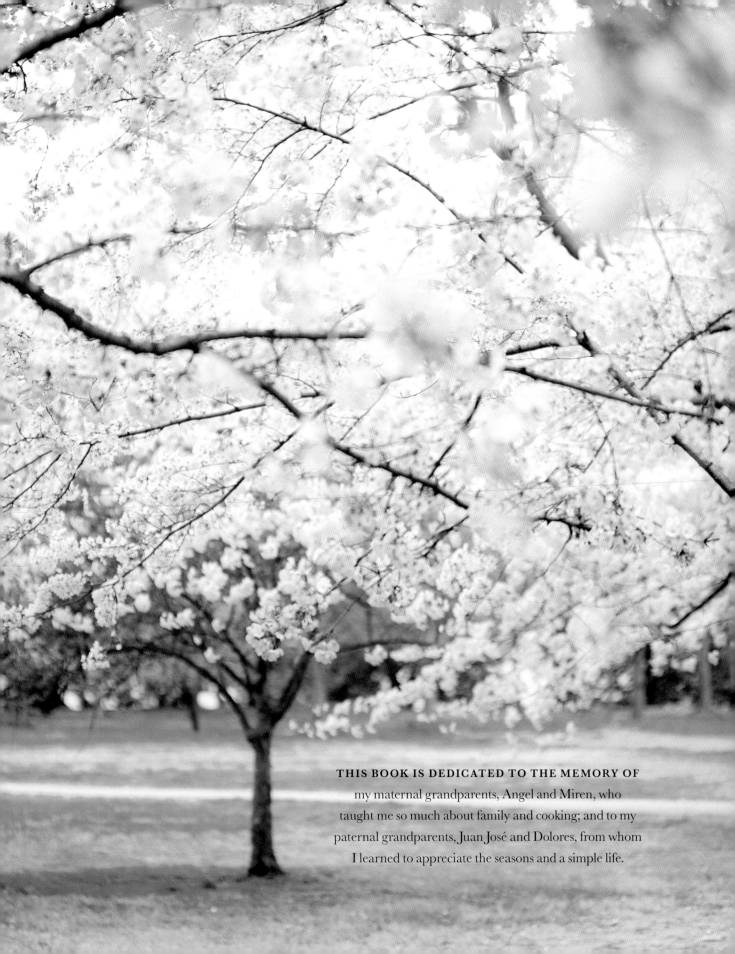

THIS BOOK IS DEDICATED TO THE MEMORY OF
my maternal grandparents, Angel and Miren, who
taught me so much about family and cooking; and to my
paternal grandparents, Juan José and Dolores, from whom
I learned to appreciate the seasons and a simple life.

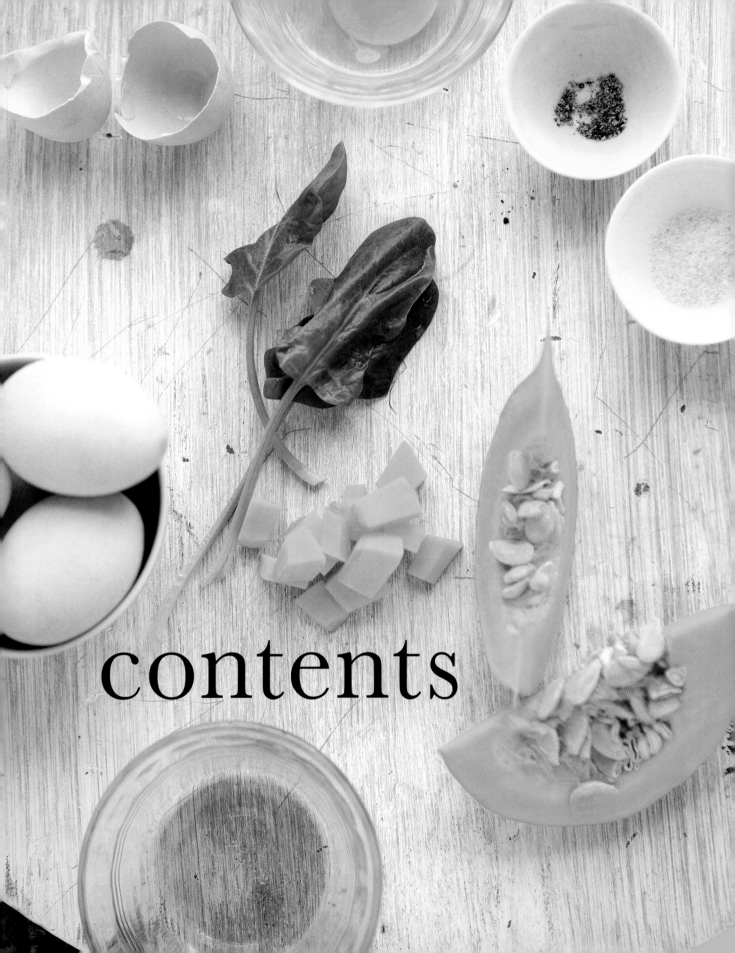

contents

autumn

small plates 23 · sweet treats 55

winter

small plates 91 · sweet treats 123

spring

small plates 155 · sweet treats 187

summer

small plates 225 · sweet treats 257

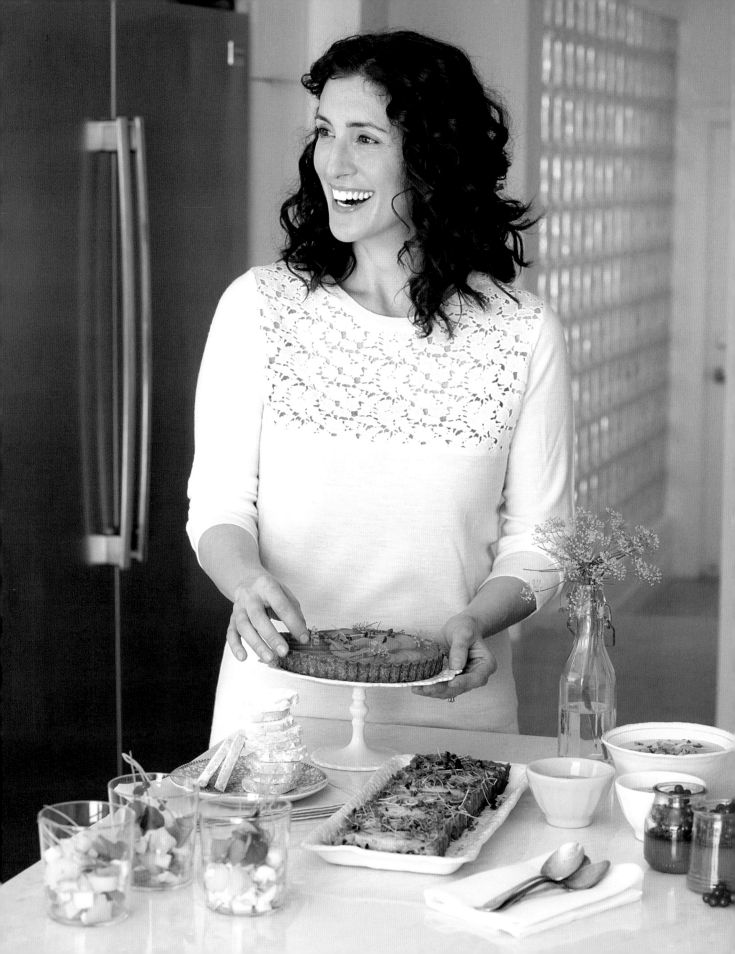

Small Plates &
Sweet Treats

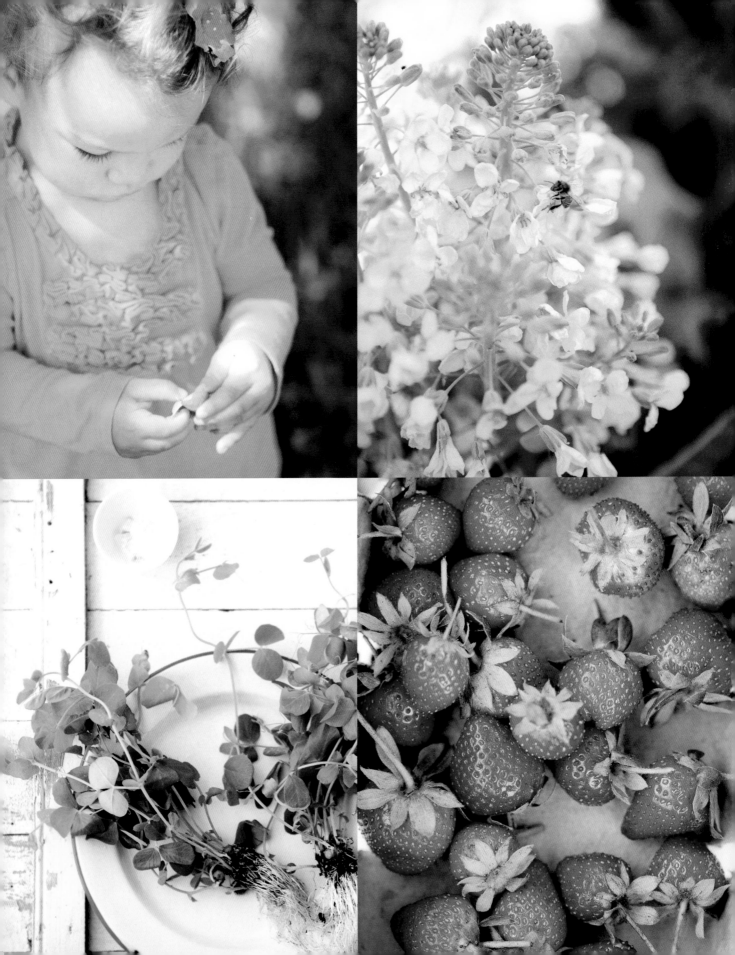

INTRODUCTION
a life in food

When I think about how I have arrived at this point in my life, writing recipes and photographing them, I can honestly say that it has been unexpected and, most likely, inevitable. My journey has had many turns, but somehow it has always led me into the kitchen. After all, I am the granddaughter, daughter, niece, and cousin of pastry chefs and farmers.

It all began in my maternal grandparents' pastry shop in the small town of Amorebieta, in the Basque Country, close to the border between Spain and France. My grandfather Angel, my grandmother Miren, and their eight children opened the shop in 1949. The place has undergone some renovations over the years, but the way I remember it is with its old wood counters and glass candy jars. There was a separate chocolate counter where we used to hide and watch the customers come and go. There were two kitchens behind the storefront. The main pastry kitchen, with all its ovens, mixers, and pastry equipment, was where most of the work was done. Right next to it there was the kitchen where my grandmother cooked. That was our main gathering place, where we ate our meals and where visitors were greeted. My grandparents built not only a family business but also a place where locals gathered.

When we weren't at school, we spent every waking minute of our days there. I remember the people coming and going, the bustling kitchen, and the sweet smell of milk simmering on the stove with cinnamon and vanilla. It was a meeting place for priests, radicals, artists, and anyone looking for great conversation and food. Tables that were used to fill cookies with buttercream and éclairs (*relámpagos* in Spanish) with pastry cream were quickly covered with flower-patterned oilcloth for an indoor picnic of *raciones* (small plates), *pintxos* (tapas), and sweet treats. Mismatched chairs and flatware scattered around the table gave a sense of casual cordiality, but food was never taken lightly.

There was also my paternal grandparents' farm in the village of Zeberio, which we visited religiously every Sunday. My grandfather Juan José took me into the chicken coop to collect eggs and into the barn to milk the cows. I loved exploring the woods behind their home and helping my grandmother Dolores in the garden, harvesting whatever the season had to offer. Calabaza squash and figs in the autumn, leeks and hearty potatoes in the winter, peas in the spring, and the sweetest wild strawberries and tomatoes in the summer were among the treasures we gathered.

I loved the feeling of cold soil in my hands and even the smell of manure—nature drew me in. From my grandparents I learned about the seasons, about foraging, and about preserving foods. They were poor and led a very modest life, but they also shared a love of food and family.

The concept of eating and entertaining with small plates is deeply rooted in Basque culture. The street where I grew up, which is no longer than 300 yards, is home to thirteen bars and restaurants. Every one of them competes to claim the best *pintxos*, *raciones*, and *bocadillos* (baguette sandwiches) in town. Sunday mornings, before lunchtime (which doesn't usually get going until 3:00 in the afternoon), people walk from bar to bar sampling the offerings of wine and food. Bar counters become mouthwatering displays of nibbles and small plates of the best produce, fish, and meat of the region. It's a kaleidoscope of fresh flavors and textures.

●

I was always obsessed with food, both eating it and making it. One of my earliest food memories is of helping my grandmother and my mom prepare Christmas Eve dinner. I stood on a green wooden stool dipping canned artichokes in egg wash and flour, handing them to my mom, who was frying them for her lamb stew. I liked working with my hands, and I liked the mood in the kitchen and how happy it made everyone feel. With time I earned my mom's trust, and I was put in charge of preparing weekend lunches for the family. At times, our kitchen table sat up to fifteen people—my grandparents, my parents, older brothers Jokin and Jon, uncles, and aunts. I loved to feed them all. Plates were my blank canvas, and I was fascinated by the shape and form of food. I stacked salads, used fresh herbs as garnishes, whisked unusual vinaigrettes, and looked for lots of texture in my food.

In spite of being very much aware of this passion for cooking, I never thought it might become my profession. I went on to study business and economics. In October 1998, after graduation from college, I packed two suitcases with some clothes and cookbooks and moved across the Atlantic to marry my love, Chad. I felt torn between my strong family ties and the new life that I had started in the United States. Cooking kept me grounded and close to my family back home.

I soon realized that this was not a mere hobby. I took a leap of faith and enrolled in culinary school. Shortly thereafter, I landed at the pastry kitchen of the Ritz-Carlton Palm Beach, where I worked for three years—the most intense, creative, and enriching years of my life. I lived and breathed flour, butter, and sugar—a dream come true.

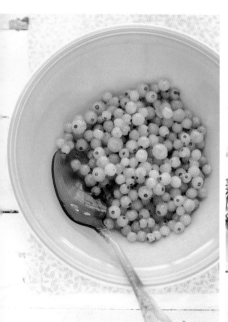
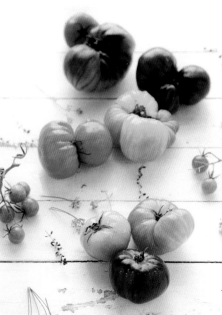
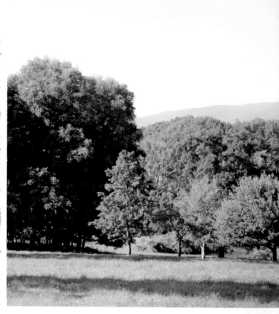

When my son, Jon, was born in the summer of 2006, I left the life of a professional cook to focus on motherhood. Of course, cooking was still a daily affair, but I missed spending time baking the way I had in a professional kitchen. However, I was extremely anxious about the idea of returning to that intense environment. Then, an e-mail I received from my friend Robyn changed the course of my life.

"Check out this blog," she wrote, followed by a link to Cupcake Bakeshop in San Francisco. I had no idea what a blog was, but I was mesmerized. "A website dedicated to recipe and story collection where people can comment? I want to do that!" In January 2008 I started my blog. I named it Cannelle et Vanille (cinnamon and vanilla) after the smells of my childhood. The blog was full of nostalgia, family stories, and baking recipes. I soon developed a small but loyal following and spent hours happily answering questions about macarons and the like. My dedication to the blog has been a constant, and I am writing this book in great part thanks to it.

becoming gluten-free

After my daughter, Miren, was born in 2009, I developed a series of debilitating health issues, vertigo being the worst of them all. I was diagnosed with Hashimoto's thyroiditis and autoimmune inner-ear disorder, which triggered the vertigo attacks followed by tinnitus and hearing loss. I was bedridden for days at a time, unable to drive or, more significantly, take care of my children. In a six-month span, my parents flew out twice to look after us. I was desperate.

After several months of weekly visits to doctors and extensive testing, I was diagnosed with gluten intolerance. I felt such relief to know that gluten—something tangible that I could eliminate from my life at once—was the cause of all these symptoms. Because there is a strong genetic component to this condition, I also tested my son, Jon. As I suspected, he was also gluten intolerant. Doctors explained to me that a person can be gluten intolerant and never show any of the typical gastrointestinal symptoms. Instead, years of inflammation caused by gluten consumption can result in chronic illness or even cancer. This put things in perspective. It was time for all of us to adopt a new lifestyle.

My best friend, Jill, and her family had been living gluten-free for years, so I was well aware of the dangers of hidden gluten. She was the person I turned to with questions. Very quickly, with her guidance, we converted our kitchen into a gluten-free space. I donated all of my wheat flours, pasta, soy sauce, oats, and anything else that contained gluten to friends and neighbors. Food labels took on a greater importance than ever before. Eating out became tricky, and I didn't trust anyone; the memory of sudden vertigo attacks was too recent. As it turned out, this has been a blessing in disguise. We cook at home more than we used to and reserve eating out for special chefs and restaurants we admire and trust.

The first time I stood in the gluten-free aisle at my local health-food store, I felt a rush of excitement. I love shopping for food more than anything else, and here was a whole new world of ingredients ready for experimentation. I loaded my shopping cart with quinoa, amaranth, buckwheat, and teff flour—I couldn't wait to bake my first cake.

Once I got into gluten-free baking there was quite a bit of trial and error, but for the most part I discovered that it was easy to convert my favorite recipes. I developed a sense for it even though I couldn't explain the science behind it. "These coconut doughnuts are some of the best I have ever had," my friend Karen said when I stopped by with a batch of freshly fried dough. "I cannot believe they are gluten-free." Hearing words like these felt like a victory.

The transition to gluten-free cooking was never too challenging for me because the Basque cooking of my childhood relies mainly on fresh ingredients cooked very simply. Besides gluten in breads and some breaded recipes, gluten rarely makes it into the dishes I grew up eating. The food I began cooking for my new family was similar—lots of legumes, vegetables, and fish. And we never felt deprived. In fact, it has always been my goal to focus on all the new foods and treats we can enjoy rather than to emphasize the things we have to give up.

When making Jon's favorite meal of pasta and crushed tomatoes, I turned to quinoa spaghetti, which closely mimics the texture of traditional wheat pasta. I found great gluten-free bread from which I made mini cheese toasties to accompany the bowls of lentil soup my kids enjoy so much.

The blog, which has always been a reflection of my life, started to mirror the shift into our new lifestyle. As I incorporated gluten-free recipes, I began to notice my readership increasing. I received e-mails from readers who were going through similar experiences, and I was happy to let them know about my personal journey. There was a whole world of people out there looking to eat healthy, and gluten-free, without compromising flavor or texture. I was delighted to take on the challenge.

This book is an homage to the endless possibilities of gluten-free cooking and baking. I have learned so much during this incredible journey, and now it is my turn to share.

how to use this book

I have structured this book to reflect the bounty of the seasons and the way we cook at home. In autumn, winter squash, heirloom apples, and hearty meat-and-bean stews make it to our table. Roasted root vegetables and dark leafy greens comfort us in winter. Spring is all about tender baby vegetables and blossoms. And summer brings a flavorful bounty of deep red berries, curly heirloom tomatoes, and fresh-caught fish. Your farmers' market should guide your cooking.

In these pages you will find ideas, techniques, and styling tips, like how to cook a perfect soft-boiled egg, a creamy and versatile risotto, or the coveted Parisian macarons. There are many notes on how to easily adapt recipes using alternative ingredients you have at hand. Nothing makes me happier than knowing my recipes inspire others to experiment in the kitchen.

I conceived the recipes to be served in smaller portions, just like the *pintxos* and small plates you will find in many restaurants and homes in the Basque Country—a symphony of small dishes with varying textures and complementary flavors. These are dishes I cook for friends or when I make lunch for myself, both of which are equally important. When I entertain a crowd, I look to serve food in such a way that I do not feel like a slave in my own kitchen. I set up a buffet-style table with individual dishes filled with soup, salads, or a paper cone filled with *patatas bravas* (spicy potatoes; page 128). Most of these recipes can be prepared ahead of time.

There is always one dish that will be the highlight of the meal, and I keep everything else around it in harmony. The whole Roasted Red Snapper with Potatoes, Shaved Fennel & Shiso (page 247) always makes an impact. I surround that with dishes that are complementary, like small bowls of Grilled Corn & Herb Chowder (page 229) and squares of Heirloom Cherry Tomato Focaccia (page 226).

The sweet treats are adaptations of some of my favorite desserts and are full of flavor and texture from the whole-grain and nut flours that I use. They are the treats we enjoy at home regularly and that always engage my children in the kitchen. They are also quick to assemble and have a strong seasonal component.

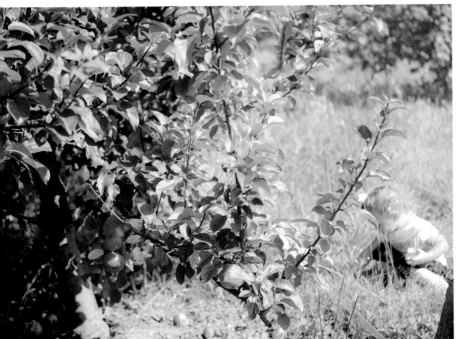
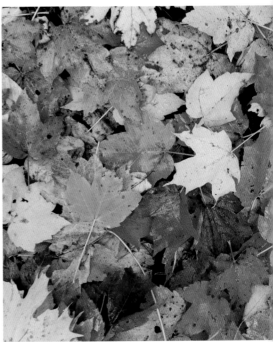

All my baking recipes use naturally gluten-free flours, but if you are in a pinch and have no issues with gluten-containing grains, you can convert the recipes by adding the gluten-free flour amounts together (by weight, not volume) and substituting your all-purpose flour for the combined amount. By doing so, the texture and color of the final dish might vary slightly from my preparation, but overall the recipes are very forgiving and will adapt easily.

rolling out tart dough

From the conversations I have had with friends and novice bakers, I sense that many people are intimidated by rolling pastry dough. The words *Do not overmix or the dough will become tough* seem to be engraved in everyone's minds. The truth is that, yes, dough should never really be worked too hard or for too long if you want to maintain the right texture. However, you should never be scared of the dough. It needs to be rolled and moved around.

As you will see, this book is filled with savory and sweet tart recipes. Before you begin cooking from this book, read these tips about how to roll pastry dough.

To get a little technical, the gluten protein in wheat flour (as well as in other grains), once combined with water, starts to form infinite strands of protein that give elasticity to dough. This is a good thing, because it allows us to roll dough without it falling apart. On the other hand, if these proteins are worked too much, too many strands of protein are formed, resulting in tough doughs and crusts. In gluten-free baking, however, the challenge can be the opposite: not having enough binding proteins to give the dough the elasticity it needs to roll. Adding gums such as xanthan gum and guar gum can help. My preference is not to add any gums to tart doughs, though. I do not like the resulting texture as much.

Sometimes when rolling out gluten-free tart dough, I find that after the dough has chilled and the butter has solidified it tends to crack a bit. If your dough is cracking too much, let it warm up a bit and simply bring it together into a ball and quickly knead it again a couple of times. This brings back a bit more elasticity. But do not let it get too warm and soft or it will just fall apart.

Chill it if needed, and then quickly roll the dough again, making sure to dust your (preferably cold) work surface and rolling pin with a bit of superfine brown rice flour. Start pressing in the center and roll outward. Turn the dough 90 degrees every couple of rolls to keep it from sticking to the work surface.

Roll the dough around the rolling pin and lift it over the tart mold. Lay it flat on top and tuck in the edges. Cut off excess dough with a paring knife, pressing it against the top of the mold. Gently press the dough against the sides of the mold.

It's very important to chill the rolled dough once it's in the mold, before baking, so that the butter solidifies.

And it's as simple as that!

ingredients

This is a list of some of the ingredients you will find throughout this book, most of which I keep in my pantry at all times.

flours, starches, and gums

ALMOND FLOUR is produced by finely grinding raw, blanched almonds. It adds protein and fat to baked goods and is great for cookies, tarts, cakes, muffins, and baking in general. You can make it at home if you wish, but make sure it is finely ground or the texture of the finished recipe will be significantly different.

AMARANTH FLOUR is produced from finely grinding amaranth, which, like quinoa, is not a true grain but rather a leafy plant that is coveted both for its seeds and its edible leaves. The flour is high in protein and fiber and adds a nutty flavor to baked goods.

BUCKWHEAT FLOUR has a rich brown color and a nutty flavor, is high in fiber, and has many nutrients. I like to blend it with milder flours. It is delicious paired with chocolate and fruit. Buckwheat is actually a fruit seed that is related to rhubarb and sorrel and is not a true grain.

CHESTNUT FLOUR can be purchased in specialty shops or online. It is widely used in Italian cooking and is quickly becoming one of my favorite ingredients. Even in small amounts it adds a warm, nutty flavor. I love it in cakes and pancakes.

CHIA SEEDS are the new superfood. They are very rich in omega-3 fatty acids, even more so than flaxseeds. And they are so rich in antioxidants that the seeds don't deteriorate and can be stored for long periods without becoming rancid. When mixed with water, they turn into a gel, which acts as a binder. It somewhat mimics xanthan gum, so I use it in yeast breads that need a bit of extra structural support.

COCONUT FLOUR is high in protein and fiber and produces very tender and flavorful baked goods. When coconut flour is added to a batter, the batter will thicken very quickly, as this flour absorbs much more water than other flours. Generally, when substituting coconut flour, the recipe's moisture content must be increased by 20 percent.

CORN FLOUR has a finer texture than cornmeal, resulting in not-so-crumbly baked goods.

FLAXSEED MEAL is rich in omega-3s and, when mixed with water, can be used in lieu of eggs in baked goods.

HAZELNUT FLOUR is produced by finely grinding hazelnuts. It has tiny brown specks from the skin, and it is my favorite nut flour.

MILLET FLOUR has a bright yellow color and a subtle, sweet taste. It's great in muffins and cakes.

OAT FLOUR is naturally gluten-free, but because of the way it is processed in the United States, it is a highly gluten-contaminated grain. Look for certified gluten-free oat flour if you are sensitive to cross-contamination. It is great for cookies, scones, and muffins.

POTATO STARCH is used as a thickener and creates great texture in baked goods.

QUINOA FLAKES are produced from steam-rolled quinoa. They add great texture to muffins, cakes, and cookies. It is also one of my go-to porridge ingredients.

QUINOA FLOUR is also one of my favorite flours because of its distinct flavor and high protein content. Made from the quinoa seed, which is a pseudo-grain or leafy plant, the flour is great in both savory and sweet baking.

SORGHUM FLOUR is a slightly sweet high-protein flour that is great in cookies and tart crusts, as it has a crumbly texture when baked. Its mildness adds no distinct flavor.

SUPERFINE BROWN RICE FLOUR is my favorite flour by far. It is very finely ground, so unlike most brown rice flours it does not yield a gritty and crumbly texture. It also adds a slightly sweet and nutty flavor. I have only been able to find it through Authentic Foods (www.authenticfoods.com). If you only have access to brown rice flour, you can use that instead, but the texture of your baked goods will be crumblier. I especially prefer superfine brown rice flour to the regular stuff for tart crusts and cookies.

SWEET RICE FLOUR, also known as glutinous flour, has a higher starch content than other rice flours. I use it predominately to thicken sauces and as the base for my roux.

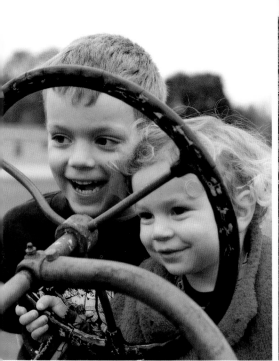

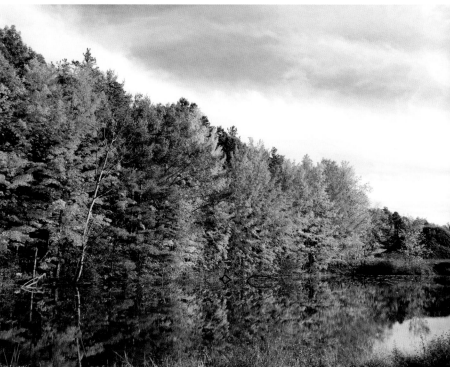

TAPIOCA STARCH is also a thickener; in baked goods it creates great crusts.

TEFF FLOUR, widely used in Ethiopian cooking, has a malty flavor and pale brown color. Because of its distinctive and deep taste, it pairs well with nuts and chocolate. I love it for muffins and quick breads.

XANTHAN GUM is a plant-based gum that mimics gluten. I personally prefer not to use it, as I find it hard to digest, and it tends to turn baked goods rather gummy. However, there are instances when a small amount is necessary and goes a long way. My basic brioche recipe on page 124 is the only recipe in this book that uses it.

sweeteners

COCONUT PALM SUGAR has the lowest glycemic index of any sugar. It has a deep caramel color, does not absorb moisture as much as light brown sugar does, and imparts a wonderful caramel taste. I like to use it in recipes with chocolate, caramel, and nuts.

DARK BROWN SUGAR is a darker variation of light brown sugar, made with additional molasses.

DARK MUSCOVADO SUGAR is an unrefined cane sugar that is darker, stickier, and coarser than brown sugar. It adds moisture and shelf life to baked goods and goes well with chocolate, coffee, and caramel.

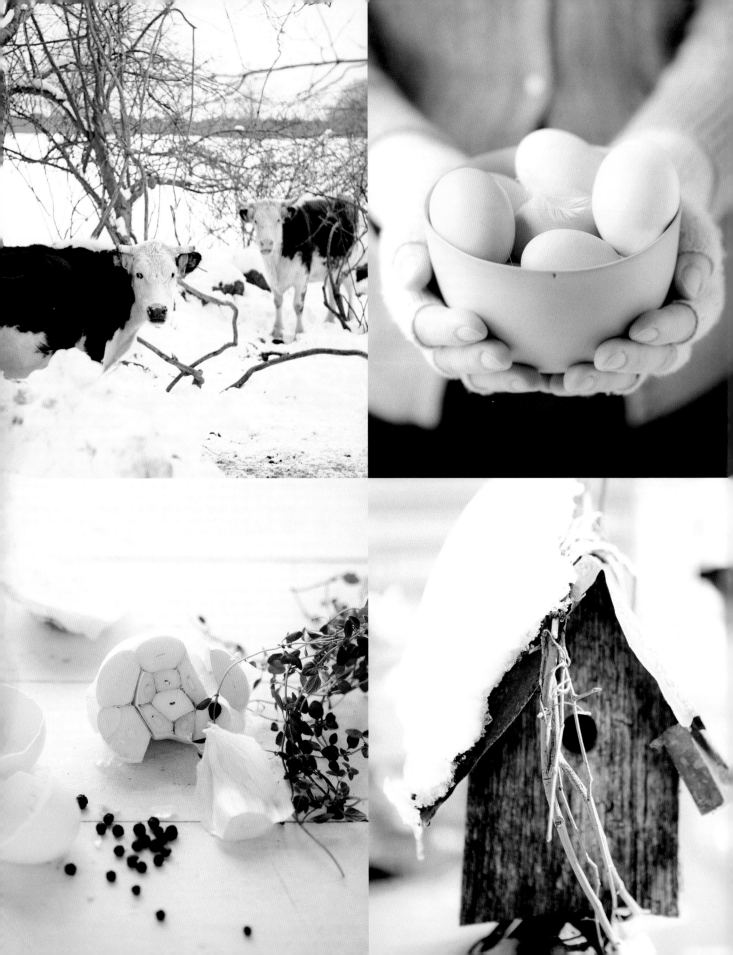

DEMERARA SUGAR, also known as *natural brown sugar*, is an unrefined cane sugar that is produced by extracting the juice from sugarcane. It has tiny, light amber–colored sugar crystals. I like to use it to make caramel or to sprinkle on top of baked goods.

HONEY is an ingredient that I purchase at the farmers' market. I like to use raw honey.

LIGHT BROWN SUGAR is refined cane sugar with molasses added back after processing. It has a light brown color and a sandy, moist texture.

NATURAL CANE SUGAR, also known as *unrefined sugar*, is my everyday sugar. It is slightly coarser than granulated white sugar, but they can be used interchangeably.

POWDERED OR CONFECTIONERS' SUGAR is a superfine sugar that usually contains a starch that works as an anti-caking agent. I use it in recipes when I need the sugar to be absorbed quickly into the other ingredients. I also like to dust some on top of finished desserts.

SUPERFINE SUGAR, also known as *caster sugar*, is a fine-grain sugar used in recipes in which sugar needs to be quickly absorbed into the rest of the ingredients. I use it mainly for meringues or ice creams when the sugar is not to be heated. It eliminates any gritty sugar particles in the finished dish.

salts

FINE SEA SALT is my everyday salt. Any time you see *salt* listed in this book, it refers to fine sea salt. Most of the time I use fine Celtic sea salt, which is harvested by hand from the Atlantic coastal region of Brittany, France. It is minimally processed and very high in minerals. It is moist and slightly gray in color. I like how evenly it distributes in baking recipes.

FLEUR DE SEL, which literally means "flower of salt," is the other salt I use, mainly as a garnish or to top finished dishes. It is harvested by hand in France, also around Brittany, by scraping only the top layer of the salt that remains from evaporating seawater. It is very delicate and flaky, and it retains its crunchy texture.

oils

COCONUT OIL is something I always have in my pantry. For baking I use refined coconut oil, as virgin coconut oil burns easily.

EXTRA-VIRGIN OLIVE OIL is the staple in my cooking. My mom always cooked with olive oil, whether it was for frying, baking, or dressing. I try to have several varieties on hand, including a good-quality all-purpose oil, and then other richer and more delicate oils for salads or for finishing dishes. I shop for Spanish oils because they are the ones I am most familiar with. Olive oil made with Arbequina olives is one of my favorite fruity oils for salads.

OTHER OILS, such as pistachio, hazelnut, truffle, or pumpkin oil, are great for drizzling over soups and salads or for finishing pasta dishes. They tend to be a bit pricey, but a little bit goes a long way.

chocolate

When I worked in pastry, I was exposed to many different chocolate makers, and I learned to appreciate the subtle differences between brands. I became accustomed to couverture, which is what most professionals use. Couverture is chocolate with a higher percentage of cocoa butter than other chocolates, and so it has a smoother mouthfeel and a better snap. It is harder to find and more expensive, but I still use it.

I buy chocolate in blocks and then I chop it as needed. I keep the blocks tightly wrapped, away from moisture and heat, and they tend to last a while, although it is true that I go through a lot of chocolate every month. Valrhona, El Rey, and Callebaut are the brands I use the most.

BITTERSWEET CHOCOLATE is chocolate liquor with cocoa butter, sugar, and sometimes lecithin added to it. It is the least sweet variety, and I like to use it when I am looking for an intense chocolate flavor.

BLACK COCOA POWDER is one of my latest finds. This super-dark, super-rich Dutch-process cocoa makes very moist and gooey cakes and cookies. It is normally used in combination with regular Dutch-process cocoa powder, but I like to use it alone as well. Expect intense black color in your baked goods.

COCOA POWDER is produced by pulverizing roasted cocoa beans. This simple process maintains the natural acidity of chocolate, and often the package in the store will be labeled *natural cocoa powder*. On the other hand, Dutch-process cocoa powder has been treated with an alkali to neutralize that acidity. The main difference is that natural cocoa powder is used along with baking soda, which reacts to an acid, while Dutch-process cocoa powder must be used with baking powder (unless there is another acid present in the recipe, in which case you can also use baking soda).

MILK CHOCOLATE has more sugar and milk powder added than other chocolates. I find that milk chocolate is great with very sour fruits, such as lemons or passion fruit.

SEMISWEET CHOCOLATE has more sugar than the bittersweet variety. Bittersweet and semisweet are great in combination.

WHITE CHOCOLATE contains no chocolate liquor. It contains, milk, sugar, and cocoa butter, and that is why sometimes it is said that it is not a true chocolate. Personally, I am not a big fan of white chocolate in large quantities, as I find it very sweet, but I think it works well paired with very tart fruits and in small amounts. Be sure to buy white chocolate with cocoa butter; some brands substitute vegetable fat.

spices and vanilla beans

SPICES should be purchased whole and in small amounts to keep them fresh and full of flavor. I like to grind them myself in a dedicated coffee grinder right before use, as this is the best way to take advantage of the fresh oils and aromas that grinding releases.

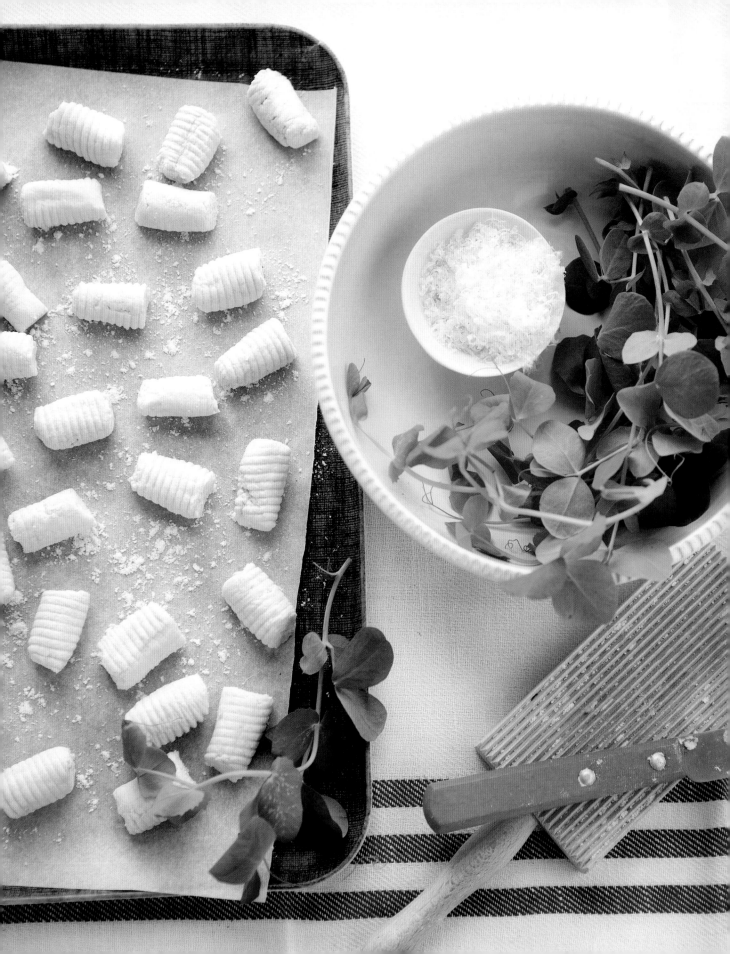

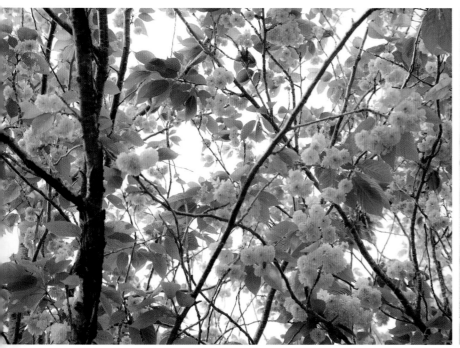
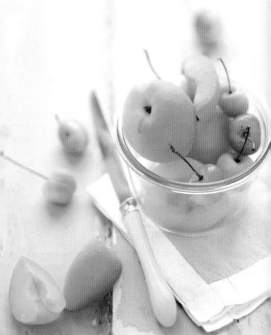

VANILLA BEANS are another luxury that I think make a world of difference in any recipe. Stay away from the small, dried-up vanilla beans sold at most major supermarkets. Buy them in bulk from specialty shops or online and store them in vacuum-sealed packages. Make sure they are deep in color, pliable, and plump. The flesh should be sticky and full of a million tiny seeds. There are many varieties, with different aromas and flavor notes depending on their country of origin. I encourage you to try different varieties to find the ones you prefer. To get the most out of your bean of choice, see Reusing Vanilla Beans (page 132).

coconut milk

COCONUT MILK is produced by combining the flesh of coconuts with water. It is very high in fat and is great to bake with and to add to soups and stews. In my recipes, I use canned, full-fat, unsweetened coconut milk. As it sits, the fat and water separate, so before opening a can of coconut milk, you must vigorously shake it to bring it back to a homogeneous mixture. I like to use it in place of heavy cream in many recipes.

dried beans

DRIED BEANS are a staple in my pantry. I cook with them at least twice a week. Beans are a great way to get protein in your diet without having to eat too much meat or fish. Because larger dried beans, such as cannellini, flageolet, or pinto, require hours of

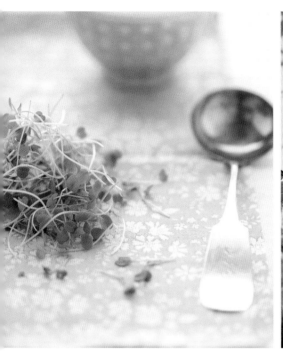
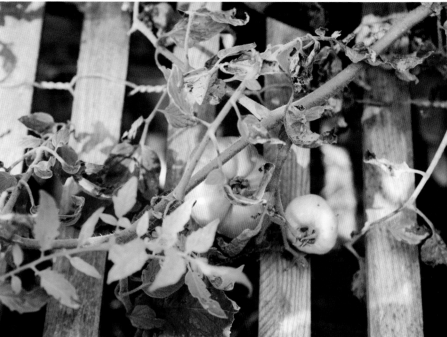

presoaking, there is some planning ahead that must be done, but they are very simple to cook and are perfect for slow cookers. On the other hand, smaller beans such as lentils do not require presoaking, which makes them great for last-minute dinners. Ivory and red lentils in particular take only about 20 minutes to cook and French green lentils approximately 40 minutes. I also cook with canned beans at home for quick dinners and dips that I can assemble in minutes, though starting with dried beans nearly always means better flavor and texture.

eggs

It is my dream to buy a little piece of land where I can raise my own chickens, where they can roam free and I can collect fresh eggs every morning. Until that becomes a reality for my family, I buy eggs from local farmers, such as the Farriss Farm in Palm Beach Country Estates, which is near my home. All the eggs used in my recipes come from Robert and Paula's free-range chickens. The eggs come in a variety of colors and sizes, and their deep orange yolks make my tortillas look golden and irresistible.

If you have access to fresh farm eggs, I encourage you to support your local farmers. The difference that fresh eggs provide in taste and color is remarkable. Although the eggs I buy are rarely identical in size, choose large eggs when buying store-bought eggs for the recipes in this book.

kitchen equipment

When I am asked what my favorite kitchen tools are, I always reply, "my sharp knives and a clean counter." I shy away from gadgets, as clutter only aggravates my obsessive-compulsive behavior in the kitchen. It is probably due to being raised in a super-organized pastry kitchen, followed by years of training under rigorous French and German chefs.

Most people probably don't know that in a professional kitchen you must bring your own knives and kitchen utensils. Everything must be clearly labeled, as there are always "kitchen thieves" who are out to steal the $100 chef's knife you just finished sharpening or the ring molds you brought back from Paris. It happens all the time. My toolbox was, and still is, a large red metal Craftsman box with four sliding drawers. Home-improvement shops can be a cook's best friend. Most of the tools we used for chocolate work, such as putty knives, large metal rulers, and sharp cutters, were from home-improvement stores. That Craftsman box was always neatly organized and always, always locked.

After my grandfather Angel passed away in 2002, the only things I really wanted that belonged to him were the old tart molds—black metal tart molds that are probably more than fifty years old. My mom was able to take some from the pastry shop and keep them for me. Seasoned with all those years of butter-filled puff pastry shells, these tart molds remain my most precious treasures.

BAKING SHEETS: I have a large stack of aluminum half sheet pans that are 13 by 18 inches. They fit perfectly in my oven and also in my refrigerator.

A FOOD PROCESSOR is helpful for making tart crusts and grinding nuts, cheese, and vegetables. Mine is a Cuisinart.

AN ICE CREAM MACHINE: I don't know what I would do without an ice cream machine, since I love homemade ice creams and sorbets. Mine is the basic Cuisinart model, the bowl of which has to be frozen for 24 hours prior to churning ice cream. It is not the fastest or most convenient, but it is a great machine for its price.

A KITCHEN SCALE, preferably digital, is one of the most important tools in a baker's kitchen. Weighing your ingredients ensures perfect results every time. Don't believe me? Try this: Give a measuring cup to three different people and ask them to measure 1 cup of quinoa flour. Each person will end up with dramatically different weights, which ultimately means that they will end up with completely different recipes. Scales are readily available and inexpensive. Try to purchase one that reads both grams and ounces. If you choose to continue baking with measuring cups and spoons, always spoon flour into the measuring cup. Do not use the measuring cup to scoop the flour, as it tends to compact it, yielding a much higher weight.

A LOAF PAN: I find that gluten-free baked goods need extra help when rising, and a loaf pan that is a bit narrower and taller than the average pan is a great help. King Arthur Flour makes one that I use the most for cakes and breads. I purchased it online (www.kingarthurflour.com), and it is 9 by 4 by 4 inches.

A MANDOLINE is a lifesaver for salads or making homemade root vegetable chips, and it's a tool that any food stylist must have. If you have never seen one, it is a utensil that consists of two parallel attachments, one of them adjustable in height, that is used to slice and cut vegetables thinly and evenly. It usually comes with different cutting attachments. The blade is extremely sharp.

PASTRY BAGS AND TIPS: I use pastry bags and tips not only to decorate cakes and cupcakes but also to pipe fillings into tarts and cake batters into baking cups. It makes the job faster and less messy. There are disposable plastic pastry bags, but I prefer the reusable plastic-coated ones. I have an assortment of pastry tips. The plain and star tips are the ones I use the most.

RING MOLDS are useful for building individual mousse cakes and *petits gâteaux*. They are not indispensable but are good to have handy. To release the cakes easily, the inside must be lined with parchment paper or acetate paper, also sold in specialty shops.

A ROLLING PIN is indispensable for making tarts. I own several different rolling pins, but my advice is to test them in the shop to see how they feel in your hands.

SILICONE MATS AND MOLDS are great for baking cookies and cakes. My silicone mats fit half sheet pans. They are easy to wash, but remember never to cut on them. I also have an assortment of mini silicone molds that I use mainly to bake *financiers* and madeleines. These are available in specialty kitchen shops or online.

A STAND MIXER is a fixture on my kitchen counter. I use it for beating eggs for cakes, whipping heavy cream, creaming butter and sugar for cookies, and kneading bread dough. If you don't have one, a handheld mixer will work. I have a white 6-quart KitchenAid that has been my loyal friend for almost ten years now.

TART MOLDS: I own every shape and size of tart mold imaginable, but as a basic rule I recommend having a 9-inch tart mold and several 4-inch individual tartlet molds, both kinds with removable bottoms. All of these molds can be found in specialty kitchen shops or online.

•

When I was writing this book, I had an electric stove. I wished for a gas one, but it just didn't happen. All the times noted in the recipes may vary depending on the stove you have. Use your judgment, trust your gut, and follow your taste buds. You will not go wrong!

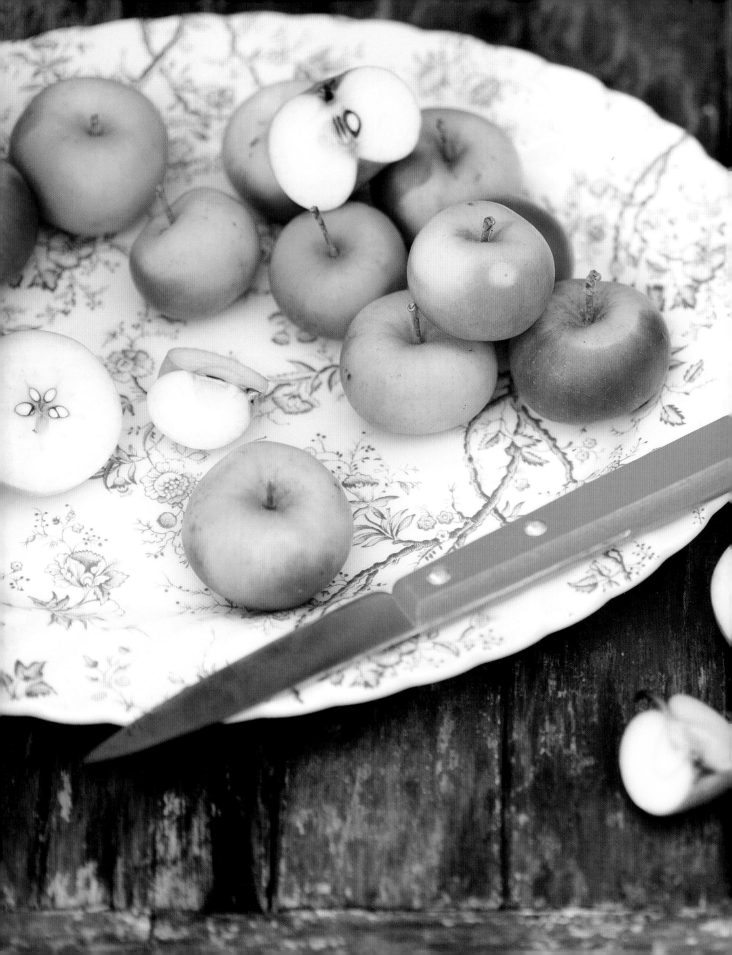

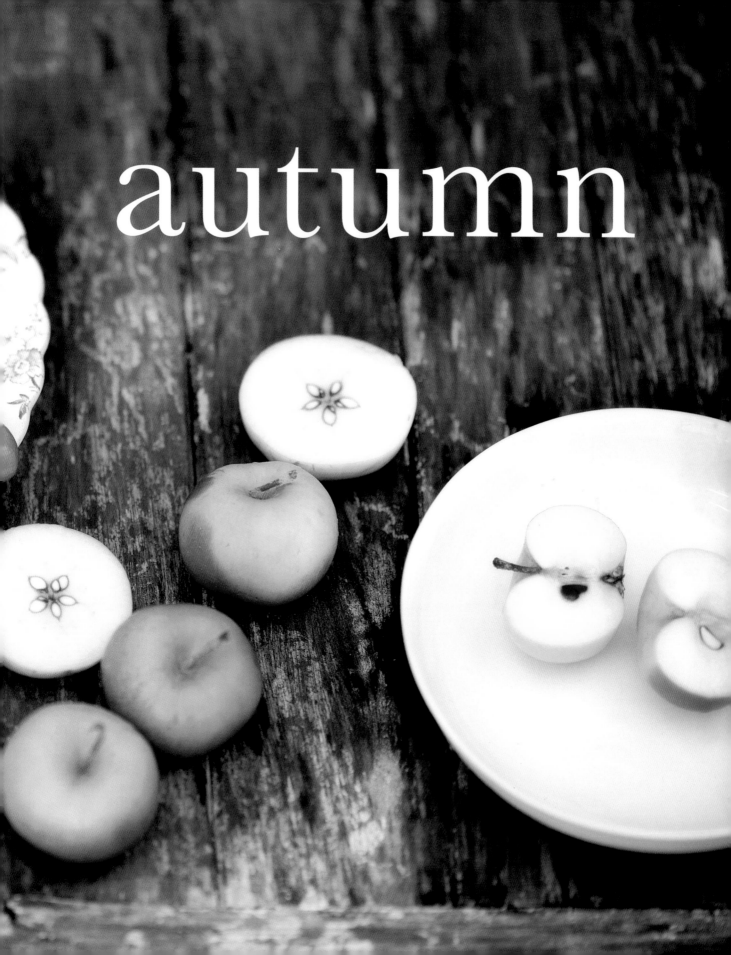

autumn

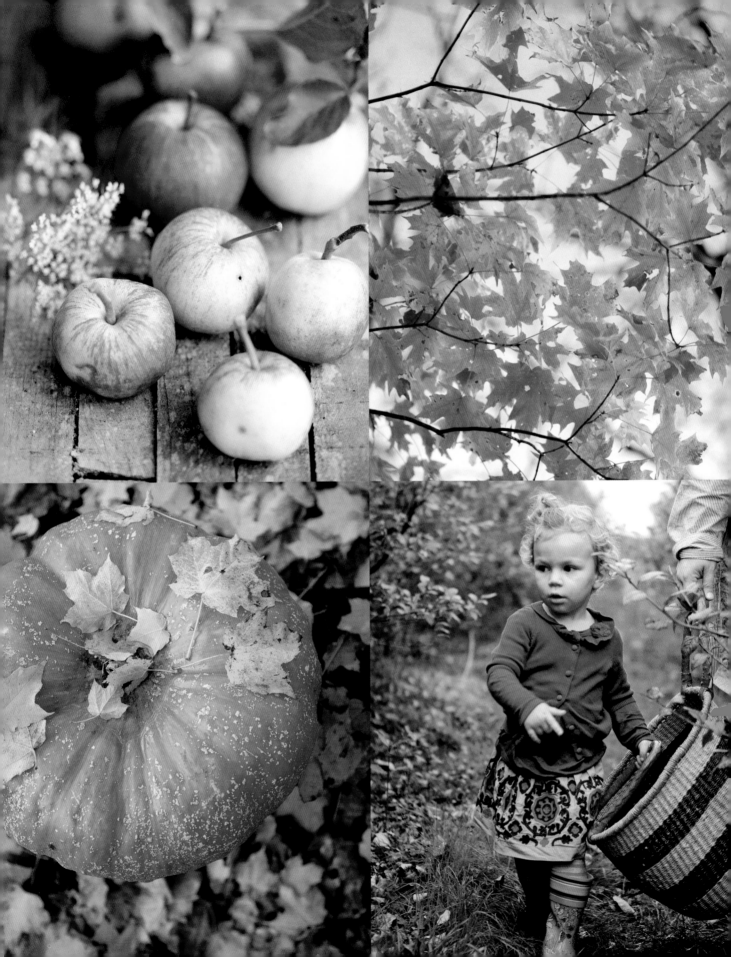

AUTUMN
small plates

I HAVE ALWAYS FELT THAT AUTUMN, not spring, is when everything feels new again, when a new cycle gets started. The cooler days after the summer heat, the beautiful foliage, and the back-to-school routine have me digging into my recipe archives in search of comfort and warmth. I return to the kitchen seeking robust flavors. Nature gives us the color wheel of winter squash, red heirloom apples, and root vegetables: deep reds, ochre, and purple. These are the colors of autumn, my favorite season.

I remember the apple and hazelnut trees that lined the street we took to school every day. A carpet of crisp, dried leaves lay under our feet, and the intense apple and chamomile-like aroma of sweet quince wafted above. My childhood friends Iratxe and Arkaitz and I were dreamers, the romantics who spent hours after school rolling around in the leaves, playing pretend in the crisp air and taking breaks to steal an apple or two from a stranger's garden. "What took you so long? It's past six o'clock already," my mom would ask with concern. "Here is your *bocadillo*. Hurry. You will be late for swimming practice." I didn't want to leave the warmth of the pastry shop kitchen, where it smelled of yeast, cinnamon, and vanilla. I knew, however, that delicious soup would await me after swimming. There was always soup in the fall.

I would not be exaggerating if I said that I could eat soup every day of the year. In fact, during the cold months, we do. A pot of simmering soup on the stove makes a home warm and brings a family to the table. "*Amatxu,*" my kids say (using the Basque term for "Mommy"), "can we have orange soup today?" So I make the Creamy Red Lentil & Squash Soup, topped with purple potato chips, and I always serve it with toasted bread or thick cheese toasties.

baked eggs with olive oil–poached tomatoes, coppa & brie

IT WAS A FOGGY, EARLY AUTUMN MORNING in Zeberio, where my paternal grandparents lived. My grandmother Dolores was hunched over the wood-burning stove holding a basket of eggs she had just collected minutes before. An old cast-iron skillet filled with olive oil, garlic, and crushed tomatoes simmered away. She kept jars of the olive oil–poached tomatoes in the attic, where it was cold. The tomatoes were harvested in late summer and preserved for the cold months.

Those tomatoes seemed to be a fixture in her cooking, I suppose because there was an abundance of them and because it made a quick meal. She cracked a few of the eggs from the basket into the tomatoes and let them gently poach in their heat. "Grab a piece of bread and let's sit at the table. Tell me about your week," she would say.

SERVES 4

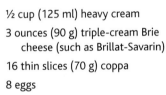

½ cup (125 ml) heavy cream

3 ounces (90 g) triple-cream Brie cheese (such as Brillat-Savarin)

16 thin slices (70 g) coppa

8 eggs

12 Olive Oil–Poached Cherry Tomatoes or 8 Olive Oil–Poached Plum Tomato halves (see below)

Freshly ground black pepper

1 Preheat the oven to 400°F (200°C). Brush 4 large ramekins (large enough to hold 2 eggs each) with olive oil and place them on a baking sheet.

2 Add 2 tablespoons of the cream to the bottom of each ramekin. Slice the Brie into ¼-inch pieces and divide them among the ramekins.

3 Place 4 slices of coppa against the sides of each ramekin. Crack 2 eggs into each ramekin and top with the tomatoes. Sprinkle the eggs with pepper.

4 Bake the eggs for 12 to 15 minutes, until the whites are set and the yolks are soft. Serve immediately.

OLIVE OIL–POACHED CHERRY OR PLUM TOMATOES

Preheat the oven to 300°F (150°C). Place 1 pound of halved plum tomatoes or whole cherry tomatoes (I like black cherry tomatoes for this, when I can find them) in a deep baking pan large enough to hold them snugly. Cover the tomatoes with olive oil. Add 2 cloves garlic and 1 large sprig rosemary. Cover the pan with aluminum foil and bake for 20 to 30 minutes, depending on the size of tomatoes used, until the skins are peeling and the tomatoes begin to burst. You do not want to turn them to mush.

Fill sterilized glass canning jars with the tomatoes, making sure they are covered with the garlic-flavored olive oil. Screw the lids on tightly. Place the jars in a pot with 2 inches of simmering water, spacing them so they do not touch each other. Simmer for 45 minutes. Carefully remove the jars from the water with kitchen tongs and let them cool completely on a rack. The tomatoes will keep for months.

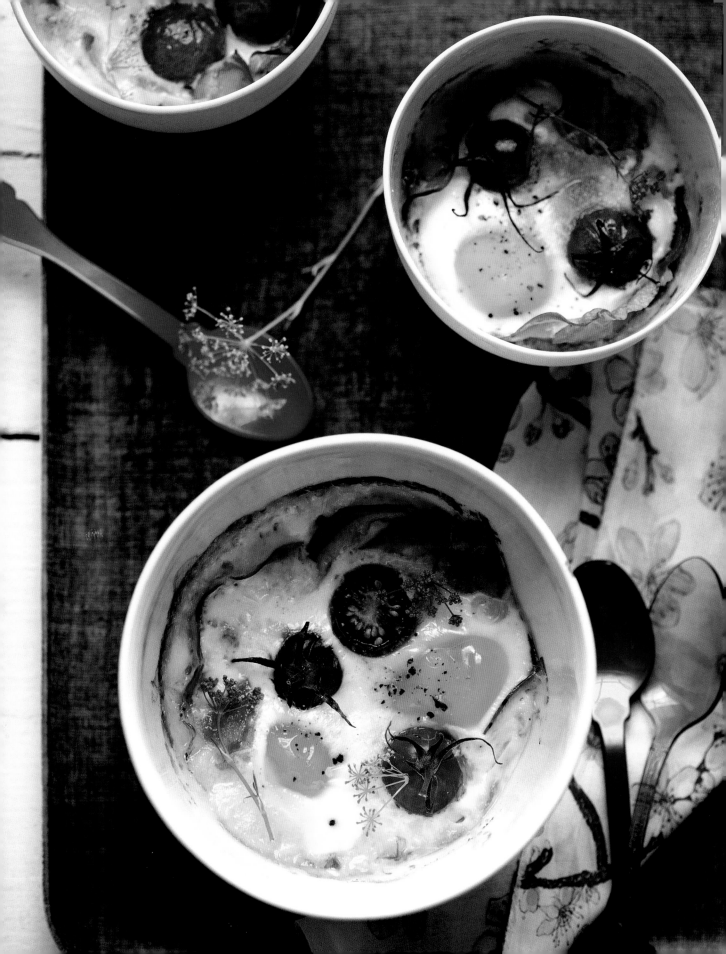

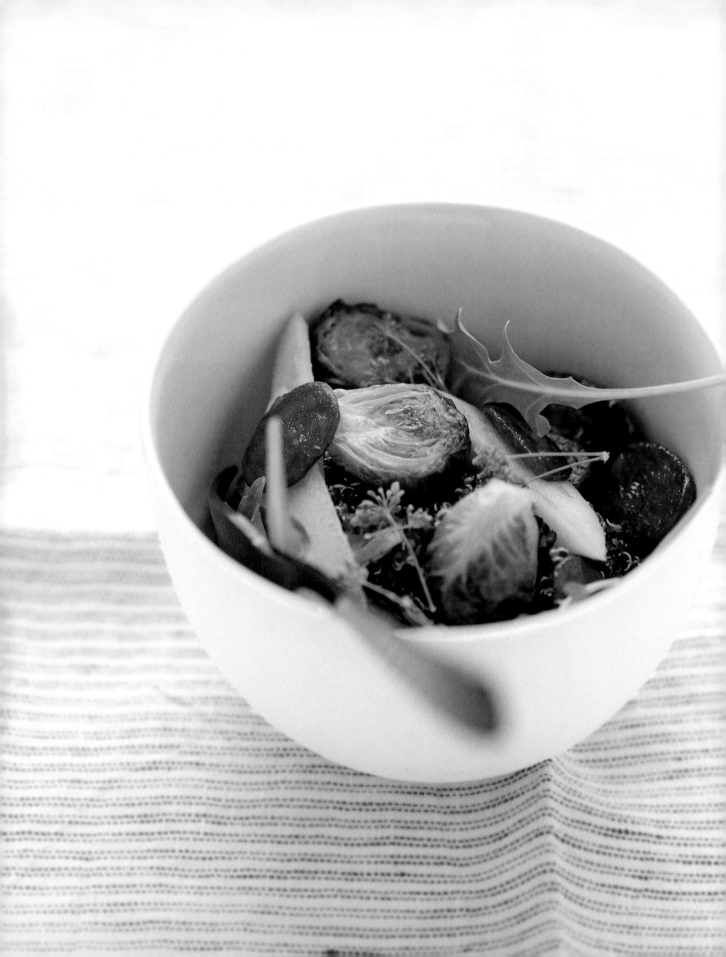

warm roasted brussels sprout, black quinoa, pear & crispy chorizo salad

THIS IS ONE OF MY FAVORITE AUTUMN lunches, and I often make it for myself with different variations. I find that black quinoa suits roasted vegetables because it has a bit of an earthier flavor and crunchier texture than white quinoa.

SERVES 6

1 Preheat the oven to 400°F (200°C). In a small saucepan, bring 1 cup (250 ml) water to a boil over medium heat. Add the quinoa and ¼ teaspoon of the salt, reduce the heat to medium-low, cover the pan, and cook for 20 to 25 minutes, until all the water has been absorbed and the quinoa is tender. Fluff it with a fork and reserve.

2 Toss the Brussels sprouts, 2 tablespoons of the olive oil, and the remaining ¼ teaspoon salt together on a baking sheet. Spread them evenly and bake for 20 minutes or until golden brown.

3 In a small saucepan, heat the remaining 1 tablespoon olive oil over medium-high heat. Add the sliced chorizo and cook until the edges are crispy, about 3 minutes.

4 In a large bowl, toss together the quinoa, roasted Brussels sprouts, chorizo, sliced pears, lemon juice, and arugula. Serve warm.

½ cup (100 g) black quinoa, rinsed

½ teaspoon salt

1 pound (450 g) Brussels sprouts, outer leaves removed and halved

3 tablespoons olive oil

3 ounces (90 g) dry Spanish chorizo, sliced into ¼-inch pieces

2 Anjou or Bosc pears, cored and thinly sliced

Juice of ½ lemon

½ cup arugula

seeded bread

THE SMELL OF FRESHLY BAKED BREAD—yeast and warmth—makes a house a home. One of my earliest childhood memories revolves around bread. I was three or four years old, lined up by my classroom door at school getting ready to go home for lunch. Every afternoon at the exact same time, the town's bread baker drove his Renault 4 in front of our school. Two honks and all the neighbors would come out to buy their baguettes.

This bread recipe is full of whole grains and seeds. Hearty yet surprisingly light, it makes wonderful toast and croutons.

MAKES one 8½ by 4½-inch loaf

¼ cup (45 g) whole millet

5 tablespoons boiling water

1 tablespoon plus 1 teaspoon chia seeds, ground

¾ cup (185 ml) water, heated to 110°F (45°C)

4 teaspoons active dry yeast

1 teaspoon natural cane sugar

1 cup (140 g) superfine brown rice flour, plus more for dusting

¾ cup (105 g) quinoa flour

½ cup (70 g) teff flour

¼ cup (40 g) potato starch

⅓ cup (35 g) almond flour

3 tablespoons tapioca starch

1 tablespoon poppy seeds

1 tablespoon sesame seeds

1 tablespoon fennel seeds

2 teaspoons salt

2 eggs, at room temperature

2 tablespoons honey

1　In a small bowl, combine the millet and 3 tablespoons of the boiling water. Let it stand for 15 minutes.

2　In a separate small bowl, stir together the ground chia seeds and the remaining 2 tablespoons boiling water. It will turn into a thick paste. Set aside.

3　In a separate bowl, whisk together the warm water, active dry yeast, and sugar. Let the yeast ferment for 10 minutes. It will become very frothy and foamy.

4　In the bowl of a stand mixer, whisk together the superfine brown rice flour, quinoa flour, teff flour, potato starch, almond flour, tapioca starch, poppy seeds, sesame seeds, fennel seeds, and salt.

5　Drain the millet and add it to the dry ingredients along with the chia seed slurry, yeast mixture, eggs, and honey. Mix on low speed for 30 seconds with the paddle attachment. Turn mixer to high speed and mix for 1 minute. The dough will be sticky and similar to a thick cake batter.

6　Transfer the dough to an oiled 8½ by 4½-inch loaf pan. Dust the top with a bit of superfine brown rice flour. Loosely cover the pan with plastic wrap and let rise until doubled in volume, 45 minutes to 1 hour.

7　Meanwhile, preheat the oven to 400°F (200°C). Bake the bread for 10 minutes and then reduce the heat to 350°F (180°C). Bake for an additional 30 minutes, until golden brown and a toothpick inserted in the center comes out clean.

8　Transfer the loaf pan to a cooling rack and let the bread cool in the pan for 15 minutes. Remove the bread from the pan and let cool completely, about 1 hour. Store at room temperature wrapped in parchment paper for 2 days or freeze tightly wrapped.

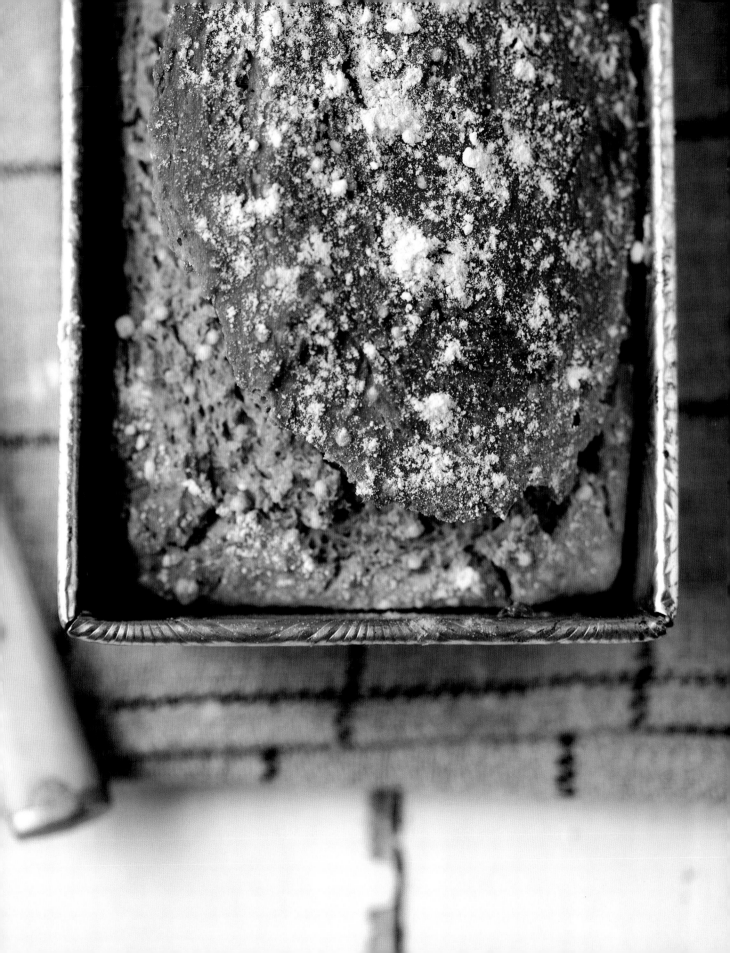

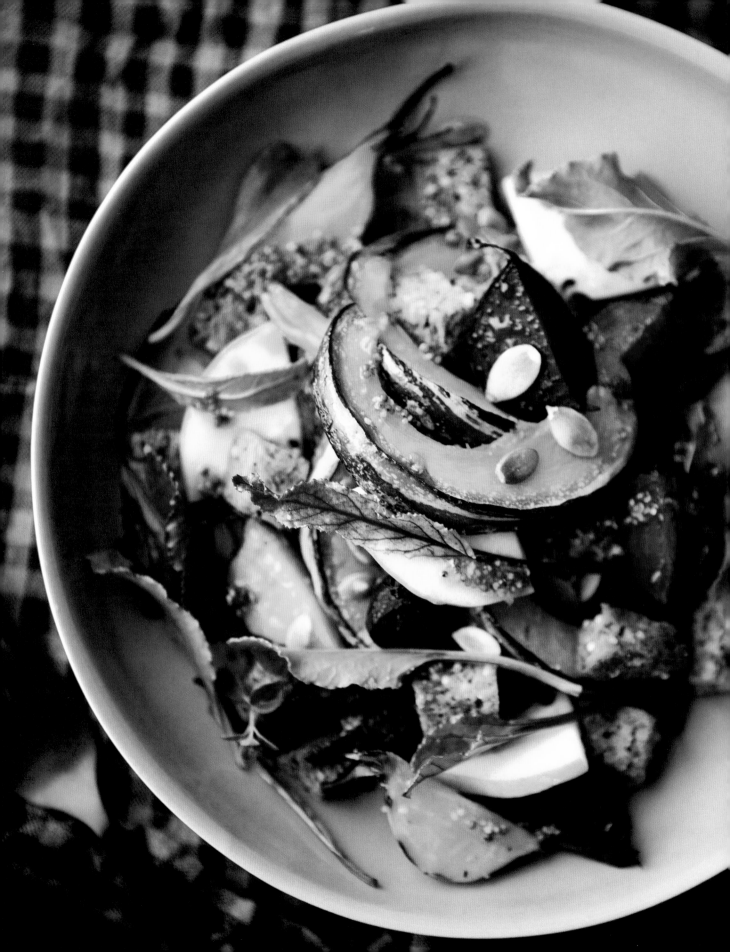

autumn panzanella salad

AS MUCH AS I LOVE A SUMMER PANZANELLA with juicy tomatoes and cucumbers, this warm autumn version is one of my all-time favorites. It's filled with hearty seeded bread croutons, creamy roasted squash, golden and red beets, crunchy slices of apple, and pumpkin seeds, all dressed with pumpkin oil and apple cider vinaigrette.

SERVES 4

make the salad

1 Preheat the oven to 325°F (160°C). Toss the cubed bread and 1 tablespoon of the olive oil on a baking sheet. Bake for 20 minutes, until dry.

2 Increase the oven temperature to 400°F (200°C). Toss the beets with 1 tablespoon of the olive oil and a pinch of salt on a deep baking pan. Cover the pan with aluminum foil and bake for 45 minutes or until fork-tender.

3 Toss the sliced squash with the remaining 1 tablespoon olive oil, a pinch of salt, and the red pepper flakes. Bake on the lower rack of the oven for 20 minutes or until fork-tender.

4 In a large bowl, toss together the croutons, roasted beets, roasted squash, sliced apple, beet greens, pumpkin seeds, sage, thyme, and oregano.

make the vinaigrette

Whisk together the mustard, vinegar, pumpkin oil, olive oil, and salt. Pour the vinaigrette over the warm salad, toss, let sit for 10 minutes so the bread absorbs the juices, and serve.

SALAD

6 (¾-inch-thick) slices Seeded Bread (page 28), cubed

3 tablespoons olive oil

5 red baby beets, peeled and quartered

5 golden baby beets, peeled and quartered

2 pinches of salt

½ medium kabocha, red kuri, or butternut squash, peeled, sliced, and seeds removed

½ teaspoon red pepper flakes

1 medium Granny Smith or Golden Delicious apple, cored and thinly sliced

1 cup (40 g) beet greens or any other leafy green

¼ cup (40 g) raw pumpkin seeds

1 tablespoon fresh sage leaves

1 teaspoon fresh thyme leaves

1 teaspoon fresh oregano leaves

VINAIGRETTE

1 teaspoon grainy Dijon mustard

2 teaspoons apple cider vinegar

2 teaspoons pumpkin oil

¼ cup (60 ml) olive oil

1 teaspoon salt

fennel & brown butter risotto with parsley pesto

RISOTTO SEEMS TO BE MY GO-TO DINNER when I am rushing to get food on the table. It is filling, versatile, and best of all, my kids love it. It is important to cook risotto with a flavorful liquid, as most rice by itself is bland. I keep pints of homemade chicken stock, which adds lots of flavor, in the freezer. The pesto here makes more than you will need for this recipe. Refrigerate leftover pesto for up to 5 days or freeze it for up to 1 month.

SERVES 4

PARSLEY PESTO (MAKES 1 CUP)

⅓ cup (55 g) pine nuts

1 clove garlic, peeled

⅔ cup (30 g) fresh parsley, tough stems removed

1 ounce (30 g) Parmesan cheese, finely grated

½ teaspoon salt

½ cup (125 ml) olive oil

FENNEL AND BROWN BUTTER RISOTTO

5 to 6 cups (1.25 to 1.5 L) chicken stock

¼ stick (2 tablespoons or 30 g) unsalted butter

1 medium fennel bulb, diced

½ medium leek, diced

½ teaspoon salt

¼ teaspoon ground coriander

1½ cups (300 g) Arborio rice

¼ cup (60 ml) dry white wine

½ cup (120 g) Parsley Pesto

2 tablespoons mascarpone cheese

Shaved Parmesan cheese, for garnish

Fresh parsley flowers, for garnish, optional

make the pesto

1 Place the pine nuts in a dry skillet. Toast them over medium heat, stirring occasionally, until fragrant and lightly golden in color, about 3 minutes. Let them cool for a few minutes.

2 Combine the pine nuts, garlic, and parsley in a food processor. Process to a fine powder. Add the Parmesan and salt and pulse to combine.

3 While the machine is running, slowly pour in the olive oil until it forms a smooth paste. Reserve.

make the risotto

1 Pour the chicken stock into a medium saucepan and bring to a low simmer over medium-high heat. Reduce the heat to low and keep it warm.

2 Melt the butter in a large pot over medium heat until the milk solids start to brown on the bottom of the pan, about 2 minutes. Do not burn the butter.

3 Add the fennel, leek, salt, and coriander. Cook over medium heat until softened but not brown, about 5 minutes. Add the rice and stir it to make sure it is well coated with the butter, about 1 minute.

4 Add the white wine and stir, deglazing the bottom of the pan. Add ½ cup (125 ml) of the hot chicken stock. Stir and cook over medium heat until the rice has absorbed the stock. Add another ½ cup (125 ml) of stock and continue to cook while stirring. Repeat, stirring constantly, until the rice is al dente, about 18 minutes.

5 Stir in the Parsley Pesto and mascarpone. Remove from the heat. Serve immediately, garnished with shaved Parmesan cheese and, if you like, parsley.

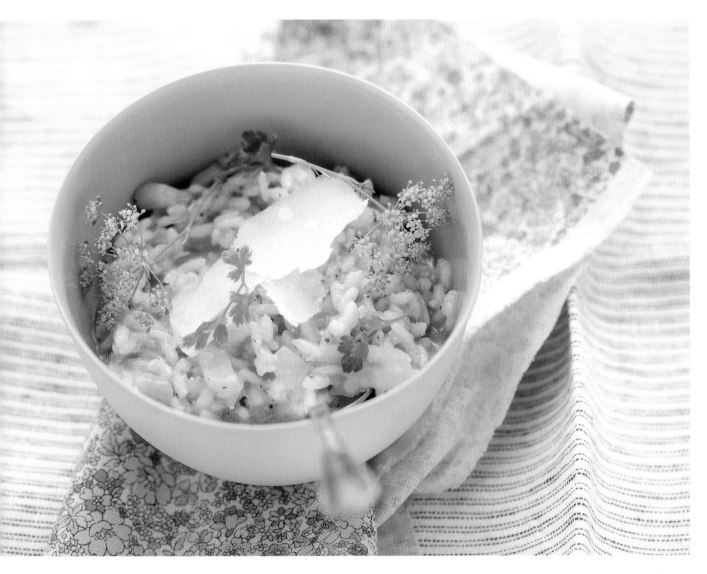

HOW TO MAKE CHICKEN STOCK AT HOME

Although making chicken stock at home takes some time, it is fairly simple and the result is gratifying. I tend to buy whole chickens and cut them up myself, but you can ask the butcher to do it for you.

Roast 1 pound (450 g) chicken bones on a baking sheet at 400°F (200°C) for 30 minutes or until the chicken pieces are brown. Let them cool for 20 minutes. Transfer the roasted bones to a large stockpot and cover them with cold water. Add a handful of aromatics such as diced carrots, onions, garlic, celery, fresh parsley, and thyme. Season the liquid with salt and pepper. Taste the water, but remember that the flavors will concentrate as the liquid reduces. Bring the liquid to a boil over high heat and then reduce the heat to medium. Skim off the impurities that collect on the top. Simmer the stock uncovered for 3 hours, but do not stir it or let it boil. Strain the stock through a fine-mesh sieve and let it cool. Divide it into containers and freeze for up to 3 months.

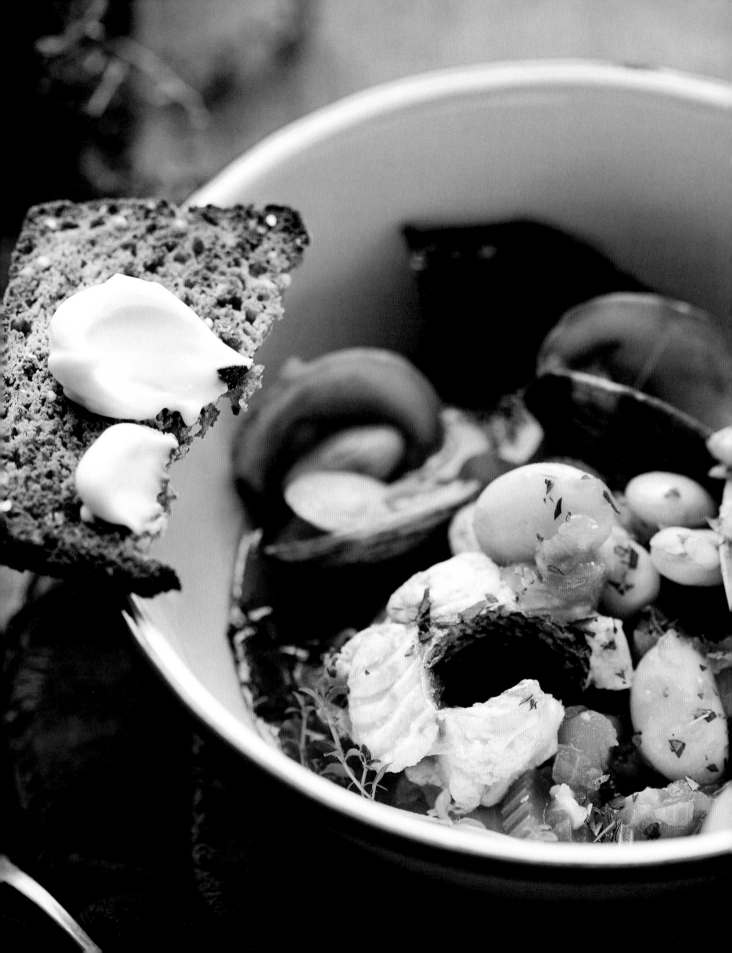

spicy fish & cannellini bean stew

THIS RECIPE IS INSPIRED BY A CLASSIC Basque dish called *potxas con almejas*—large white beans cooked with clams and lots of garlic and parsley. In this version I add tomatoes, red pepper, and red snapper. I use Rancho Gordo heirloom cannellini beans, which are a bit larger than traditional cannellini. Cooking time will depend on the size and variety of beans you use.

SERVES 4 to 6

1   Rinse the cannellini beans in cold water. Place them in a bowl and cover them with 2 inches of cold water. Soak them in the refrigerator overnight.

2   In a large pot, heat the olive oil over medium heat. Add the onion, garlic, and celery. Cook for 3 minutes or until soft.

3   Add the diced tomatoes, bay leaf, thyme sprigs, and red pepper flakes. Add the soaked beans with their soaking water and the white wine. Make sure the beans are covered by 1 inch of water; you might need to add some more water.

4   Bring the liquid to a boil over medium to high heat. Reduce the heat to low, cover the pot, and simmer the beans for 1½ to 2 hours or until tender. Season the stew with salt once the beans are tender.

5   Increase the heat to medium-high and bring it to a low boil. Add the clams and the snapper. Cover the pot and cook for 5 minutes or until the clams open. Remove the pot from the heat immediately.

6   Garnish with parsley and serve with aioli and toasted bread.

1 cup (190 g) dried cannellini beans

3 tablespoons olive oil

1 small yellow onion, diced

2 cloves garlic, minced

1 celery stalk, diced

1 cup (220 g) fresh or canned diced tomatoes

1 dried bay leaf

3 sprigs thyme

½ to 1 teaspoon red pepper flakes, depending on how spicy you like it

¼ cup (60 ml) dry white wine

½ teaspoon salt

1 pound (450 g) littleneck clams

8 ounces (225 g) yellowtail or red snapper fillet, cut into bite-size pieces

Chopped fresh parsley, for garnish

Aioli (page 112)

Toasted Seeded Bread (page 28)

ABOUT CLAMS

There are a few tricks for cleaning clams that I have learned from my mom:

• When buying clams, always make sure they are closed. Sometimes, they tend to open a bit, which doesn't always mean the clams are dead. To make sure the clams are still alive, take two of them and gently tap them against each other. If they are alive, they should close back up immediately. If they remain open, discard them.

• The best way to clean clams is to cover them with cold water in a bowl. Add enough salt to make the water taste like seawater. Refrigerate them for at least 30 minutes prior to cooking them. They will release sand. Rinse them one more time before cooking.

• If any of the clams do not open during the cooking process, discard them.

rustic fig, serrano ham & hazelnut tartines

A TARTINE IS AN OPEN-FACED SANDWICH usually composed of a slice of crusty artisan bread topped with a spread, vegetables, and sometimes meat or fish. They are usually served along with a soup or a salad to make a complete meal—definitely one of my favorites. In this recipe, figs, Serrano ham, goat cheese, and greens are piled on top of a savory hazelnut crust.

SERVES 4 to 6

HAZELNUT AND HERB CRUST

¾ cup (105 g) superfine brown rice flour, plus more for dusting

¼ cup (35 g) millet flour

3 tablespoons hazelnut flour

2 tablespoons tapioca starch

2 teaspoons ground chia seeds

1 teaspoon chopped fresh parsley

1 teaspoon fresh thyme leaves

¾ teaspoon salt

¼ teaspoon freshly ground black pepper

1 stick (8 tablespoons or 110 g) cold unsalted butter, cut into ½-inch cubes

6 to 8 tablespoons ice water

FIG, SERRANO, AND WATERCRESS TOPPING

2 tablespoons hazelnuts

4 ounces (110 g) creamy goat cheese

8 ounces (225 g) Black Mission figs, halved

6 thin slices (3 ounces or 90 g) Serrano ham

1 cup (40 g) watercress, tough stems removed

¼ small red onion, thinly sliced

1 tablespoon olive oil

2 teaspoons balsamic vinegar

make the crust

1 Combine the first nine ingredients in a food processor. Pulse three times to aerate. Add the cold butter and pulse ten times, until the butter is the size of small peas. Add 6 tablespoons of ice water and pulse. The dough does not need to form a ball. Simply press the dough and see if it comes together. If it seems crumbly, add another tablespoon of ice water.

2 Transfer the dough onto a work surface and knead it a couple of times. Quickly form it into a 6-inch square. Do not handle the dough too much, and don't worry if it isn't a perfect square. Wrap the dough in plastic wrap, flatten it, and refrigerate it for 30 minutes.

3 Preheat the oven to 375°F (190°C). Remove the dough from the refrigerator. It is best to work on a cold surface, such as marble. Dust your surface and your rolling pin with a little bit of superfine brown rice flour. Roll the dough to a rectangle that is approximately 7 by 10 inches and ¼ inch thick. Again, it doesn't have to be perfect. Work quickly so the dough doesn't become too soft. If it cracks, pinch it back together.

4 Transfer the rolled dough to a baking sheet lined with parchment paper. Trim the edges with a pie cutter if desired. Chill the dough for 20 minutes or until firm.

5 Bake for 20 to 25 minutes, until golden brown. Remove from the oven and let the crust cool while preparing the topping (leave the oven on). I recommend arranging the topping while the crust is slightly warm, as the warmth brings out all the flavors.

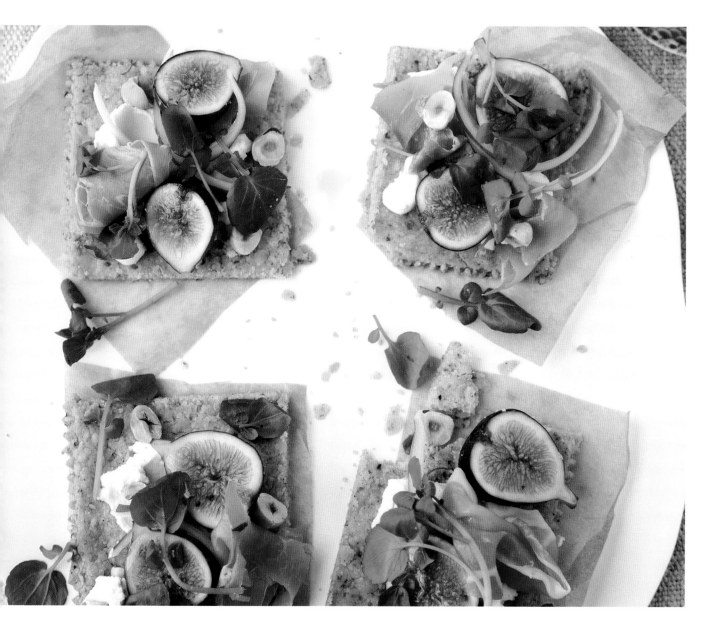

prepare the topping

1 Reduce the oven temperature to 350°F (180°C). Place the hazelnuts on a baking sheet and toast them for 5 to 7 minutes or until golden and the skin begins to loosen. Transfer them to a kitchen towel and rub them together to remove their skins. Let them cool. Coarsely chop them.

2 Place the goat cheese in a bowl and quickly stir it to loosen it. Spread over the warm tart.

3 Arrange the figs, ham, watercress, red onion, and toasted hazelnuts over the goat cheese. Drizzle the olive oil and balsamic vinegar over the top. Cut into squares and serve immediately.

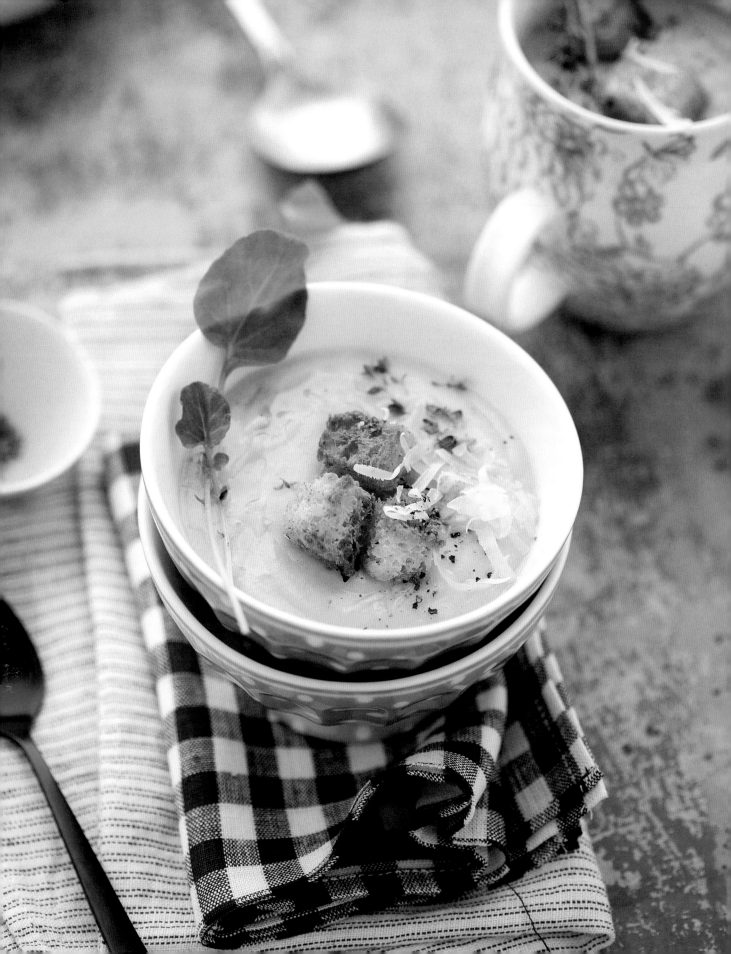

roasted parsnip & apple soup
with mustard croutons

PARSNIPS HAVE BECOME A BIT OF an obsession for me, especially when they are fried or roasted, as they are here. They are sweet yet peppery and enhance every soup, stew, or roast imaginable.

SERVES 6 to 8

1 Preheat the oven to 400°F (200°C). Toss the diced parsnips, 1 tablespoon of the olive oil, ¼ teaspoon of the salt, and ¼ teaspoon of the black pepper on a baking sheet. Bake for 30 minutes, turning the parsnips halfway through the cooking process.

2 Heat 2 tablespoons of the olive oil in a large pot over medium heat. Add the onion, garlic, and celery. Cook the vegetables for 5 minutes, stirring occasionally, or until tender but not brown.

3 Add the roasted parsnips, apples, potatoes, chicken stock, coriander, remaining ½ teaspoon salt, and remaining ¼ teaspoon black pepper. Bring the liquid to a boil, reduce the heat to medium-low, cover the pot, and simmer for 15 minutes or until the vegetables are tender.

4 Meanwhile, reduce the oven temperature to 350°F (180°C). In a small bowl, whisk together the Dijon mustard, remaining 3 tablespoons olive oil, and thyme leaves. Add the diced bread cubes and toss them in the dressing. Lay the croutons on a baking sheet and bake for 15 minutes, until golden and crispy.

5 Puree the soup in a blender. Serve the soup with the croutons, olive oil, and Gruyère. The soup will keep in the refrigerator for up to 3 days, or it can be frozen for up to 1 month.

1 pound (450 g) parsnips, peeled and diced into ½-inch pieces

¼ cup plus 2 tablespoons (90 ml) olive oil, plus more for garnish

¾ teaspoon salt

½ teaspoon freshly ground black pepper

1 medium yellow onion, diced

2 cloves garlic, minced

1 celery stalk, diced

2 medium Pink Lady or Granny Smith apples, peeled, cored, and diced

2 medium russet potatoes, peeled and diced

5 cups (1.25 L) chicken stock

1 teaspoon ground coriander

1 teaspoon Dijon mustard

1 teaspoon fresh thyme leaves

3 slices Seeded Bread (page 28) or gluten-free bread, cut into ½-inch cubes

Grated Gruyère cheese, for garnish

cheesy mushroom, rutabaga & parsnip *parmentier*

MY FRIEND SANDRA'S MOM was known for her beef *parmentier*, a shepherd's pie of sorts with layers of slow-cooked beef, mashed potatoes, and cheese baked in a glass baking dish. In our high-school years we had many sleepovers at Sandra's, where leftover *parmentier* often served as a hangover cure. It was our medicine and worked every time. This is a lighter version with cheesy mashed rutabaga, parsnips, and potatoes topped with mushrooms and cooked in wine and tomato.

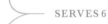

SERVES 6

12 ounces (340 g) assorted wild or cultivated exotic mushrooms, stems removed and sliced (reserve stems)

1 medium rutabaga, peeled and cut into 1-inch pieces

2 medium parsnips, peeled and cut into 1-inch pieces

2 medium russet potatoes, peeled and cut into 2-inch pieces

½ cup (125 ml) crème frâiche, at room temperature

2 ounces (60 g) Comté or Gruyère cheese, grated

1¾ teaspoons salt

3 tablespoons olive oil

1 large shallot, minced

2 cloves garlic, minced

3 medium scallions, diced

¼ teaspoon freshly ground black pepper

½ teaspoon fresh thyme leaves

½ teaspoon chopped fresh sage leaves

¼ cup (55 g) strained canned tomatoes

2 teaspoons sweet rice flour

¼ cup (60 ml) dry red wine

¼ cup (15 g) finely chopped fresh parsley

Microgreens, for garnish

1   Combine the mushroom stems and 2 cups (500 ml) water in a small saucepan. Bring the liquid to a boil over medium-high heat, reduce the heat to medium-low, cover the pot, and cook for 10 minutes. Strain the liquid into a bowl and discard the stems. Return the liquid to the pot and reduce it by half (to 1 cup) over medium-high heat. Reserve the stock.

2   Meanwhile, place the rutabaga, parsnips, and potatoes in a medium pot. Cover the vegetables with cold water. Bring the liquid to a boil over medium-high heat, reduce the heat to medium, cover the pot, and cook the vegetables for 15 minutes or until tender. Drain well, return them to the pot, and immediately mash them in a food mill or by hand. Add the crème frâiche, grated cheese, and 1 teaspoon of the salt. Stir until combined. Adjust the liquid and seasoning, if needed. Keep warm.

3   Heat the olive oil in a large sauté pan. Add the shallot, garlic, and scallions. Cook over medium heat for 3 minutes or until soft. Add the mushrooms, remaining ¾ teaspoon salt, black pepper, thyme leaves, and sage leaves and cook until soft but not mushy, about 3 minutes.

4   Add the tomatoes and sweet rice flour. Cook for 1 minute, stirring constantly. Add the mushroom stock and red wine. Simmer for 3 minutes or until the sauce has thickened. Add the chopped parsley.

5   Divide the root vegetable mash among six bowls and top with the mushrooms. Serve immediately topped with microgreens.

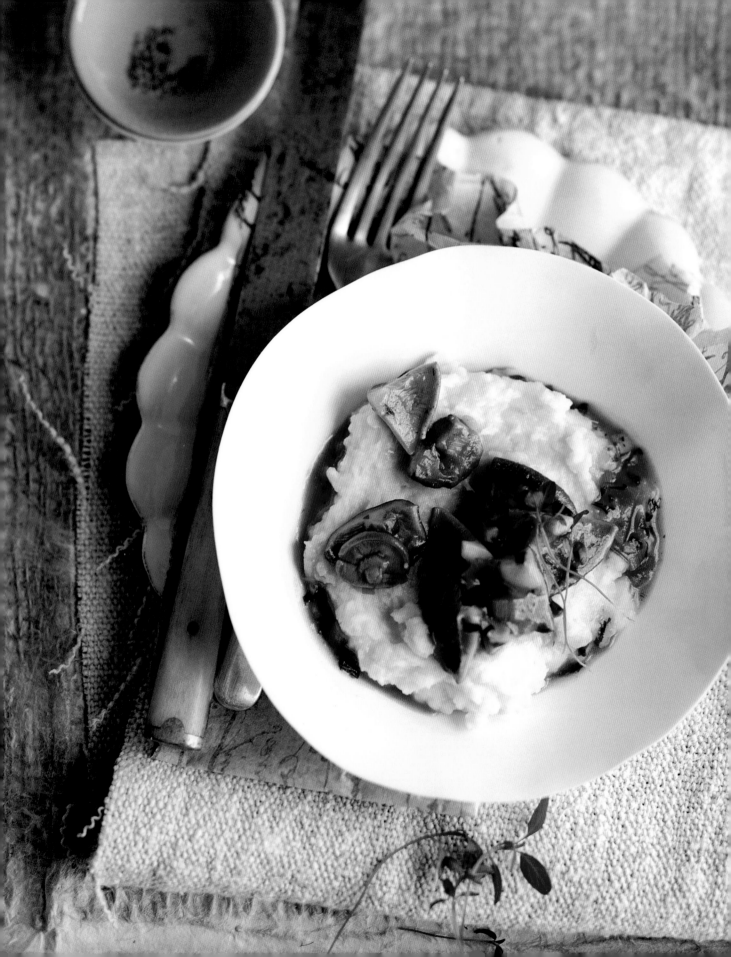

sweet potato, goat cheese
& herb soufflé

WARM AND LIGHT PUFFS OF SALTY GOAT cheese and sweet potato puree:
What could be nicer? These soufflés are perfect as a starter or served with a salad for lunch.

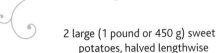

MAKES eight 6-ounce soufflés

2 large (1 pound or 450 g) sweet
  potatoes, halved lengthwise

4 eggs

3 tablespoons unsalted butter
  (45 g), plus more at room
  temperature for ramekins

⅓ cup (30 g) gluten-free bread
  crumbs

3 tablespoons sweet rice flour

1 cup (250 ml) whole milk or
  unsweetened coconut milk,
  at room temperature

3 ounces (90 g) goat cheese,
  at room temperature

1 tablespoon finely chopped fresh
  parsley

2 teaspoons finely chopped fresh
  chives

1¼ teaspoons salt

½ teaspoon ground cumin

¼ teaspoon freshly ground black
  pepper

⅛ teaspoon ground nutmeg

Shaved Manchego cheese, optional

Fresh parsley flowers, optional

1   Preheat the oven to 400°F (200°C). Place the sweet potatoes on a
baking sheet cut side down. Bake for 25 to 30 minutes or until fork-tender.
Let them sit for a few minutes, until they are cool enough to handle. Peel
them and puree them in a food processor. Measure out 1¼ cups (280 g)
sweet potato puree. Reserve. Reduce the oven temperature to 350°F
(180°C).

2   Separate the egg whites from the egg yolks and let them come to
room temperature. Brush the inside of 8 ramekins with soft butter. Add
some bread crumbs to 1 ramekin. Turn the ramekin so that the crumbs
coat the inside completely. Turn the crumbs into another ramekin and
repeat. Coat all the ramekins with the crumbs. Gently pat the ramekins
upside down to remove excess bread crumbs. Set aside.

3   Melt the 3 tablespoons butter in a small saucepan over medium-
high heat. Add the sweet rice flour and stir with a wooden spoon for 1 minute.
Add the milk and whisk to remove any lumps. Cook the mixture until it
comes to a boil. It will thicken immediately. Transfer to a large bowl.

4   Add the egg yolks, sweet potato puree, goat cheese, parsley, chives,
salt, cumin, black pepper, and nutmeg. Stir all the ingredients together.

5   Place the egg whites in the bowl of a stand mixer and whip them on
medium-high speed until they form medium peaks. Do not overmix them
or they will be dry and too lumpy to fold.

6   Fold one-third of the whipped egg whites into the sweet potato
mixture until no egg white is visible. Gently fold the rest of the egg whites
into the base, being careful not to deflate the batter too much.

7   Divide the batter among the buttered ramekins. Bake for 15 to
20 minutes or until the soufflés have puffed up and the tops are lightly
golden. Serve immediately. I like to top them with shaved Manchego
cheese and parsley flowers.

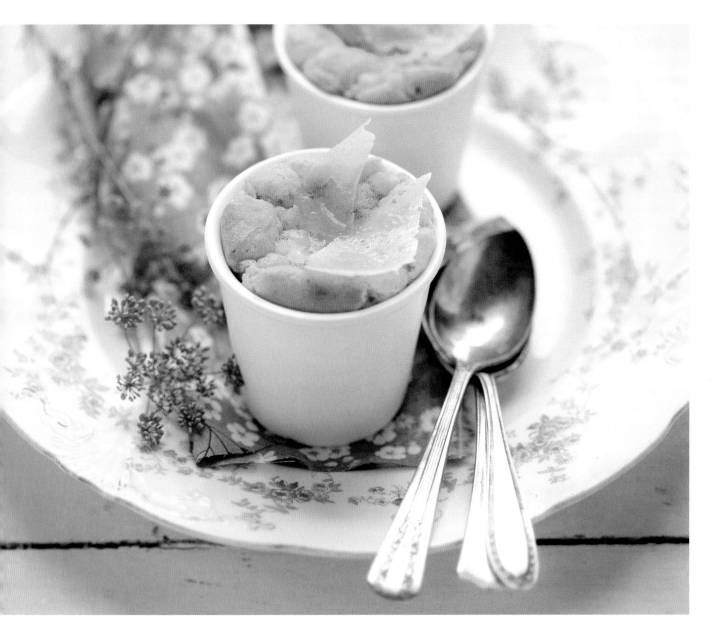

HOW TO MAKE GLUTEN-FREE BREAD CRUMBS

Udi's makes my favorite commercial gluten-free sandwich bread. It is light with large air pockets, which I always consider a good characteristic in bread. This makes it perfect for bread crumbs.

Start by preheating your oven to 325°F (160°C). Lay 6 slices of bread on a baking sheet. Bake them for 15 minutes or until dry. The purpose is not to toast them but to dry them. Let them cool to room temperature and then pulse them in a food processor until you reach the texture that you like. I prefer chunky bread crumbs, but you could turn them into a fine powder if you like. You could also add seasonings such as dried oregano, garlic powder, or black pepper. Store them in an airtight container for up to 1 month.

creamy red lentil & squash soup with purple potato chips & scallops

I DISCOVERED RED LENTILS ONLY A few years ago. Because they do not require presoaking and because of their short cooking time, I resort to them when I am in need of a last-minute soup or am rushing to get dinner on the table. They break down to mush quickly, which is why I like to puree them after cooking. They make great creamy soups, full of protein. A larger serving of this recipe can easily be a main course, loaded as it is with purple potato chips and sautéed sea scallops.

SERVES 6

¼ cup plus 2 tablespoons (90 ml) olive oil

1 medium shallot, diced

2 cloves garlic, minced

2 medium carrots, peeled and diced

1 celery stalk, diced

1 teaspoon fresh thyme leaves

1 teaspoon salt, plus more for seasoning the scallops

½ teaspoon freshly ground black pepper, plus more for seasoning the scallops

1 cup (200 g) red lentils, rinsed

1 small (1½ pounds or 680 g) kabocha or butternut squash, peeled, halved, seeded, and diced (about 3 cups diced)

1 medium russet potato, peeled and diced

6 cups (1.5 L) chicken stock

2 small purple or Yukon gold potatoes, very thinly sliced

4 ounces (110 g) small sea scallops

Pumpkin oil, optional

Fresh parsley flowers, optional

1 In a large pot, heat 2 tablespoons (30 ml) of the olive oil over medium heat. Add the shallot, garlic, carrots, celery, thyme leaves, ½ teaspoon of the salt, and ½ teaspoon of the black pepper. Cook the vegetables, stirring occasionally, for 5 minutes or until tender but not mushy.

2 Add the red lentils, squash, russet potato, chicken stock, and remaining ½ teaspoon salt. Cover the pot. Bring the liquid to a boil over medium-high heat. Reduce the heat to low and simmer for 20 minutes or until all the vegetables are tender. Puree the soup in a blender. Adjust the seasoning if needed and keep warm.

3 In a small sauté pan, heat the remaining ¼ cup (60 ml) of olive oil over medium heat. Add the thinly sliced potatoes in batches and cook until golden. Drain them on paper towels. Reserve.

4 Remove most of the oil from the sauté pan. Season the scallops with salt and pepper and cook them over medium heat for 30 seconds to 1 minute per side, depending on their size.

5 Serve the soup warm topped with the potato chips, scallops, a few drops of pumpkin oil, parsley flowers, and black pepper. The soup will keep for up to 3 days in the refrigerator, or it can be frozen for up to 1 month.

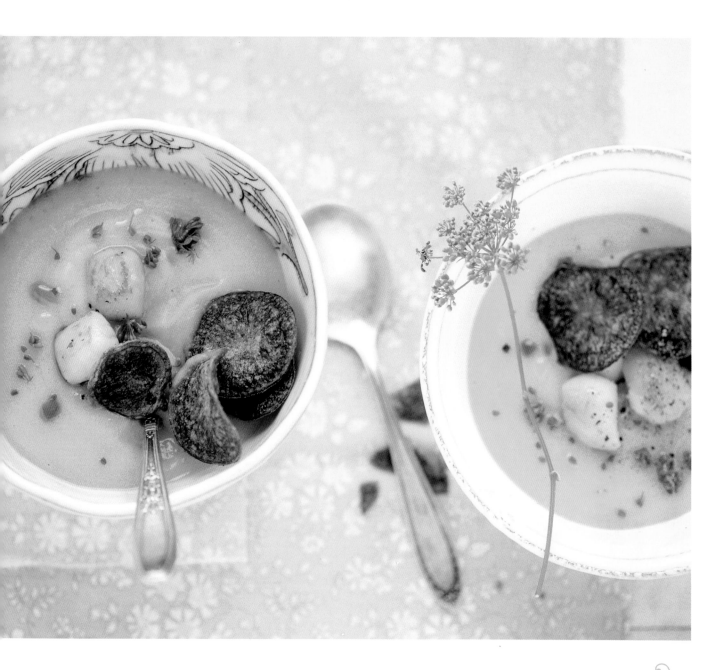

WHAT TO DO WITH ALL THAT WINTER SQUASH

If you are anything like me, once autumn comes around you are loading up on all varieties of winter squash. Red kuri, kabocha, hubbard, butternut squash, and acorn are usually in my kitchen, ready to be added to any dish. But peeling and cutting all this squash is not always easy, especially the larger, hard varieties. For these, I use a time-saving trick my mother taught me. Peel and dice the entire squash at once. Divide the diced squash among individual freezer bags and freeze them for up to 3 months. The frozen squash can be added to any soup as is without the need to thaw it. This saves a tremendous amount of prep time when you are ready to cook.

shiitake mushroom & leek quiche

FORAGING AND MUSHROOM PICKING are important parts of Basque culture. When I go home to visit my family, I enjoy following my father around forests looking for the coveted chanterelles and russulas. Wicker basket in hand and Wellies on my feet, I walk for miles listening to him talk about the different varieties and the best places to find them. There's something so Zen about it all. Once home, the bounty is shared with other family members, and there are endless debates about where the best mushrooms can be found, favorite preparations, and so on. As always, food is the center of the conversation.

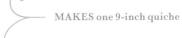

MAKES one 9-inch quiche

PASTRY CRUST

⅔ cup (90 g) superfine brown rice flour, plus more for dusting

⅓ cup (45 g) quinoa flour

¼ cup (40 g) potato starch

½ teaspoon salt

¼ teaspoon freshly ground black pepper

1 teaspoon finely chopped fresh rosemary

1 teaspoon fresh thyme leaves

1 stick (8 tablespoons or 110 g) cold unsalted butter, cut into ½-inch cubes

6 to 8 tablespoons ice water

SHIITAKE MUSHROOM AND LEEK FILLING

1 tablespoon olive oil

1 medium leek, diced (white and tender green part only)

8 ounces (225 g) shiitake mushrooms, sliced and stems removed

2 cloves garlic, minced

1 teaspoon finely chopped fresh rosemary

1 teaspoon finely chopped fresh sage

¾ teaspoon salt

¼ teaspoon freshly ground black pepper

¼ cup (60 ml) dry white wine

make the crust

1   Mix the first seven ingredients in a food processor. Pulse three times to aerate. Add the cold butter and pulse ten times, until the butter is cut into the flour in pea-size pieces.

2   Add 6 tablespoons of ice water and pulse until the mixture comes together. It will not form a ball. Simply press the dough together in your hand. If it's too crumbly and will not hold together, add a bit more water.

3   Turn the dough out onto a work surface, knead it a couple of times, and form a disk. Wrap it in plastic wrap, flatten it, and refrigerate for 1 hour.

4   Dust your (preferably cold) work surface with a bit of superfine brown rice flour. Roll the dough to a ⅛-inch thickness. If the dough cracks, pinch it back together. Fill a 9-inch tart pan with the dough. Cut excess dough with a paring knife and chill the dough for another 30 minutes while preparing the filling.

prepare the filling and bake the quiche

1   Preheat the oven to 400°F (200°C). In a medium sauté pan, heat the olive oil over medium heat. Add the leek and cook for 3 minutes or until tender but not brown.

2   Add the sliced shiitakes, garlic, rosemary, sage, ½ teaspoon of the salt, and black pepper. Cook for 5 minutes, stirring occasionally, until tender.

3   Add the white wine and stir to pick up the bits on the bottom of the pan. Let the wine cook and reduce for about 1 minute. Let the filling cool slightly.

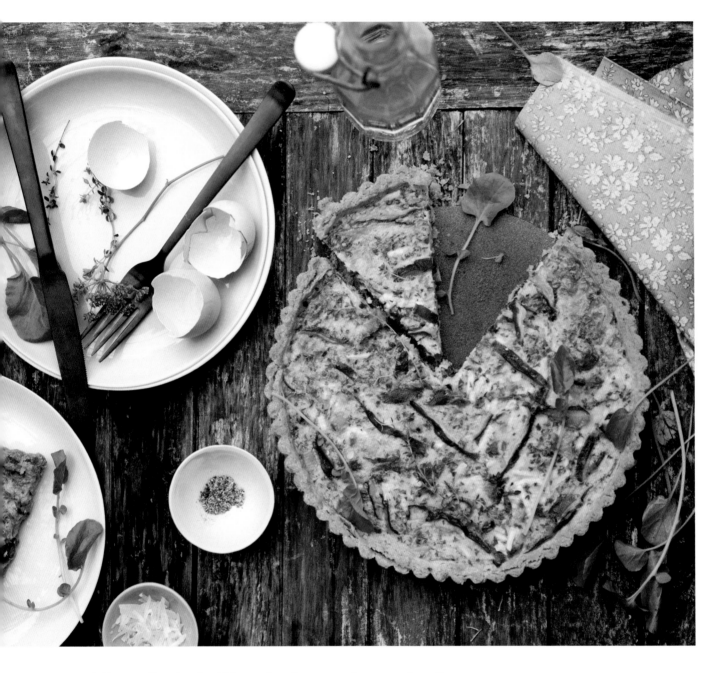

4 In a medium bowl, whisk together the eggs and cornstarch until lump-free. Add the half-and-half, Gruyère, remaining ¼ teaspoon salt, parsley, and thyme leaves. Whisk until smooth.

5 Fill the tart pan with the cooled mushroom and leek mixture. Pour the egg mixture over the filling; make sure to spread it evenly. Bake for 25 to 30 minutes or until golden brown. Let the quiche cool for 20 minutes before cutting.

2 eggs

2 tablespoons cornstarch

1 cup (250 ml) half-and-half or unsweetened coconut milk

1 ounce (30 g) Gruyère cheese, grated

2 tablespoons finely chopped fresh parsley

1 teaspoon fresh thyme leaves

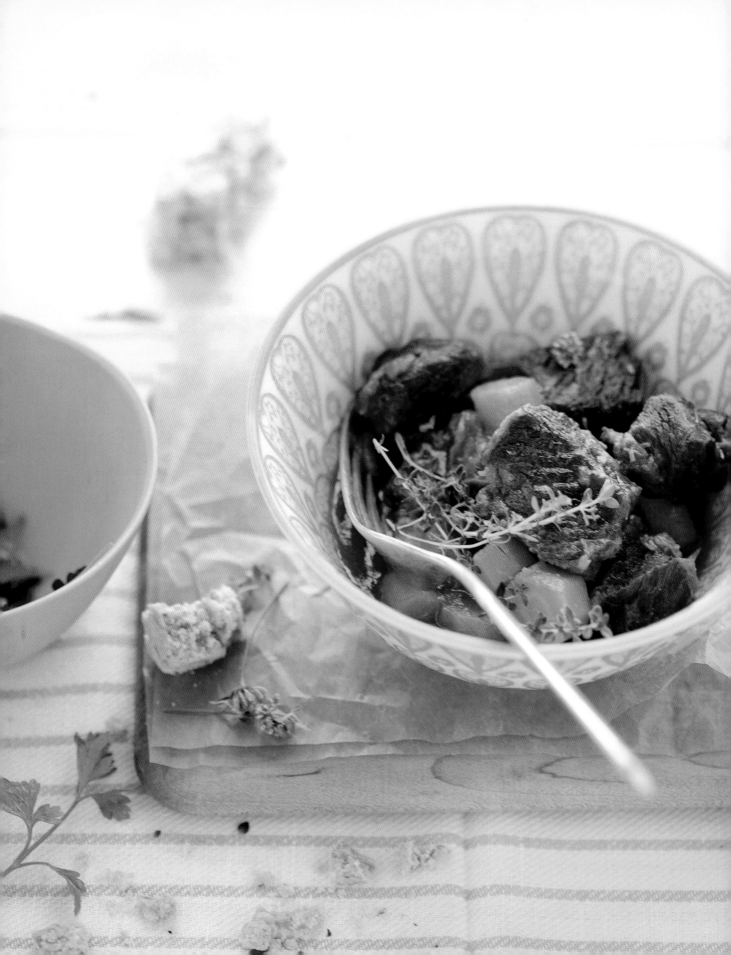

sunday beef stew

I KNOW IT MIGHT SEEM AS THOUGH beef stew could hardly be considered a small plate. We think of it as hearty and heavy. However, in the Basque Country, when temperatures start to drop, all *pintxo* bars offer some kind of slow-cooked beef plate. They serve tongue, tripe, and all the other tough cuts of meat. These plates are small in size but hearty and flavorful nonetheless.

"I am going to walk to the pastry shop for an *hamaiketako* [mid-morning snack]," I told my brother Jokin one lazy Sunday morning. It was that magical hour when everyone took a break from work and ate a bite of whatever my grandmother Miren was cooking. The smell of the simmering stew drew me in. "Come have a taste," she said as she offered me the old wooden spoon. The broth was rich with tomato, slowly broken down onions, and the freshness of herbs. It was the perfect mid-morning snack.

SERVES 6

1   Pull the meat out of the refrigerator at least 30 minutes before starting to cook. Season the meat with 1 teaspoon of the salt and the black pepper. Sprinkle the sweet rice flour over the meat and toss to coat it.

2   Heat a heavy cast-iron pot over medium-high heat. Add the olive oil. Add the meat (in two batches) and brown on all sides. Once the meat touches the oil, do not turn it until it browns, as it will tend to stick to the bottom of the pan. This is good and actually essential for caramelization to happen. When the first batch is browned on all sides, transfer it to a bowl. Finish cooking all the meat and set it aside.

3   Add 1 more tablespoon of olive oil to the pan, if needed. Add the onion, bell pepper, garlic, and remaining ½ teaspoon salt. Stir the vegetables while scraping the brown bits up off the bottom of the pan. Cook the vegetables over medium heat until tender, about 5 minutes.

4   Add the tomato paste and cook, stirring regularly, for 1 minute. Add the red wine and let it cook for about 1 minute. Add the meat back into the pot, along with 1½ cups (375 ml) water, the parsley, and thyme. Bring the liquid to a boil over medium-high heat, reduce the heat to medium-low, cover the pot, and simmer for 1 hour.

5   Add the diced carrots and potatoes. Give the stew a stir, cover the pot, and continue simmering for another hour or until the meat is fork-tender. Adjust the seasoning if needed.

6   Serve the stew warm with fresh herbs sprinkled over the top. The stew will keep in the refrigerator for up to 3 days. In fact, I believe it is better the next day.

2½ pounds (1.2 kg) grass-fed, boneless chuck roast or other stew meat, fat trimmed and cut into 1½-inch cubes

1½ teaspoons salt

1 teaspoon freshly ground black pepper

2 tablespoons sweet rice flour

2 tablespoons olive oil, plus more if needed

1 medium yellow onion, diced

½ medium green bell pepper, diced

2 cloves garlic, peeled

2 tablespoons tomato paste

¼ cup (60 ml) dry red wine

2 tablespoons finely chopped fresh parsley, plus more for serving

4 sprigs thyme, plus more for serving

4 medium carrots, peeled and diced

2 medium russet potatoes, peeled and diced

Fresh mixed herbs, for garnish

roasted garlic, celery root & saffron soup with curried shrimp

THIS SIMPLE ROOT VEGETABLE SOUP takes on a new dimension with the addition of the right spices. At home, I have a small coffee grinder that I use exclusively as a spice grinder. Sometimes I lightly toast the spices before grinding to bring out their flavor, and I always work with small quantities to preserve freshness.

SERVES 4

1 head garlic

2 tablespoons plus 2½ teaspoons (40 ml) olive oil

1 medium yellow onion, diced

1 celery stalk, diced

¾ teaspoon salt

¼ to ½ teaspoon saffron threads, depending on your taste

½ teaspoon ground coriander

1 large (1 pound or 450 g) celery root, peeled and diced

2 medium russet potatoes, peeled and diced

3½ cups (875 ml) chicken stock

½ cup (125 ml) unsweetened coconut milk, plus more for serving

8 ounces (225 g) wild-caught pink shrimp, peeled and deveined

½ teaspoon curry powder

Unsalted natural pistachios, chopped, for garnish

1   Preheat the oven to 400°F (200°C). Cut off the top part of the garlic, leaving the flesh exposed. Peel most of the outer layers of skin. Drizzle ½ teaspoon of the olive oil on top of the garlic. Wrap it in aluminum foil and bake it for 55 minutes to 1 hour, or until the flesh has turned golden. Remove the foil and let it cool until you are able to handle it. Squeeze out all of the roasted garlic flesh into a bowl. Reserve.

2   In a medium pot, heat 2 tablespoons of the olive oil over medium heat. Add the onion, celery, and ¼ teaspoon of the salt. Cook the vegetables until tender, about 5 minutes, while stirring occasionally.

3   Add the saffron and coriander and cook while stirring for about 30 seconds. Add the roasted garlic, celery root, potatoes, chicken stock, and the remaining ½ teaspoon salt. Bring the liquid to a boil over medium-high heat, reduce the heat to medium-low, cover the pot, and cook for 15 minutes or until the vegetables are tender.

4   Puree the soup in batches in a blender. Add the coconut milk and stir. Adjust the liquid and seasoning if necessary.

5   Right before serving, cut the shrimp into bite-size pieces. Toss with the curry powder. Heat the remaining 2 teaspoons olive oil in a medium sauté pan over medium-high heat. Add the shrimp and cook for 1 minute or until no longer translucent.

6   Serve the soup with the curried shrimp, a drizzle of coconut milk, and the chopped pistachio garnish.

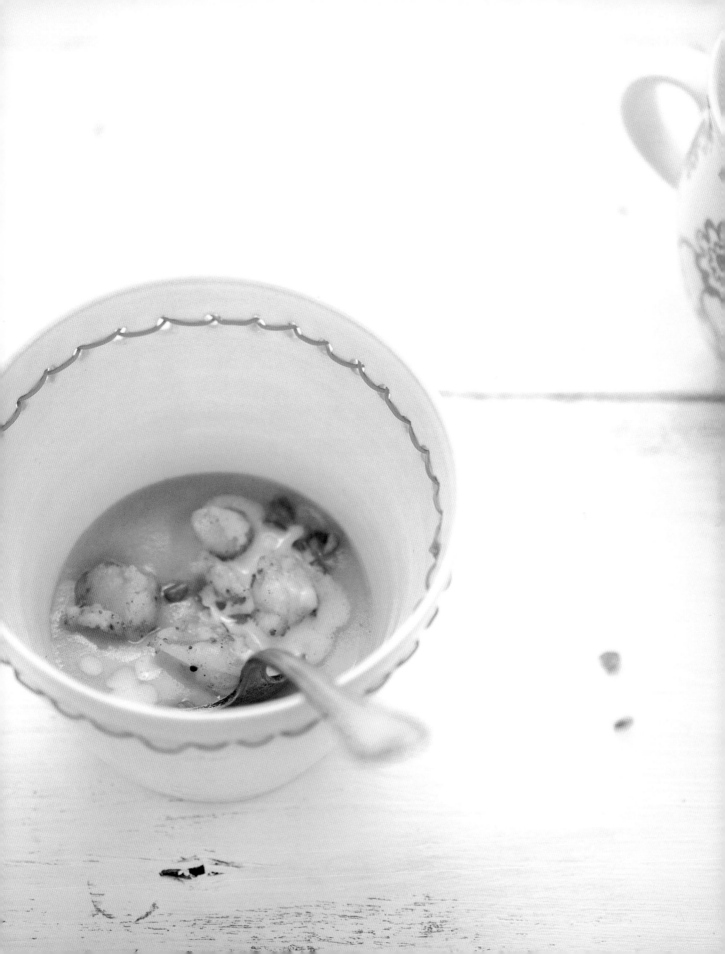

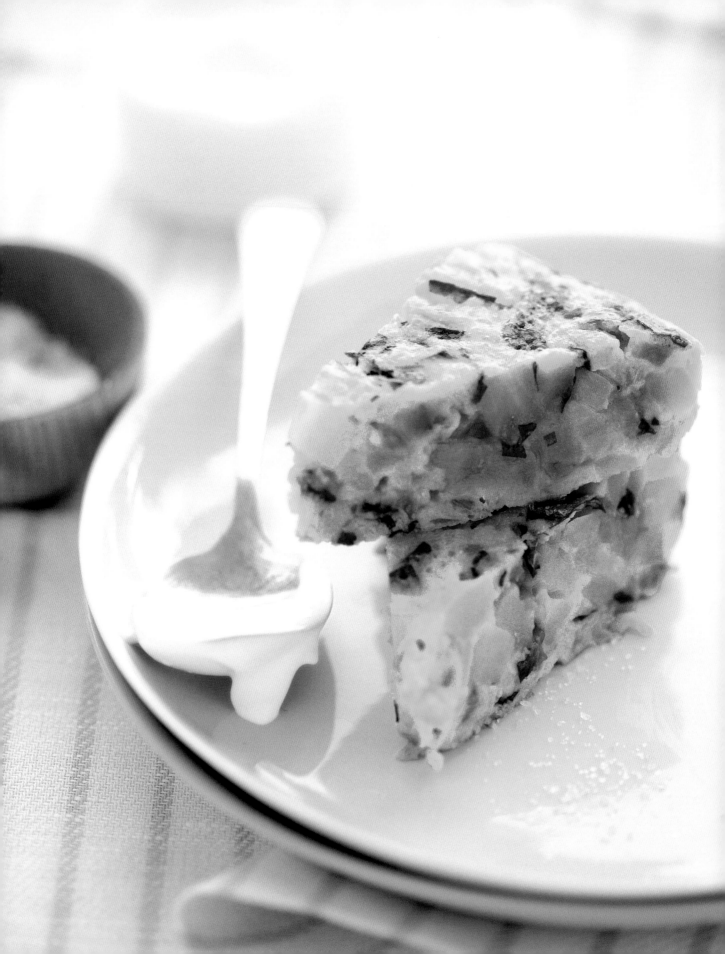

red kuri squash & spinach tortilla

SPANISH TORTILLA IS A FRITTATA-LIKE DISH OF onions, potatoes, and eggs cooked on the stovetop rather than in the oven. It is one of the most classic *pintxos* and is always present in bars and restaurants. It is the dish we grew up eating and making. It is the dish my mom cooked for us for school fundraisers, what we packed for the beach, and the salty bite we craved after a night of too much wine and dancing.

Red kuri squash is one of my favorite varieties of winter squash. Also known as Hokkaido squash, it tends to be smaller than a pumpkin, with thin skin that is edible once roasted. I love it for its chestnut-like aroma and the creaminess of its flesh. In this recipe, I combine potatoes with diced red kuri squash and spinach for a colorful and slightly sweeter version of the classic tortilla.

SERVES 4

1 Locate a plate or pan lid that measures about 8 inches or the same circumference as the nonstick skillet you will be using. This will help you flip the tortilla.

2 In a deep 8-inch nonstick pan, heat the olive oil over medium heat. Add the potato and ½ teaspoon of the salt, and cook for 5 minutes while stirring occasionally. You don't want the potato to brown.

3 Add the squash and the remaining ½ teaspoon salt. The pan might look overcrowded with vegetables, but do not worry; they will cook down. Continuing to stir occasionally, cook for another 7 minutes or until the vegetables are soft.

4 Meanwhile, whisk the eggs in a medium bowl. Drain the vegetables from the oil and add them to the beaten eggs, along with the spinach. Give the mixture a quick stir. Pour out most of the oil from the sauté pan into another bowl. I keep this flavorful oil for up to 3 days and use it for other soups or stews; however, be careful not to overheat it, as it has been heated previously.

5 Increase the heat to medium-high. Add the egg mixture back into the nonstick pan. Stir the center of the tortilla in a circular motion with a wooden spoon. When the center is lightly coagulated, stop stirring and let the eggs cook for 1 minute. Place the plate that is the same size as the pan over it. Carefully flip the pan over and transfer the tortilla onto the plate. Slide the tortilla back into the pan to finish cooking on the other side, 1 to 2 minutes depending on how runny you like it.

6 Gently slide the tortilla out of the pan onto a clean plate. Let it cool for 10 minutes before cutting into it. Serve warm or at room temperature.

½ cup (125 ml) olive oil

1½ cups (225 g) peeled and medium-diced russet potato (about 1 medium potato)

1 teaspoon salt

1½ cups (225 g) peeled and medium-diced red kuri or acorn squash (about ½ small squash)

4 eggs

1 cup (60 g) coarsely chopped spinach leaves

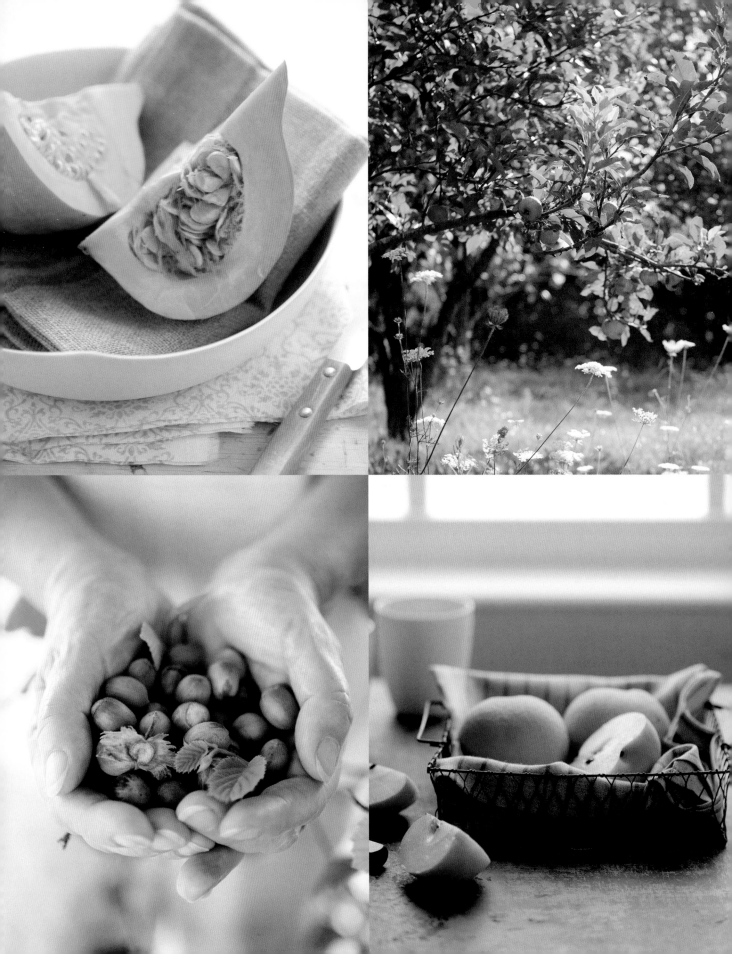

AUTUMN
sweet treats

ONE OF MY FAVORITE THINGS TO DO once the days become shorter and the leaves begin to turn is to take long walks in the forest. I seek fresh air and the smell of rain. I'll bring along a Thermos with hot chocolate and a small treat: something sweet and sticky, with the aroma of warm spices, the color of caramel, and the crunch of nuts. Perhaps a slice of upside-down apple, yogurt, and olive oil cake, as my mom used to make when I was growing up.

In my family, autumn means there are always baskets of apples and pears on the kitchen table, ready to be eaten throughout the day. Heirloom Reineta apples, widely available in Europe, are soft, tart, crisp, and sandy and are my preferred baking variety. In the United States I usually substitute Pink Lady apples. "Is it ready yet?" my son, Jon, asks impatiently every time my mom bakes the olive oil cake with Reinetas for us now. We know she will never cut into a warm cake regardless of how anxiously and irrationally we behave. She just will not, yet we beg every single time. "Take it out onto the balcony. The cold air will cool it faster." The neighbors must love the aroma of cinnamon and sugar.

When I moved to the United States, I learned to bake with cranberries, pumpkins, and sweet potatoes. They had not been part of my upbringing, but I soon came to love them. They speak of comfort and warmth. As Halloween approaches, baking takes on the color of caramel with sweet treats like Hazelnut Butter Toffee (page 68). Jon begs for Roasted Pumpkin Ice Cream (page 80) and Chocolate & Sweet Potato Doughnuts (page 77)—his sister, Miren, is never far behind. It is my goal that they learn to understand the seasons through the aromas in our kitchen.

red plum & rosemary tarte tatin

PLUMS OUTLAST THE DAYS OF SUMMER, surviving into early autumn. Many varieties can still be found at the farmers' markets, with their deep-colored skin and sweet flesh. The first time I tasted plums, caramel, and rosemary together I thought I had died and gone to heaven. This unexpected combination made so much sense to my palate—it was sweet, woodsy, and tart all at once.

Make sure to use plums that are ripe yet hold their shape; otherwise they will turn to mush.

MAKES one 9-inch tart

PASTRY CRUST

¾ cup (105 g) superfine brown rice flour, plus more for dusting

¼ cup (35 g) sorghum flour

3 tablespoons tapioca starch

1 tablespoon natural cane sugar

¼ teaspoon salt

1 stick (8 tablespoons or 110 g) cold unsalted butter, cut into ½-inch cubes

6 to 8 tablespoons ice water

PLUM AND ROSEMARY FILLING

½ cup (100 g) natural cane sugar

¼ stick (2 tablespoons or 30 g) unsalted butter, at room temperature

2 sprigs rosemary, cut into 2-inch pieces

1 vanilla bean, split lengthwise and seeds scraped

9 or 10 ripe yet firm large red plums (about 1½ pounds or 675 g), halved and pits removed

make the crust

1 Combine the first five ingredients in a food processor. Pulse three times to aerate. Add the cold butter and pulse ten times, until the butter is the size of peas. Add the 6 tablespoons of ice water and pulse. The dough should come together when pressed between your fingers. If too dry, add a bit more ice water.

2 Transfer the dough to a work surface, knead it a couple of times, and form into a disk. Wrap it in plastic wrap, flatten it, and refrigerate for 1 hour.

3 Roll the dough out on a cold surface dusted with superfine brown rice flour. Roll to a ¼- to ⅛-inch thickness. Cut a 9½-inch circle. Transfer the dough to a baking sheet lined with parchment paper, lightly dock it with a fork, and chill for another 20 minutes.

prepare the filling and bake the tart

1 Preheat the oven to 400°F (200°C).

2 Line the bottom of a 9-inch cake pan with parchment paper.

3 Heat a medium sauté pan over medium-high heat. Evenly sprinkle half of the sugar into the pan. Let this melt and then add the rest of the sugar. If some of the sugar turns to caramel quicker in some spots than others, gently stir the caramel with a spatula. When the caramel turns amber (do not burn the caramel!), add the butter, rosemary, and vanilla bean and seeds. Swirl the pan around until the butter is melted.

4 Place the plums cut side down over the caramel. Immediately reduce the heat to medium and cook for 5 minutes. You want them soft but not mushy. Remove the pan from the heat. Discard the rosemary and vanilla bean pod.

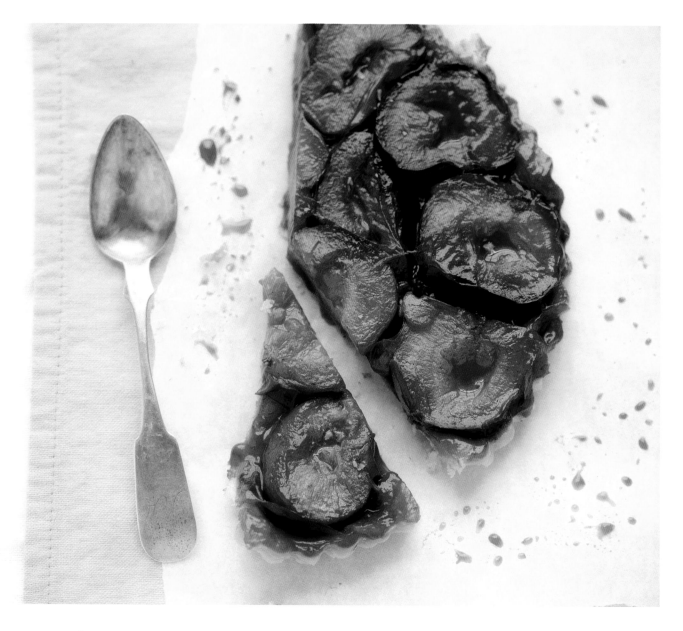

5   Carefully (the caramel is very hot!) transfer the cooked plums to the prepared cake pan, cut side down. Tightly arrange the plums in a circle and pour the leftover caramel on top.

6   Lay the pastry over the plums and tuck in the edges. If the dough cracks, pinch it back together.

7   Bake for 35 minutes, until the pastry is golden brown and juices are bubbling over. Carefully invert the tart over a cooling rack that is placed over a baking sheet. The caramel will run over the sides. Remove the parchment paper from the tart. Let it cool completely on the cooling rack before cutting. Serve warm or at room temperature.

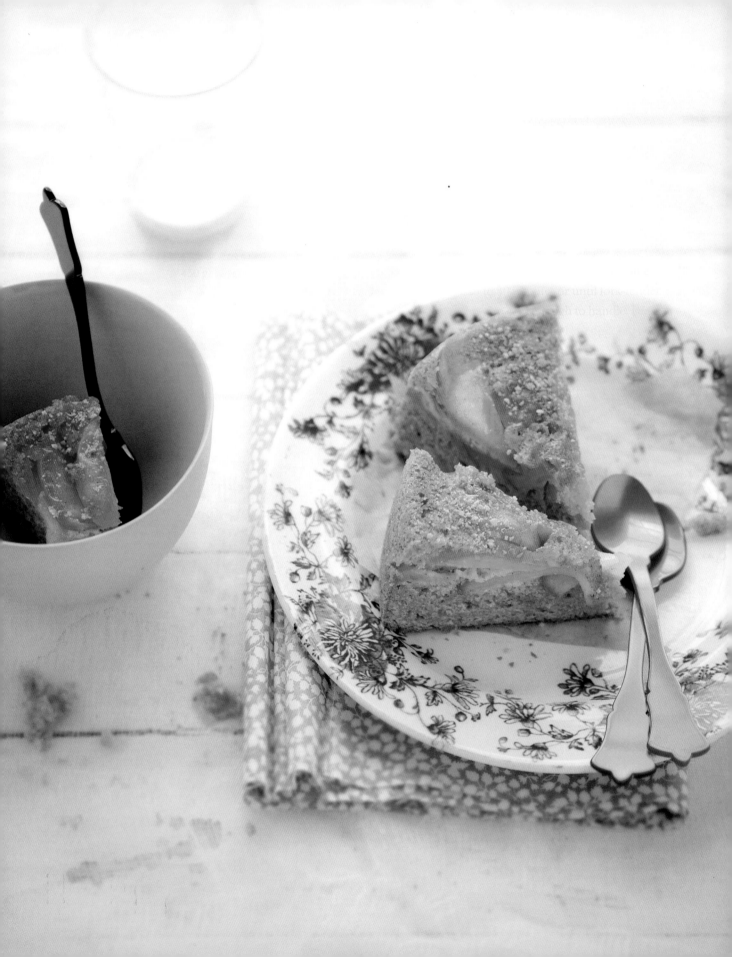

apple, yogurt & olive oil
upside-down cake

MOST FAMILIES HAVE A SWEET TREAT or dessert that can always be found on the kitchen counter. For us it was my mom's olive oil cake. This was a pound cake–like loaf baked in a red nonstick pan that my mom still uses today. She never really followed a recipe. It was 1 container of yogurt, 2 jars of sugar, 4 eggs. . . . We couldn't wait for it to cool to start cutting into it.

The recipe here is inspired by my mom's cake. Sliced Pink Lady apples sautéed in butter and sugar top this moist and dark loaf—pretty healthy, if you ask me!

MAKES one 8-inch cake

1   Preheat the oven to 350°F (180°C). Lightly grease an 8 by 3-inch round cake pan and line the bottom with a circle of parchment paper.

2   Core the apples, quarter them, and cut each quarter into fourths. Heat the butter, 2 tablespoons of the natural cane sugar, and the vanilla pod (save the seeds for the batter) in a large sauté pan over medium heat until the butter has melted. Add the sliced apples and cook for 7 minutes or until they are tender but still hold their shape. The sugar should not caramelize. Let the apples cool for 15 minutes.

3   Arrange the apples tightly on the bottom of the cake pan in a circular pattern.

4   In a large bowl, whisk together the superfine brown rice flour, almond flour, potato starch, millet flour, tapioca starch, baking powder, baking soda, cinnamon, ginger, and salt.

5   In a separate bowl, whisk together the eggs, remaining ½ cup (100 g) natural cane sugar, muscovado sugar, yogurt, olive oil, and vanilla seeds. Pour the wet ingredients over the dry and whisk until the batter comes together. Pour the batter into the cake pan.

6   Bake for 1 hour or until a toothpick inserted in the center of the cake comes out clean. Let the cake cool in the pan for 15 minutes. Carefully invert it onto a cooling rack and cool completely.

7   Store in the refrigerator, tightly wrapped, for up to 3 days. You can also freeze it for up to 1 month.

3 Pink Lady apples, or any other crisp apple you like

2 tablespoons (¼ stick or 30 g) unsalted butter

½ cup plus 2 tablespoons (130 g) natural cane sugar

1 vanilla bean, split lengthwise and seeds scraped

¾ cup (105 g) superfine brown rice flour

⅓ cup (35 g) almond flour

¼ cup (40 g) potato starch

¼ cup (35 g) millet flour

2 tablespoons tapioca starch

1 tablespoon baking powder

½ teaspoon baking soda

½ teaspoon ground cinnamon

¼ teaspoon ground ginger

¼ teaspoon salt

3 eggs

½ cup (100 g) packed muscovado or dark brown sugar

½ cup (125 ml) whole-milk plain yogurt

½ cup (125 ml) olive oil

cranberry & quinoa scones

I WAS TWELVE THE FIRST TIME I VISITED London. My brother Jon and I stayed with our family friends Giovanni and Iziar, while my older brother Jokin stayed with another family across the street. We attended English classes in the morning and discovered the city in the afternoons and on weekends. Giovanni was a maitre d' at a fine-dining Italian restaurant in the city, and Iziar worked at a proper English teahouse and bakery.

Every evening, Iziar came home with leftovers from the bakery. The blueberry muffins were always a breakfast favorite, and the scones were packed in our school lunch sacks for afternoon tea break, a tradition I have kept ever since.

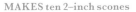

MAKES ten 2–inch scones

1¼ sticks (10 tablespoons or 140 g) unsalted butter

½ cup (125 ml) cold unsweetened coconut milk

1 teaspoon freshly squeezed lemon juice

1 cup (100 g) cranberries

1 cup (140 g) superfine brown rice flour

1 cup (90 g) quinoa flakes, plus more for topping

⅓ cup (45 g) quinoa flour

⅓ cup (40 g) tapioca starch

⅓ cup (70 g) natural cane sugar

1 tablespoon baking powder

½ teaspoon baking soda

½ teaspoon salt

Zest of 1 orange

2 eggs

1 tablespoon demerara sugar, for topping

1 Place the butter in the freezer at least 30 minutes before beginning.

2 Preheat the oven to 400°F (200°C).

3 Mix the coconut milk and lemon juice in a bowl and chill for 5 minutes.

4 Coarsely chop the cranberries in a food processor and set them aside.

5 In a large bowl, whisk together the superfine brown rice flour, quinoa flakes, quinoa flour, tapioca starch, sugar, baking powder, baking soda, salt, and orange zest. Take the butter out of the freezer and grate it using the large holes in a box grater. Gently toss the butter into the flour mixture, but try not to touch it too much, as the warmth from your hands can melt it.

6 Whisk 1 egg into the coconut milk mixture. Add this mixture to the flour-and-butter base and fold with a wooden spatula until it comes together. Fold in the chopped cranberries.

7 Transfer the dough to a work surface and knead it a few times until it comes together. Form a disk, pat it down, and roll it out to a ¾-inch thickness. Using a 2-inch round cookie cutter dipped in superfine brown rice flour, cut out the scones and place them on a baking sheet lined with parchment paper. Re-roll scraps once and cut again.

8 Whisk the remaining egg in a small bowl. Using a pastry brush, brush the tops of the scones with the egg wash. Sprinkle demerara sugar and quinoa flakes on top of each scone.

9 Bake the scones until golden brown, about 18 minutes. Let them cool on the baking sheet for 15 minutes and then cool them completely on a wire rack. They keep well at room temperature for 2 days, or they can be frozen for up to 1 month.

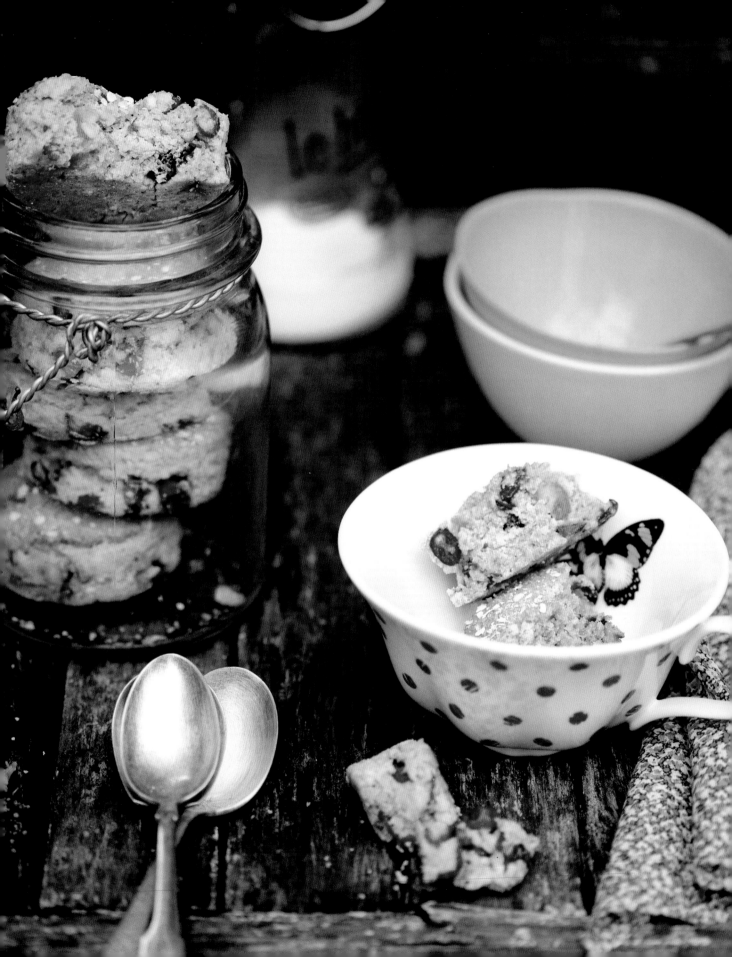

chocolate, hazelnut &
fleur de sel pots de crème

VANILLA AND CHOCOLATE CUSTARD POTS are a staple in our house. I make sure we always have some baked and in the refrigerator for an afternoon snack when the kids come home from school. It is a nutritious treat and I never feel guilty serving it. This custard recipe is made with coconut milk and eggs flavored with bittersweet chocolate, hazelnut butter, and *fleur de sel*.

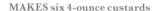 **MAKES** six 4-ounce custards

¼ cup (30 g) hazelnuts

2 cups (500 ml) unsweetened coconut milk

1 vanilla bean, split lengthwise and seeds scraped

1 egg

2 egg yolks

¼ cup (50 g) coconut palm sugar

2 tablespoons hazelnut butter

2 ounces (60 g) milk chocolate, finely chopped

2 ounces (60 g) bittersweet chocolate, finely chopped

½ teaspoon *fleur de sel*

1 Preheat the oven to 350°F (180°C). Roast the hazelnuts on a baking sheet for 5 to 7 minutes, until golden and fragrant. Place them in a dry kitchen towel and rub them together to remove their skins. Let the hazelnuts cool and then chop them coarsely. Reduce the oven temperature to 300°F (150°C).

2 In a medium saucepan, heat the coconut milk, the vanilla bean, and its seeds over medium heat. Bring to a low simmer.

3 Meanwhile, in a medium bowl, whisk together the egg, egg yolks, coconut palm sugar, and hazelnut butter until almost lump-free.

4 When the coconut milk has come to a simmer, remove the pan from the heat. Remove the vanilla bean pod and add the milk and bittersweet chocolates. Stir to melt the chocolates into the milk.

5 Pour a little bit of the hot coconut milk mixture over the eggs while whisking to keep the eggs from coagulating. Add the rest of the mixture and whisk. Strain the mixture through a fine-mesh sieve into a clean bowl. Add the *fleur de sel* and stir.

6 Pour the custard into 6 (4-ounce) oven-safe ramekins or jars. Place the ramekins in a deep baking pan and place the pan on the oven rack. Add enough hot water to the pan to come halfway up the sides of the ramekins, creating a water bath.

7 Bake the custard for 30 to 40 minutes or until the center is set. Let the ramekins cool to room temperature. They can be served at room temperature or chilled.

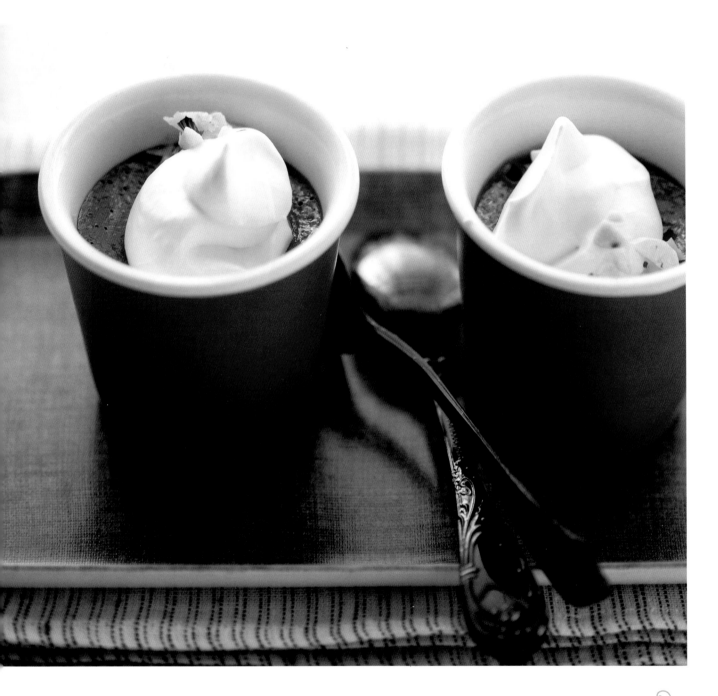

MAKING YOUR OWN NUT BUTTER

It is easy to make nut butters at home. Spread 2 cups of your favorite nuts on a baking sheet (I love hazelnuts). Bake the nuts at 350°F (180°C) for 5 to 10 minutes or until fragrant and golden. Transfer them to a food processor or high-speed blender and process them until they turn into a paste. Add 1 tablespoon vegetable oil or nut oil (hazelnut, almond, or pistachio) and a pinch of salt and process until smooth. You can sweeten the nut butter with 1 tablespoon honey or leave it plain.

spiced pear & brown butter muffins

RADIATING A WARM AROMA FULL OF autumn spices, these muffins satisfy any midafternoon sweets craving. Serve them with a cup of ginger tea for breakfast or turn them into cupcakes with a swirl of cane sugar buttercream.

MAKES 12 muffins

1¼ sticks (10 tablespoons or 140 g) unsalted butter

1 cup (140 g) superfine brown rice flour

½ cup (50 g) almond flour

2 tablespoons tapioca starch

1½ teaspoons baking powder

½ teaspoon salt

½ teaspoon ground cinnamon

¼ teaspoon ground ginger

⅛ teaspoon ground nutmeg

⅛ teaspoon ground cardamom

2 eggs, at room temperature

⅓ cup (100 g) dark amber maple syrup

⅓ cup (60 g) packed light brown sugar

1 vanilla bean, split lengthwise and seeds scraped

2 medium-size ripe Bartlett pears

2 tablespoons chopped natural pistachios, for garnish

1 Preheat the oven to 350°F (180°C).

2 In a small saucepan, cook the butter over medium heat until it starts to bubble and the milk solids start to brown on the bottom of the pan. It will take about 5 minutes and will smell like roasting nuts. Remove the pan from the heat and transfer the brown butter to a clean bowl to cool.

3 In a large bowl, whisk together the superfine brown rice flour, almond flour, tapioca starch, baking powder, salt, cinnamon, ginger, nutmeg, and cardamom.

4 In a separate bowl, whisk together the eggs, maple syrup, brown sugar, vanilla seeds, and brown butter. Add the wet ingredients to the dry and mix until combined.

5 Grate the pears using a box grater, skin and all. Fold the grated pear into the batter.

6 Line a muffin pan with paper liners and, using an ice cream scoop, fill the liners with the batter about three-quarters of the way full. Sprinkle the tops with chopped pistachios.

7 Bake the muffins for 20 to 25 minutes or until a toothpick inserted in the center comes out clean. Transfer the muffins to a cooling rack and let them cool completely. They will keep in the refrigerator, tightly wrapped, for up to 3 days.

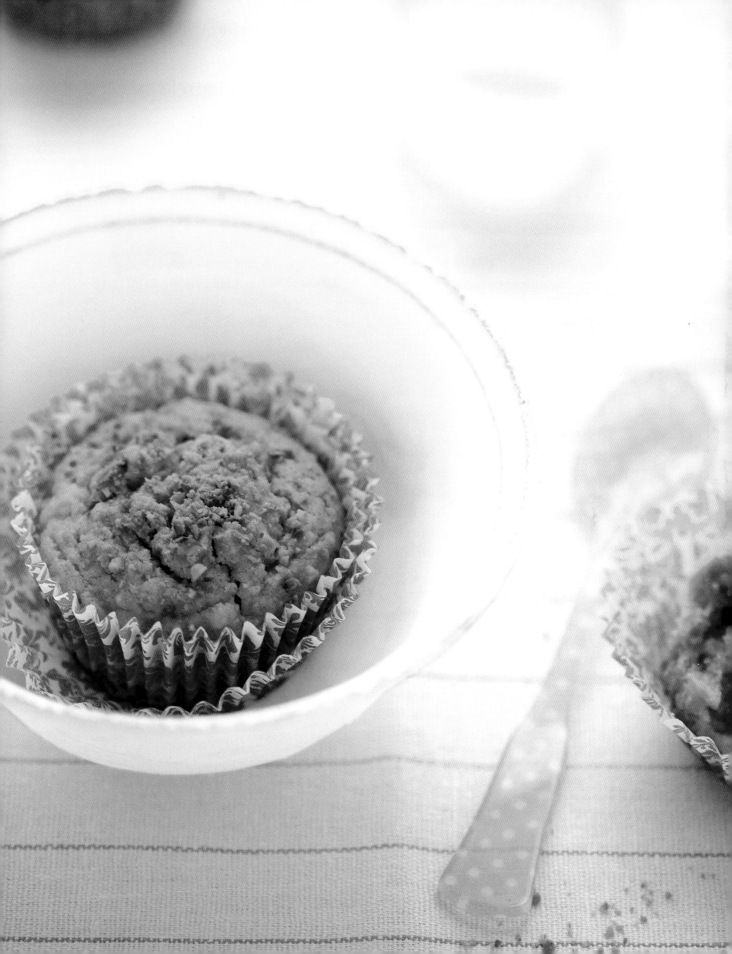

caramel-poached pears with crushed chocolate chip meringue

ONE OF THE THINGS THAT I THINK ABOUT when developing a recipe is the texture combination. In this case, I was looking for something soft, crunchy, and creamy. Sound plays a part too. I love to be able to "hear" all the textures as I take a bite. The poached pears are wonderfully creamy, and the meringue adds the crunchy element as well as the soft and gooey one. Serve with softly whipped cream, if you like.

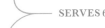

SERVES 6

CHOCOLATE CHIP MERINGUE

4 egg whites, at room temperature

Pinch of salt

1 cup plus 2 tablespoons (225 g) superfine sugar (caster sugar)

2 ounces (60 g) bittersweet chocolate, finely chopped

CARAMEL-POACHED PEARS

2¼ cups (450 g) demerara sugar

1 vanilla bean, split lengthwise and seeds scraped

1 teaspoon whole pink peppercorns

2 whole star anise

Peel of 1 lemon

12 small ripe Forelle or Bartlett pears, peeled, stems on

make the meringue

1   Preheat the oven to 250°F (120°C).

2   Place the egg whites in the bowl of a stand mixer. Add the pinch of salt. Whip on medium-high speed until soft peaks form. Slowly, and while continuing to whip, add the sugar, a little at a time to prevent the meringue from deflating. Finish adding all the sugar and continue whipping until glossy and stiff peaks form, about 10 minutes.

3   Turn the mixer off and gently fold in the finely chopped chocolate.

4   Line a baking sheet with parchment paper. Using a spoon, drop 12 mounds of meringue on the baking sheet, about 1 inch apart. Bake the meringues for 40 to 45 minutes, until they do not stick to the paper. You want them to be crispy on the outside yet soft on the inside. Let them cool until ready to assemble.

5   You can store the meringues in an airtight container for 1 week. They are great to have handy to eat alone or to crumble on top of ice cream or any creamy dessert.

make the caramel and poach the pears

1   Evenly sprinkle the bottom of a 6-quart pot with roughly one-third of the demerara sugar. Turn the heat to medium-high and let the sugar melt. No need to stir at this point. When that first layer of sugar has melted, sprinkle in another one-third and let that melt as well. Then add the last of the sugar. Stir until there are no lumps or undissolved granules.

2   Pour in 4 cups (1 L) water. Be careful when doing so, because the caramel will splatter. The sugar might harden. Do not worry; let it melt back into the caramel.

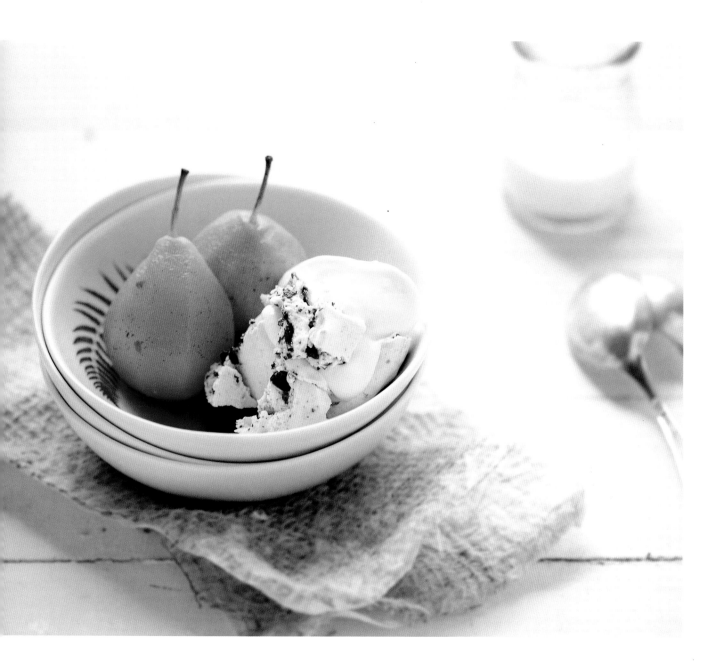

3 Add both the vanilla seeds and the pod to the caramel. Add the pink peppercorns, star anise, and lemon peel.

4 Add the peeled pears to the caramel. Let them simmer, covered, on low heat for about 8 minutes or until tender. Remove the pot from the heat and let the pears cool in the syrup for about 4 hours.

5 Serve the poached pears warm or at room temperature; crumble the meringues over the top. You can store the pears in the caramel syrup, covered, in the refrigerator for up to 5 days.

hazelnut butter toffee

THIS HAZELNUT BUTTER TOFFEE is wonderful on its own, sprinkled over ice cream, or folded into a mousse. In this case, I divided the amount to make two delicious desserts (recipes follow).

MAKES 1 cup

⅓ cup (45 g) hazelnuts

⅓ cup (70 g) natural cane sugar

½ stick (4 tablespoons or 55 g) unsalted butter

¼ teaspoon salt

1 Preheat the oven to 350°F (180°C). Place the hazelnuts on a baking sheet. Toast for 5 to 7 minutes or until golden. Place them inside a cloth towel while still warm and rub them together to remove their skins. Reserve.

2 Combine the sugar, butter, 2 tablespoons water, and salt in a small saucepan. Cook on medium-high heat while stirring until the sugar dissolves and the butter melts. Stop stirring and cook until a candy thermometer reads 300°F (150°C). Add the toasted hazelnuts and stir. Pour the toffee onto a baking sheet lined with parchment paper or a silicone mat. Let it cool completely.

3 Coarsely chop the toffee. Store in an airtight container for up to 1 week.

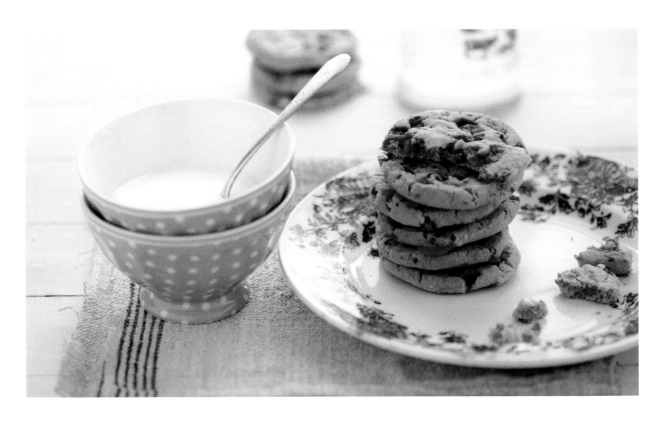

hazelnut butter toffee–chocolate chip cookies

THIS IS PROBABLY MY CHILDREN'S favorite cookie. Soft and chewy, served with a glass of milk on a chilly afternoon . . . need I say more?

MAKES about 24 cookies

1 In the bowl of a stand mixer, mix together the butter, brown sugar, and cane sugar with the paddle attachment on medium speed until light, about 2 minutes. Add the vanilla extract and the egg. Mix until combined.

2 In a separate bowl, whisk together the superfine brown rice flour, potato starch, tapioca starch, salt, and baking soda. Add the dry ingredients to the butter mixture and mix until it comes together. Add the chopped hazelnut butter toffee and chocolate chips. Mix until well combined.

3 Scrape the dough onto a sheet of parchment paper; it will be sticky. With the help of the parchment paper, shape the dough into a round log that is about 13 inches long and 2 inches in diameter. Roll the parchment around the log and refrigerate for at least 1 hour.

4 Preheat the oven to 350°F (180°C). Line two baking sheets with parchment paper or silicone mats.

5 Cut the cookie log into ½-inch-thick disks. Place them on the baking sheets, spaced 2 inches apart. Bake for 15 minutes, until golden. Let the cookies cool on the baking sheet for 10 minutes before lifting them. Store them in an airtight container for up to 3 days (if they last that long!).

1 stick (8 tablespoons or 110 g) unsalted butter, at room temperature

½ cup plus 2 tablespoons (125 g) light brown sugar

¼ cup (50 g) natural cane sugar

½ teaspoon vanilla extract

1 egg, at room temperature

1 cup (140 g) superfine brown rice flour

⅓ cup (55 g) potato starch

⅓ cup (40 g) tapioca starch

½ teaspoon salt

½ teaspoon baking soda

½ cup (70 g) chopped Hazelnut Butter Toffee (facing page)

½ cup (90 g) mini semisweet chocolate chips

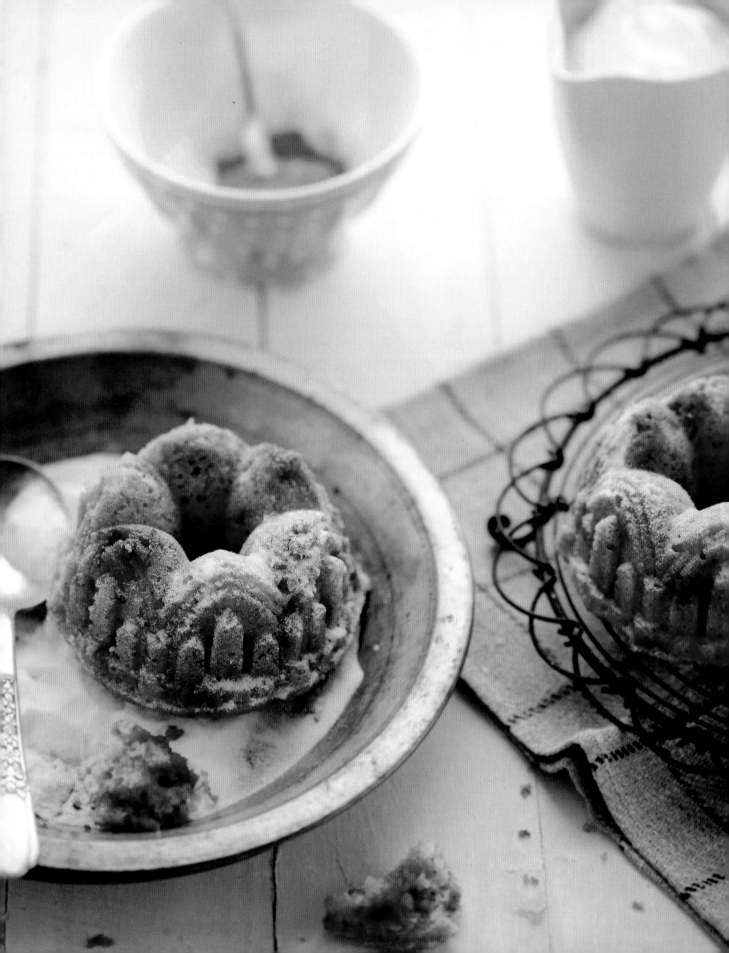

asian pear & hazelnut butter toffee cake

THIS RECIPE IS A VARIATION ON MY MOTHER'S yogurt and olive oil cake, the cake we grew up eating. I use that recipe often as a base for many adaptations. In this case, crisp Asian pears and salty toffee are folded into the batter, creating a swirl of caramel throughout the cake.

In case you have never had an Asian pear, they look similar to apples, but don't let that fool you—they are not a cross between an apple and a pear. They have a very crunchy texture, similar to apples, but a much higher water content. They are great thinly sliced in salads.

MAKES 8 mini Bundt cakes or 1 large Bundt cake

4 eggs

½ cup (100 g) natural cane sugar

½ cup (100 g) demerara sugar

1 vanilla bean, split lengthwise and seeds scraped

½ cup (125 ml) whole-milk plain yogurt

½ cup (125 ml) olive oil

¾ cup plus 1 tablespoon (115 g) superfine brown rice flour

½ cup (70 g) sorghum flour

¼ cup (30 g) tapioca starch

¼ cup (25 g) hazelnut flour

1 tablespoon baking powder

½ teaspoon salt

1 Asian pear, peeled and cut into ½-inch pieces

½ cup (70 g) chopped Hazelnut Butter Toffee (page 68)

1   Preheat the oven to 350°F (180°C). Grease 8 mini (1-cup) Bundt pans or a 10-cup Bundt pan with butter. In a large bowl, whisk together the eggs, cane sugar, demerara sugar, vanilla seeds, yogurt, and olive oil.

2   In a separate large bowl, whisk together the ¾ cup (105 g) superfine brown rice flour, sorghum flour, tapioca starch, hazelnut flour, baking powder, and salt.

3   Add the wet ingredients to the dry mixture and whisk. In a small bowl, toss the pears and toffee with the remaining 1 tablespoon of superfine brown rice flour and fold them into the batter.

4   Pour the batter into the greased pan(s). Bake for 25 to 30 minutes for the mini Bundt pans or 45 to 50 minutes for the large Bundt pan, until a wooden skewer inserted in the center comes out clean. Let cool in the pan(s) for 15 minutes before inverting onto a cooling rack to cool completely. The cake will keep, tightly wrapped at room temperature, for 3 days, or it can be frozen for up to 1 month.

brown butter–candied apple clafoutis

CLAFOUTIS IS A CLASSIC FRENCH DESSERT, somewhere between a custard and a cake. Lots of eggs, milk, and a little bit of flour are the traditional ingredients. It is an easy recipe to convert using gluten-free flours, as it relies mostly on eggs and milk. I make many versions with seasonal fruits. I was browsing through the pages of Thomas Keller's *The French Laundry Cookbook* when I came across his candied apple ice cream. I am up for candied apple anything, and with those flavors in mind I created this clafoutis with brown butter and the intense flavor of reduced apple juice.

SERVES 6

2 cups plus 1 tablespoon (515 ml) unsweetened apple juice

¼ stick (2 tablespoons or 30 g) unsalted butter, plus more for lining pie dish

4 medium Granny Smith apples (2 pounds or 1 kg), peeled, cored, and sliced into ¼-inch pieces

½ cup plus 3 tablespoons (140 g) natural cane sugar

1 vanilla bean, split lengthwise and seeds scraped

3 eggs

⅓ cup (35 g) almond flour

¼ cup (30 g) tapioca starch

½ teaspoon salt

¾ cup (185 ml) unsweetened coconut milk

1   Preheat the oven to 400°F (200°C). Butter a 10-inch deep-dish pie pan.

2   Pour 2 cups of the apple juice into a small saucepan. Cook over high heat for 12 minutes, until the juice is reduced to ½ cup (125 ml). Let the reduced juice cool.

3   In a large sauté pan, cook the butter over medium-high heat until the milk solids start to brown, about 3 minutes. Add the sliced apples, 3 tablespoons of the sugar, half of the vanilla seeds, and the remaining 1 tablespoon apple juice. Cook the apples over medium heat, stirring occasionally, for 5 to 8 minutes or until the apples are soft but not mushy. Set aside.

4   In a medium bowl, whisk together the eggs, remaining ½ cup (100 g) sugar, remaining vanilla seeds, almond flour, tapioca starch, and salt until smooth. Add the coconut milk and reduced apple juice, and whisk to combine.

5   Pour the custard into the prepared pan. Top with the cooked apples and their released juices. Bake the clafoutis for 35 to 40 minutes, until the center is set and the edges are golden brown. Serve warm or at room temperature.

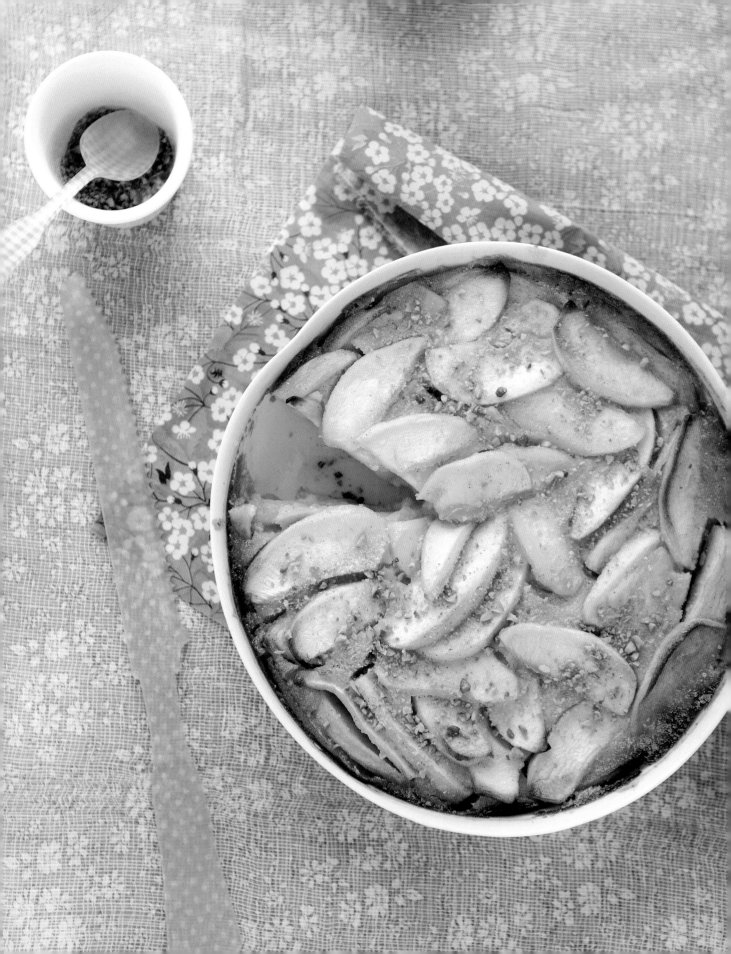

sweet buttermilk risotto
with apple compote

I COULD EAT THE ENTIRE POT OF THIS sweet risotto in one sitting. It's the perfect balance of sweet and tangy, creamy and crunchy. For the apple compote, the amount of sugar and apple juice can be adjusted depending on the tartness and juiciness of the apples you are using. A great tip is to always taste your fruit before starting to cook with it. This will give you control over the sweetness of the final dish.

SERVES 4 to 6

APPLE COMPOTE

3 medium Granny Smith, Pink Lady, or Reineta apples, peeled, cored, and sliced

¼ cup (60 ml) unsweetened apple juice

2 tablespoons freshly squeezed lemon juice

2 tablespoons natural cane sugar

½ vanilla bean, split lengthwise and seeds scraped

1 cinnamon stick

2 tablespoons golden raisins

2 tablespoons diced dried apricots

SWEET BUTTERMILK RISOTTO

4½ cups (1.125 L) whole milk, plus more if needed

¼ cup plus 2 tablespoons (75 g) natural cane sugar

1 vanilla bean, split lengthwise and seeds scraped

1 cinnamon stick (from the compote)

¼ teaspoon salt

¼ stick (2 tablespoons or 30 g) unsalted butter

¾ cup (150 g) Arborio rice

1 cup (250 ml) full-fat buttermilk or crème fraîche

Unsalted natural pistachios, chopped, for garnish

make the compote

Combine all the ingredients in a medium saucepan. Cook over medium heat, stirring occasionally, for 10 to 12 minutes or until the apples are soft but still have a bite and the liquid has evaporated. Remove the pan from the heat. Pick out the cinnamon stick and vanilla bean. Reserve the cinnamon stick for use in the risotto.

make the risotto

1 In a small saucepan, combine the whole milk, sugar, vanilla bean and seeds, cinnamon stick, and salt. Bring to a low simmer over medium-high heat, but do not boil. Reduce the heat to low and keep the mixture warm while cooking the risotto.

2 In a medium saucepan, melt the butter over medium heat. Add the rice and cook for 1 minute, until it is well coated with the butter.

3 Add about 1 cup (125 ml) of the warm milk mixture to the rice. Stir it constantly for 2 minutes, until the rice starts to thicken. Add a ½-cup ladle of the warm milk and continue cooking while stirring constantly. When the milk has been absorbed, add some more. Continue cooking the risotto, stirring constantly, until the rice is al dente and all the liquid has been absorbed. It will take 20 to 25 minutes.

4 Remove the pan from the heat and stir in the buttermilk. It should be creamy and loose, but it will thicken as it sits. If needed, you could add some more milk.

5 To serve, spoon some of the risotto into a bowl or glass. Top with Apple Compote and pistachios.

6 If you have leftovers, which I doubt you will, refrigerate them. To serve again, heat the risotto over low heat in a saucepan and loosen it with additional milk as needed.

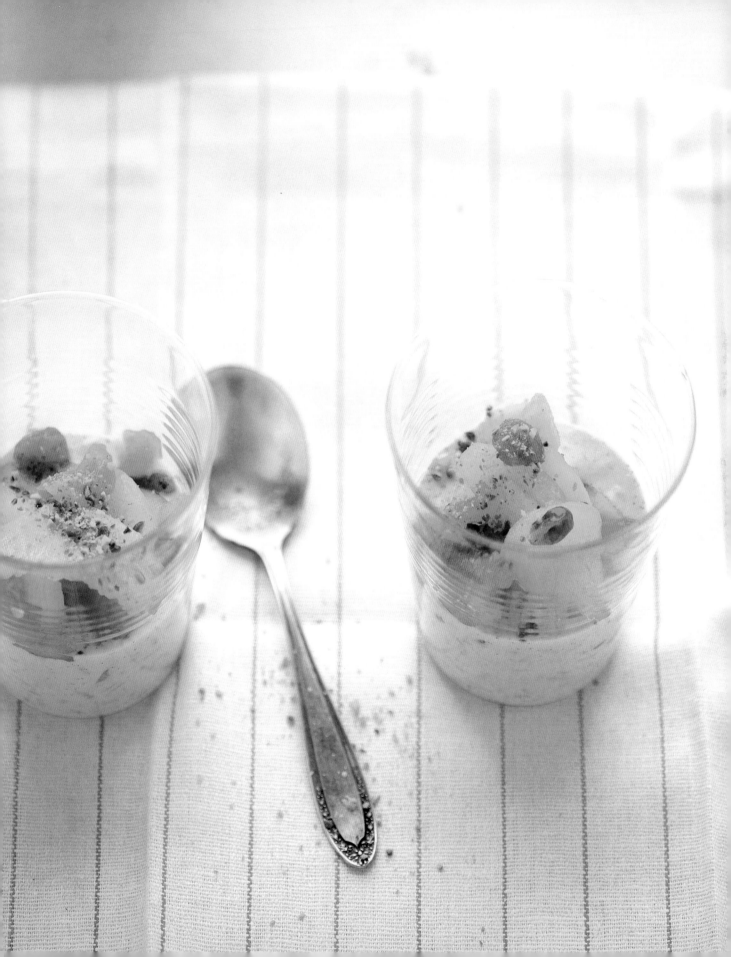

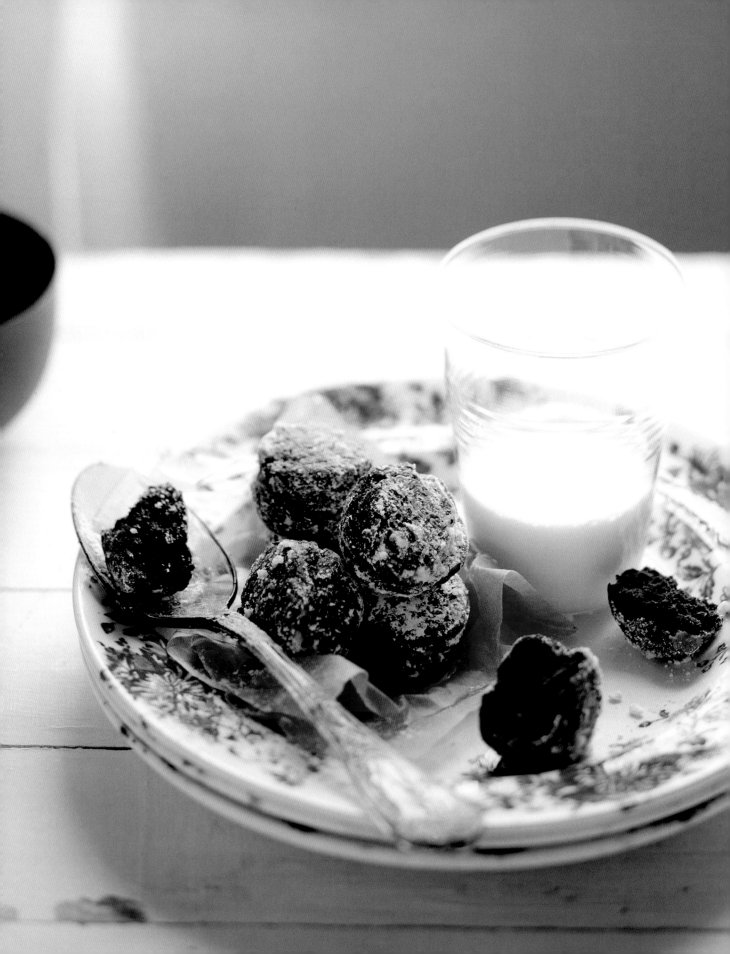

chocolate & sweet potato doughnuts

MY GRANDFATHER SELDOM MADE DOUGHNUTS, or *buñuelos*, at the pastry shop. I used to count down the days to November 1, All Saints Day—the day we celebrated the dead and also, year after year, indulged in *buñuelos*. People lined up out the door waiting anxiously for the annual batch of cinnamon Chiboust cream–filled doughnuts, and I had to beat them all to it before the *buñuelos* were gone.

MAKES 80 doughnut holes

1 Preheat the oven to 400°F (200°C). Place the sweet potato halves on a baking sheet, cut side down. Bake for 30 minutes or until tender. Remove the skin and mash the flesh with a fork. Measure ½ cup (125 g) packed puree.

2 In a large bowl, whisk together the superfine brown rice flour, sorghum flour, potato starch, hazelnut flour, tapioca starch, cocoa powder, baking powder, salt, baking soda, and cinnamon.

3 In a separate bowl, whisk together the eggs, sugar, coconut milk, olive oil, vanilla extract, and sweet potato puree. Add the wet ingredients to the dry and mix. Knead the dough together with your hands a few times, until it comes together.

4 Lightly dust a work surface with superfine brown rice flour. Transfer the dough to your work surface and pat it down with your hands. It will be a sticky dough and you might be tempted to add more flour, but it will not be necessary. As the dough sits, it becomes more compact. Roll to a ½-inch thickness. Cut 1½-inch circles with a cookie cutter. Dip the cookie cutter in superfine brown rice flour to make it easier. Place the doughnut holes on a baking sheet lined with parchment paper. Re-roll the scraps of dough once and cut more circles. Chill the doughnut holes for 30 minutes.

5 Fill a cast-iron Dutch oven with 2 inches of vegetable oil and heat to 325°F (160°C) over medium heat. Gently add a few doughnuts at a time without overcrowding the pan. They will sink to the bottom and then slowly rise to the top. When they rise to the top, flip them over and let them fry for another 30 seconds to 1 minute. Transfer them to a baking sheet lined with paper towels. Finish frying all the doughnuts and let them cool slightly, then roll them in powdered sugar. The fried doughnuts are best eaten the day they are made, but they can be frozen, tightly wrapped, for up to 1 month.

1 medium sweet potato, halved lengthwise

1 cup (140 g) superfine brown rice flour, plus more for dusting

¾ cup (105 g) sorghum flour

½ cup (80 g) potato starch

½ cup (50 g) hazelnut flour

½ cup (60 g) tapioca starch

3 tablespoons unsweetened black cocoa powder or Dutch-process cocoa powder

2 teaspoons baking powder

1 teaspoon salt

1 teaspoon baking soda

¼ teaspoon ground cinnamon

2 eggs, at room temperature

½ cup (100 g) natural cane sugar

½ cup (125 ml) unsweetened coconut milk

¼ cup (60 ml) olive oil

1 teaspoon vanilla extract

Vegetable oil, for frying

Powdered sugar, for rolling

everything cookies

THESE COOKIES EMBODY EVERYTHING that my senses long for. Chewy in the center and crispy on the outside, they are mildly sweet and full of chocolate pieces, pecans, oats, and coconut. Cinnamon and nutmeg add warmth and the smell of autumn.

MAKES 32 cookies

1 stick (8 tablespoons or 110 g) unsalted butter, at room temperature

½ cup (100 g) natural cane sugar

½ cup (100 g) dark muscovado or dark brown sugar

1 teaspoon vanilla extract

1 egg, at room temperature

½ cup (70 g) superfine brown rice flour

⅓ cup (45 g) buckwheat flour

¼ cup (30 g) tapioca starch

2 teaspoons baking powder

2 teaspoons baking soda

1 teaspoon salt

1 teaspoon ground cinnamon

⅛ teaspoon ground nutmeg

¾ cup (150 g) mini chocolate chips

½ cup (50 g) gluten-free rolled oats

½ cup (60 g) coarsely chopped pecan pieces

½ cup (35 g) unsweetened coconut flakes, cut into small pieces

1   Combine the butter, natural cane sugar, and muscovado sugar in the bowl of a stand mixer. Mix with the paddle attachment on medium speed for 3 minutes.

2   Add the vanilla extract and egg and mix until combined. Scrape the sides of the bowl and mix one more time.

3   Add the superfine brown rice flour, buckwheat flour, tapioca starch, baking powder, baking soda, salt, cinnamon, and nutmeg. Mix on medium speed until the dough comes together.

4   Add the chocolate chips, oats, pecans, and coconut. Mix until the ingredients come together; it will be a sticky dough.

5   Transfer the dough to a piece of parchment paper and roll it into a log that is 16 inches long and 2 inches in diameter. Use the parchment to help you roll the log. Wrap the log in the parchment paper and refrigerate for 1 hour.

6   Preheat the oven to 350°F (180°C). Cut the cookie dough log into ½-inch-thick disks. Place the cookies on baking sheets lined with parchment paper, spaced 2 inches apart. Bake two sheets at a time for 8 to 10 minutes. The cookies might still look soft and not fully baked, but don't worry. Let them cool completely on the baking sheets and they will harden as they cool. The cookies become very crispy and hard when overbaked, and you want to avoid that.

7   The baked cookies will keep in an airtight container for up to 5 days. The raw cookie dough will keep in the refrigerator for up to 5 days, or it can be frozen, tightly wrapped, for up to 1 month.

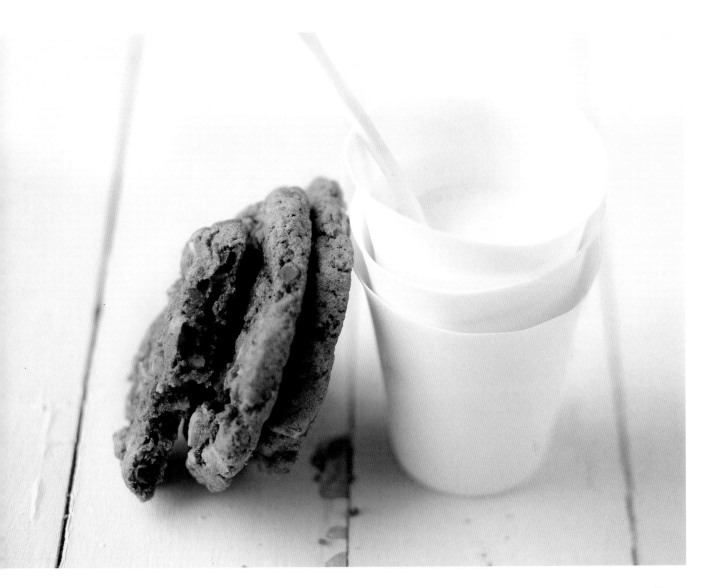

FREEZING COOKIE DOUGH

One of the tricks that I learned while working in professional kitchens, and that I have now integrated into my everyday life, is always to have a batch of freshly baked cookies on hand. It is one of the easiest things to do and will get you out of many "I want dessert now!" situations.

At the Ritz-Carlton, where we had intricate and layered desserts, cookies were by far the most frequently requested sweets. I cannot recall exactly how many pounds of cookie dough we mixed in a week's time, but it was plenty. It took two people to lift the 60-quart mixer onto the work table, where we would make batch after batch after batch. All the doughs were rolled into logs, tightly wrapped, and then frozen for days to come. Our freezer was always stocked full of chocolate chip, oatmeal raisin, blueberry white chocolate chunk, and my favorite, the cowboy cookies.

Simply thaw the cookie dough in the refrigerator for a couple of hours, slice it, and bake it for freshly baked cookies anytime.

roasted pumpkin ice cream sundae

I FIND THAT I STILL CRAVE ICE CREAM in the cooler days of autumn. This is when I turn to heartier concoctions with lots of nuts and homemade caramel. "Be careful not to burn that caramel," Jon says from across the room. He has seen me leave caramel unattended on the stove before. "Not this time," I assure him. Three scoops of roasted pumpkin ice cream, some broken pecan shortbread, candied pecans, and a few nice dollops of soft-peak whipped cream—we sit and share.

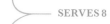

SERVES 8

1 large sugar pumpkin, red kuri, or butternut squash (2½ pounds or 1.25 kg)

1 cup (250 ml) heavy cream

1 cup (250 ml) whole milk

¾ cup (150 g) light brown sugar

1 teaspoon finely grated fresh ginger

5 egg yolks

1 teaspoon ground cinnamon

¼ teaspoon salt

⅛ teaspoon ground nutmeg

Pecan Shortbread Cookies (follow the Pistachio & Vanilla Bean Shortbread Cookies recipe on page 128, substituting pecans for pistachios)

Caramel Sauce, for serving (page 82)

Candied Pecans, for serving (page 82)

Whipped cream, for serving

make the ice cream

1 Preheat the oven to 400°F (200°C). Meanwhile, cut the squash in half lengthwise. Scoop out the seeds, peel each piece, and cut them in half lengthwise. Place the squash on a baking sheet and bake until the pieces are fork-tender and the outside is slightly caramelized, 45 minutes to 1 hour.

2 Transfer the roasted squash to a food processor and puree to a smooth paste. You should have about 2½ cups (625 g) puree. Measure out 1 cup (250 g) pumpkin puree and reserve. The rest can be refrigerated for up to 3 days or frozen for up to 3 months, for other uses.

3 Combine the heavy cream, milk, ½ cup (100 g) of the light brown sugar, and ginger in a medium saucepan. Bring the mixture to a simmer over medium-high heat.

4 Meanwhile, in a separate bowl, whisk together the egg yolks, remaining ¼ cup light brown sugar, cinnamon, salt, and nutmeg until frothy. When the cream mixture reaches a simmer, pour it slowly into the yolk mixture while whisking. Be careful not to scramble the eggs. Pour this back into the saucepan and cook over medium heat while constantly stirring until it thickens, 2 to 3 minutes.

5 Remove the ice cream base from the heat and whisk in the pumpkin puree. Strain this mixture through a fine-mesh sieve into a clean bowl. Place this bowl over an ice bath and stir occasionally until it chills, about 30 minutes. Cover the bowl with plastic wrap and refrigerate the mixture for at least 2 hours.

recipe continues

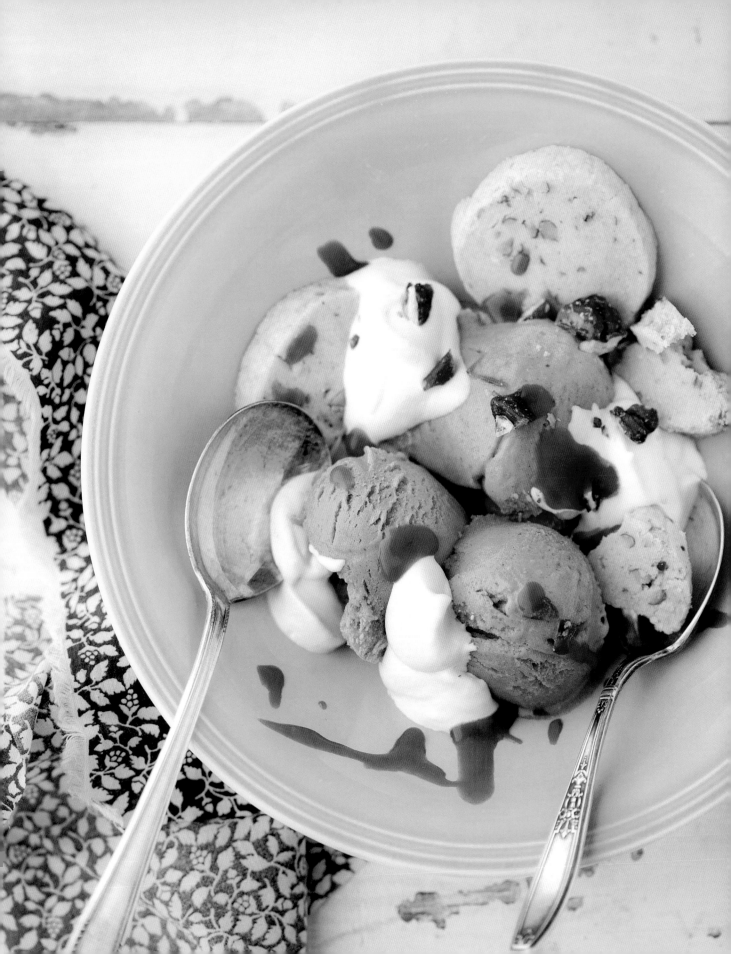

CARAMEL SAUCE

1 cup (200 g) natural cane sugar

1 cup (250 ml) heavy cream, at room temperature

½ vanilla bean, split lengthwise and seeds scraped

½ teaspoon salt

CANDIED PECANS

⅓ cup (70 g) natural cane sugar

½ cup (60 g) halved pecans

6 Transfer the pumpkin ice cream base to an ice cream maker. Churn the ice cream according to the manufacturer's instructions. Transfer to a freezer-safe container and freeze until solid.

7 Serve the ice cream with Pecan Shortbread, Caramel Sauce, Candied Pecans, and whipped cream.

make the caramel

1 Sprinkle half the sugar in a large pan. Heat over medium-high heat and let the sugar melt. Add the rest of the sugar in an even layer and let this melt. Continue cooking until the sugar turns amber. You can gently swirl the pan to evenly caramelize the sugar, but do not stir too much.

2 When the sugar has turned a deep amber color, add the heavy cream and vanilla seeds. The caramel will bubble up and splatter, so be careful not to get burned. The sugar might harden, but continue to cook it and stir it until smooth. You can also strain the caramel if you want it completely smooth.

3 Add the salt and stir. Serve immediately or let cool slightly and store it in a glass jar until ready to use. The caramel can be refrigerated for up to 1 month.

make the pecans

1 Evenly sprinkle the sugar in a medium saucepan. Heat it over medium-high heat until the sugar dissolves and starts to turn amber. Add the pecans and stir them in the caramel constantly until the caramel turns deep amber and the pecans begin to toast, about 2 minutes.

2 Transfer the pecans to a baking sheet lined with parchment paper or a silicone mat. Spread evenly and let cool completely. Coarsely chop them when cool.

3 Store in an airtight container for up to 1 week.

vanilla-poached quince & flan tartlets

QUINCES ARE AMONG THE MOST fragrant of fruits, and they remind me of my childhood years. Quince trees surrounded our school, and the fruit was often found scattered on the grass. Boys loved to use them as projectiles against us girls. I can honestly say I have endured many quince-induced injuries.

Raw quince is hard and unpalatable, which is why it needs to be cooked, long and slow, before being eaten. If you cannot find quinces for this recipe, pears will work. Poach them as directed below, but note that they will cook in less time.

MAKES five 4½-inch tartlets

prepare the quinces

1 Have a bowl filled with water ready before you start prepping the quinces. Squeeze the juice of the lemon into it.

2 Quarter the quinces, then peel and core each quarter. Cut each quarter in half. Be careful when peeling quinces, as they are very tough. Submerge the quince pieces in the lemon water as you are working to stop the oxidizing process.

3 Meanwhile, combine 6 cups (1.5 L) water, sugar, and the vanilla bean seeds in a large pot. Bring the liquid to a boil over medium-high heat. Add the quince pieces and reduce the heat to medium-low. Cut a circle of parchment paper that is the same diameter as the pot. Cover the quinces with the parchment.

4 Cook the quinces in the syrup over medium-low heat for 1½ to 2 hours or until tender. Let cool in the syrup. The quinces can be poached in advance and stored in the syrup in the refrigerator for up to 7 days.

make the pastry

1 Combine the first seven ingredients in a food processor and pulse to aerate. Add the cold butter and pulse ten times or until the butter is cut into pea-size pieces.

2 In a small bowl, whisk together the egg yolk and 2 tablespoons ice water. Add to the dough and mix. It will not form a ball. Simply press the dough between your fingers to see if it holds together. If not, add 1 more tablespoon of ice water at a time.

recipe continues

VANILLA-POACHED QUINCES

1 lemon

4 quinces

2 cups (400 g) natural cane sugar

1 vanilla bean, split lengthwise and seeds scraped

SPICED PASTRY

¾ cup (105 g) superfine brown rice flour, plus more for dusting

¼ cup (40 g) potato starch

¼ cup (35 g) sorghum flour

4 teaspoons natural cane sugar

¼ teaspoon ground cinnamon

⅛ teaspoon ground ginger

⅛ teaspoon salt

1 stick (8 tablespoons or 110 g) cold unsalted butter, cut into ½-inch cubes

1 egg yolk

2 to 4 tablespoons ice water

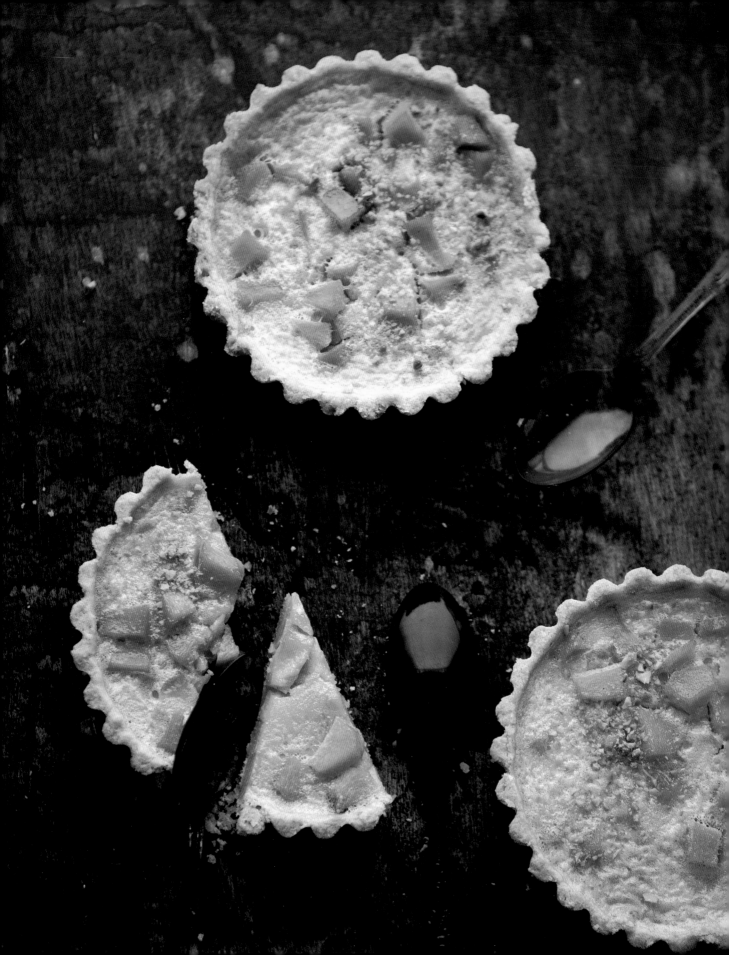

3 Transfer the dough to a work surface, knead it a couple of times, and form it into a disk. Wrap it in plastic wrap, flatten it, and refrigerate for 1 hour.

4 Dust your (preferably cold) work surface with a little bit of superfine brown rice flour. Roll the dough to a $\frac{1}{4}$- to $\frac{1}{8}$-inch thickness. If the dough cracks, simply press it back together. Cut four disks that are approximately 5 inches in diameter. Fill 4 ($4\frac{1}{2}$-inch) tartlet molds with the dough and cut off the excess. Re-roll scraps of dough and fill the last tart mold. Cut off excess dough. Refrigerate them for 20 minutes.

make the flan and bake the tartlets

1 Preheat the oven to 400°F (200°C). In a medium bowl, whisk together the eggs, egg yolk, sugar, cornstarch, and honey until smooth. Add the coconut milk and whisk to combine.

2 Place the prepared tartlet shells on a baking sheet. Fill the tartlet molds with the diced poached quince. Pour the flan mixture over the fruit.

3 Bake for 15 minutes, and then reduce the heat to 350°F (180°C) and continue baking for an additional 25 minutes or until golden. Cool the tartlets for 20 minutes before cutting.

FLAN

2 eggs

1 egg yolk

¼ cup (50 g) natural cane sugar

3 tablespoons cornstarch

1 tablespoon honey

¾ cup (185 ml) unsweetened coconut milk

2½ cups (375 g) diced Vanilla-Poached Quinces

OTHER WAYS TO ENJOY POACHED QUINCES

If you have a large pot of poached quinces, here are some other serving ideas:

- Cut them into small pieces and mix them into your favorite pancake batter. Serve the pancakes with warm maple syrup and toasted hazelnuts.

- Serve warm poached quinces with softened vanilla ice cream and crushed baked meringue as a last-minute dessert.

- Make a quick poached-quince galette with any leftover pastry dough you might have in the freezer. Roll the pastry out, sprinkle the bottom with almond flour, and pile the poached quince slices on top. Fold the pastry over the quinces and bake at 425°F (220°C) for 30 minutes.

chocolate, beet &
almond butter molten cakes

THESE MOLTEN CHOCOLATE CAKES ARE RICH and gooey. The beet puree
adds a touch of earthiness and a red tint that I love. A little goes a long way with these
cakes. Serve them warm with a dollop of whipped cream or vanilla ice cream.

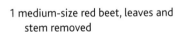

MAKES four 4-ounce cakes

1 medium-size red beet, leaves and
   stem removed

6 ounces (170 g) bittersweet
   chocolate, chopped

¼ cup (60 g) smooth almond
   butter

2 eggs

2 egg yolks

¼ cup (50 g) dark muscovado
   sugar

2 tablespoons superfine brown
   rice flour

¼ teaspoon *fleur de sel*

1 Fill a small pot with water. Bring the water to a boil over high heat.
Add the beet and cook until tender, 30 to 45 minutes. Insert a knife in the
center to see if it is cooked all the way through. Drain the water and let
the beet cool enough to handle. Peel the beet and cut it into chunks. Puree
it to a smooth paste in a food processor or blender. Measure out ¼ cup
(60 g) of the puree and reserve. The rest can be refrigerated or frozen for
another use.

2 Preheat the oven to 425°F (220°C). In a medium bowl, combine
the chocolate and almond butter. Place the bowl over a pot of simmering
water and let the chocolate melt slowly over medium-low heat. Stir
occasionally to ensure that the chocolate doesn't burn on the bottom.
Transfer the bowl to a rack and let cool slightly.

3 Meanwhile, combine the eggs, egg yolks, and muscovado sugar in
the bowl of a stand mixer. Whip on high speed for 5 minutes or until thick
and pale. Add the chocolate mixture, beet puree, superfine brown rice
flour, and *fleur de sel*. Whip over medium speed until it comes together into
a smooth batter. Make sure to scrape the sides and bottom of the bowl.

4 Divide the batter among 4 (4-ounce) greased ramekins. Bake for 8 to
10 minutes, until the edges are set but the center is still soft. Serve warm.

TIP: If you are craving molten chocolate cake but have no
beets or almond butter at home, you can still make this recipe.
Simply omit the beets and use unsalted butter in place of the
almond butter. It works every time.

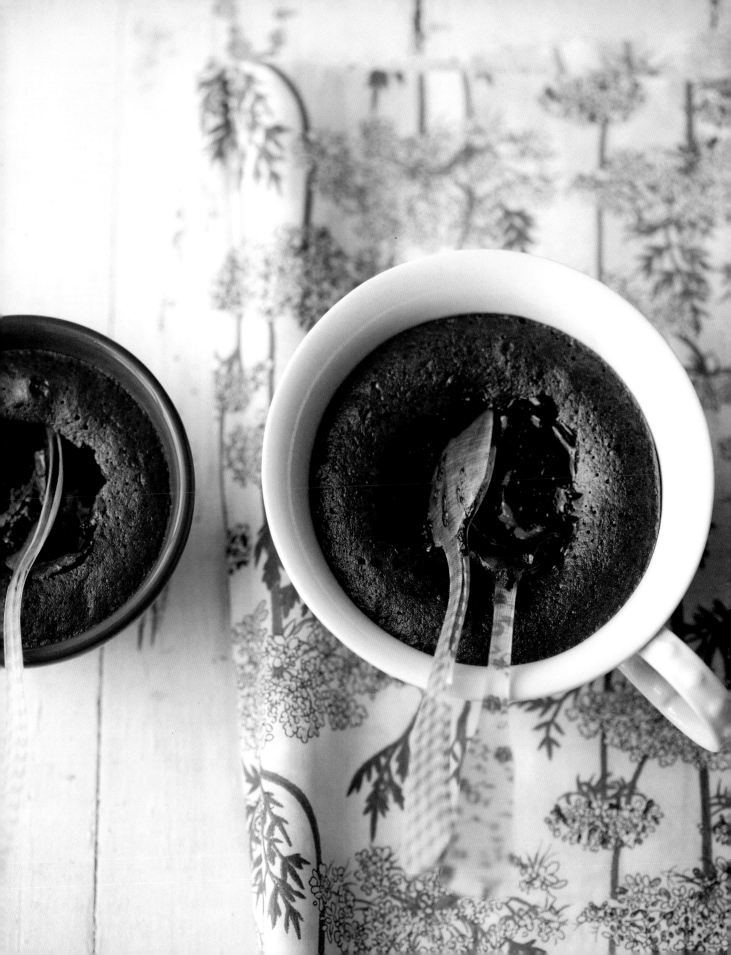

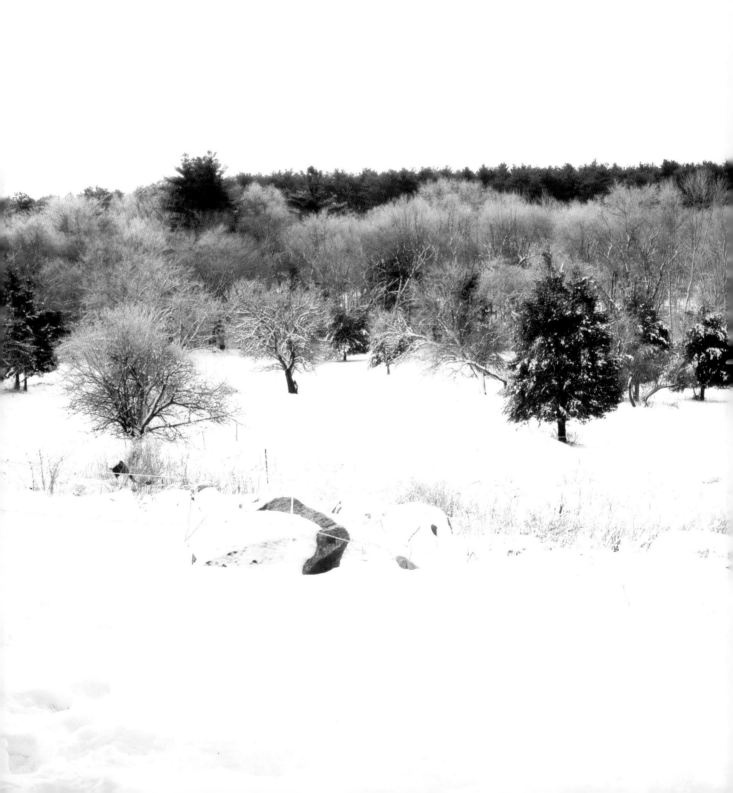

winter

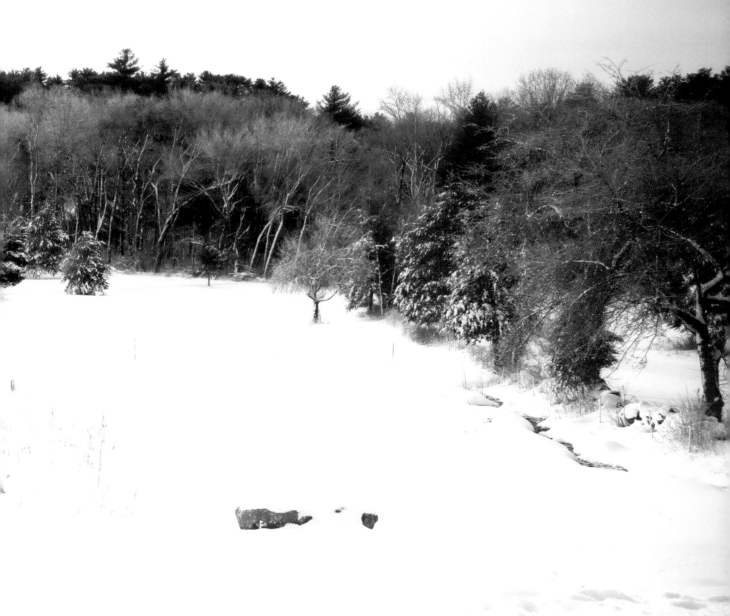

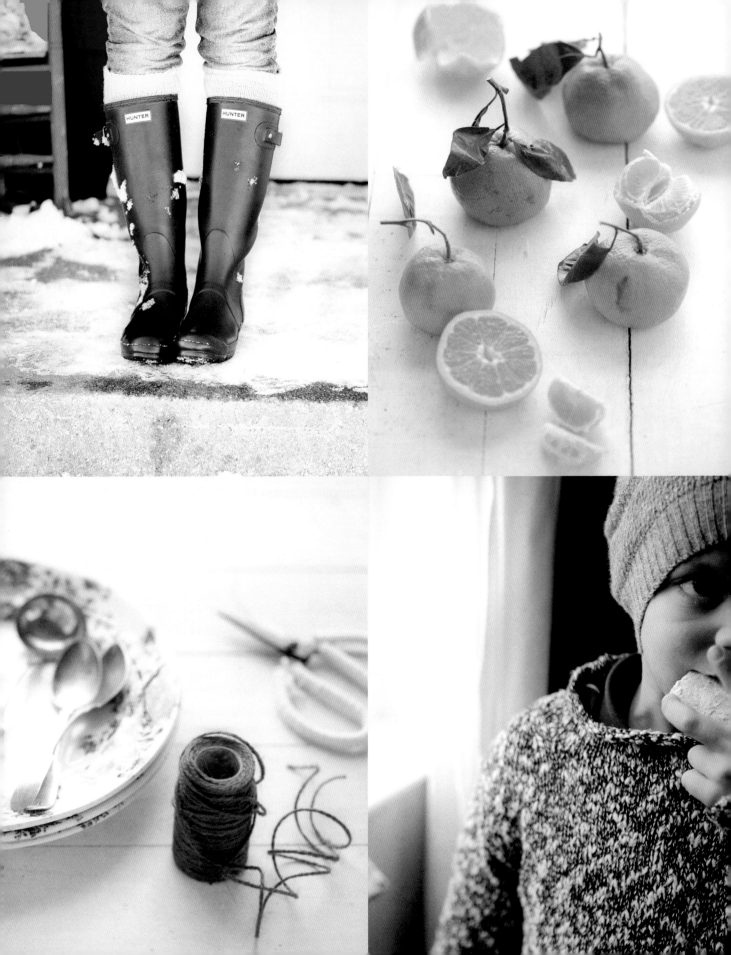

WINTER
small plates

"BE HOME BY TWO," MY MOM SAID as we were running out the door with our rain boots on. We were excited. It was Sunday morning, and as on every Sunday morning, my dad, my brothers, and I were driving to see my grandparents at their farm in the small town of Zeberio, about fifteen miles from our home.

Tucked away at the bottom of a hill, the farm was surrounded by pine, beech, and oak trees, with Mount Gorbea to the south. It was cold and damp, as are most winters in the Basque Country, and we were looking forward to seeing the animals and playing in the dirt. "Let's go harvest some leeks," my grandmother said. Her rain boots were old and worn, but nothing was ever disposed of unless absolutely necessary. Hunched over with age, she walked us into the rain-soaked garden. We pulled leeks right out of the ground. "These should last you all through the week," she said. *"Bai, amama."* ("Yes, Grandma.")

When I think of winter, I see gray yet peaceful skies, and I smell the intense aroma of those leeks with the cold and damp dirt attached to their roots, chestnuts roasting, and my mom's red bean soup simmering on the stove. Winter was filled with hearty dishes, stews, and legumes that were considered peasant food and everyday fare.

Here I compile some of my favorite winter recipes, dishes that we often cook for ourselves on cozy family nights or for friends for holiday parties. I like to keep the recipes simple and to add an element of surprise by incorporating a special ingredient or a touch of unexpected styling.

red bean, chorizo & short rib stew

IF THERE IS ONE DISH THAT DESCRIBES my childhood winter weekends, it is this red bean stew. Every Saturday it simmered on my mom's stove from early morning until early afternoon, when we would sit down at the table to enjoy our family lunch. Often we added chorizo, ribs, a slab of salty bacon, and sometimes stewed cabbage. This was serious comfort food. Because the stew is so nourishing and naturally gluten-free, I continue to make it for my own family on chilly winter weekends and, I must admit, even well into spring.

The red beans of Gernika or Tolosa are my favorites for it, but since they are nearly impossible to find in the United States, you can use red calypso or pinto beans, which also work well. When cooking dried beans, it is important not to season them until the very end so that they remain tender. This stew cooks slowly, but it is worth the wait.

SERVES 4 to 6

12 ounces (340 g) heirloom red calypso or pinto beans

3 tablespoons olive oil

½ medium yellow onion, diced

½ medium leek, diced

½ medium green bell pepper, diced

½ medium red bell pepper, diced

1 medium carrot, peeled and diced

1¾ teaspoons salt

1 tablespoon tomato paste

1½ ounces (45 g) Spanish chorizo, sliced

12 ounces (340 g) grass-fed short ribs

1 medium russet potato, peeled and diced

1 medium pink turnip, peeled and diced

1   Place the beans in a large pot and cover them with 2 inches of cold water. Soak the beans overnight. The following day, make sure the beans are still covered by 1 inch of water, topping it up if necessary. Place the pot over medium-high heat and bring the water to a low simmer.

2   In a separate large cast-iron pan, heat the olive oil and add the onion, leek, peppers, and carrot. Add ½ teaspoon of the salt and cook the vegetables for 5 minutes or until soft but not brown. Add the tomato paste, chorizo, and short ribs.

3   Add the beans with their simmering water to the cast-iron pan. Bring the mixture to a boil. Reduce the heat to low, cover the pot, and simmer for 1½ hours.

4   Add the diced potato and turnip and cook for another hour or until the beans are tender. Season with the remaining 1¼ teaspoons salt and adjust the amount of liquid by adding more water if needed. Serve warm.

TIP: To cut down the cooking time, use canned pinto beans and omit the short ribs, which take longer to cook. Make sure to rinse the beans under water and add 4 cups (1 L) of water after the potato and turnip are incorporated. Cook the stew for 30 minutes and serve.

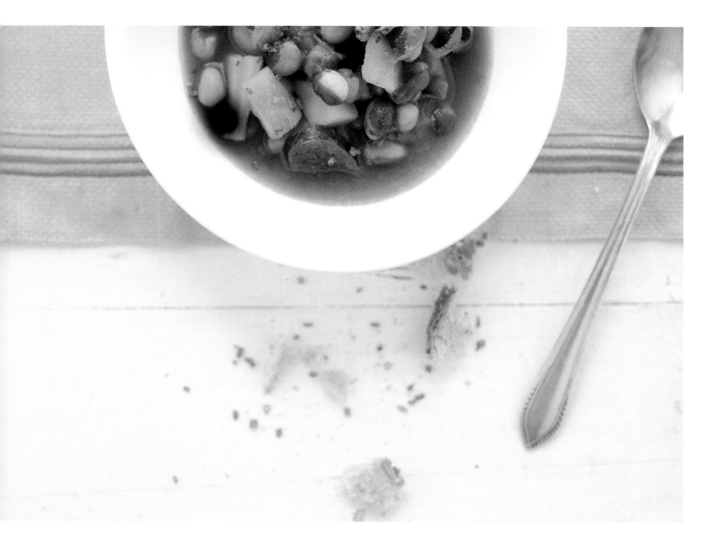

CHORIZO

Spanish chorizo is a cured and air-dried sausage made with coarsely chopped pork and pork fat, and seasoned with Spanish *pimentón* (paprika) and salt. It is sold in most butcher shops, where you will often see it hanging from the ceiling. It is eaten sliced with bread, cooked in stews and soups, or fried in olive oil.

Many families, including mine, take pride in making their own chorizo. My paternal grandparents raised one or two pigs every year. The pigs were slaughtered in midwinter, always taking into account the lunar cycles, and the meat fed many families for the entire year. No animal part was ever wasted, and there was always a sense of gratitude for having this food.

Making chorizo was the ultimate family gathering, and everyone participated. The meat and the spices were mixed by hand, encased in long strands, and then air-dried for months in the cold attic of my grandparents' farm. They kept their dry chorizo covered in extra-virgin olive oil in large clay barrels. My grandmother often sent me to the attic to retrieve a slice for her stews. Those chorizo-making days often ended with an *alubiada* (a large feast of bean and pork stew) and endless bottles of red Rioja-Alavesa wine.

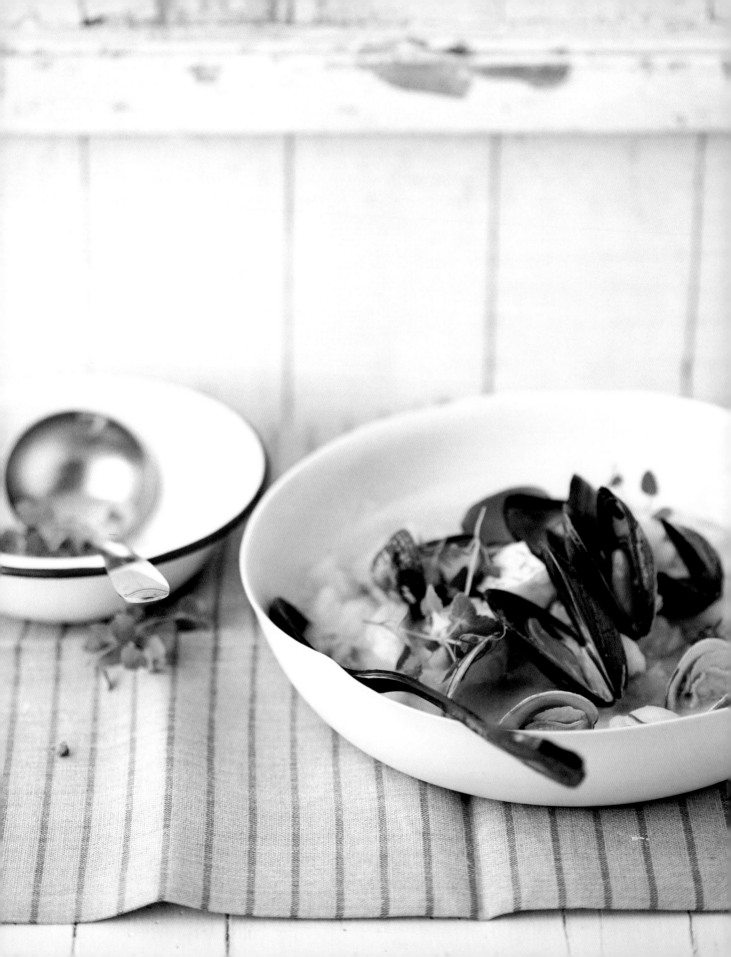

coconut milk &
saffron seafood stew

WHEN THE COLD MONTHS ARRIVE, I crave soup. I serve it with every meal, even if it's just a simple puree of vegetables flavored with broth. This one is creamy and aromatic, loaded with shellfish and flavored with fennel, saffron, and coconut milk. Make sure you have some toasted bread to dip into the juices.

SERVES 4

1 Place the mussels and clams in a large bowl. Cover them with cold water and add a small handful of salt. Refrigerate and let them soak for 30 minutes, which will help remove any sand. Drain the salted water and rinse them under cold water. Discard any mussels or clams that are open.

2 Transfer the mussels and clams to a large pot. Add 1 cup (250 ml) water, the white wine, saffron, and thyme. Cover and cook over medium-high heat for 3 to 5 minutes, until all the mussels and clams are open. Mussels tend to open quicker than clams, so you might have to remove those from the pot first. Discard any that have not opened. Strain the released juices and reserve. You should have approximately 1¾ cups (435 ml) of juice.

3 In a large pot, heat the olive oil over medium heat and cook the pancetta until golden. Add the onion, garlic, fennel, and red pepper flakes and cook until tender, about 5 minutes.

4 Add the potato, reserved juice from the mussels and clams, and coconut milk. Bring to a boil. Reduce the heat to medium-low, cover, and simmer for 10 to 15 minutes, until the potatoes are tender.

5 Add the scallops and the snapper to the pot and simmer for 3 to 5 minutes, until cooked. Season with the salt and pepper. Add the clams and mussels to the pot, quickly stir, and serve immediately.

1 pound (450 g) mussels

1 pound (450 g) clams

½ cup (125 ml) white wine

1 teaspoon saffron threads

4 sprigs thyme

2 tablespoons olive oil

6 thin slices pancetta, chopped

1 large yellow onion, diced

2 cloves garlic, minced

½ medium fennel bulb, diced

Small pinch of red pepper flakes

1 large russet potato, peeled and diced

1½ cups (375 ml) unsweetened coconut milk

8 ounces (225 g) bay scallops, or sea scallops cut into bite-size pieces

10 ounces (290 g) scaled and boned red snapper, cut into chunks (I like to keep the skin on, but you could remove it)

½ teaspoon salt, plus more to clean the clams

¼ teaspoon freshly ground black pepper

chestnut crêpes
with creamy mushrooms

THIS IS A VERY SIMPLE RECIPE FOR CRÊPES that can be filled with all kinds of savory ingredients or turned into a sweet dessert by omitting the herbs and black pepper and adding a touch of honey. I like them sweet-savory: Spread a little bit of sweetened yogurt over a Chestnut Crêpe, roll it, and drizzle with honey. It makes the perfect snack.

If you cannot find chestnut flour, use a combination of ½ cup (70 g) superfine brown rice flour and ¼ cup (35 g) buckwheat flour.

SERVES 4 to 6

CHESTNUT CRÊPES (MAKES FIFTEEN 8-INCH CRÊPES

2 eggs, at room temperature

1 cup (100 g) chestnut flour

1 cup (250 ml) whole milk, at room temperature

1 tablespoon finely chopped fresh parsley

¼ teaspoon salt

Pinch of freshly grated nutmeg

¼ stick (2 tablespoons or 30 g) unsalted butter, melted, plus more melted butter for the pan

CREAMY MUSHROOMS

3 tablespoons olive oil

2 cloves garlic, peeled

8 ounces (225 g) exotic mushrooms, such as cremini, oyster, and shiitake

4 sprigs thyme

½ teaspoon salt

¼ teaspoon freshly ground black pepper

2 tablespoons crème fraîche or whole-milk sour cream

1 tablespoon finely chopped fresh parsley

make the crêpes

1 Combine all the ingredients in a blender and mix until a thin batter forms. Chill the batter for at least 1 hour before using. It can be stored in the refrigerator for up to 24 hours.

2 Heat an 8-inch nonstick sauté pan over medium heat. Brush the bottom and sides of the pan with some of the melted butter reserved for this purpose.

3 Stir the chilled batter. Add about 2 tablespoons of batter to the pan while swirling it. This ensures a thin layer of the batter all over the pan. You want thin crêpes. Let the crêpe cook for about 30 seconds or until it gets lightly golden. Tuck in the sides with a rubber spatula. Using a spatula or even your hands (careful!), quickly flip the crêpe over and finish cooking. The first crêpe is usually a test one, so don't worry if it sticks. Transfer it to a plate and repeat with the rest of the batter. Stack all the crêpes. They should not stick together.

4 At this point, you can fill them with anything or freeze them, stacked and tightly wrapped, for up to 1 month.

prepare the mushroom filling

1 In a medium sauté pan, heat the olive oil over medium heat. Add the cloves of garlic and gently let the garlic infuse the oil for 1 to 2 minutes; then remove it. Do not burn the garlic.

2 Add the mushrooms and thyme. Cook for another couple of minutes, until soft and slightly caramelized. Season with the salt and pepper. Remove from the heat and add the crème fraîche.

3 Add about 2 tablespoons of filling and a sprinkle of parsley to each crêpe and roll them up. Serve immediately.

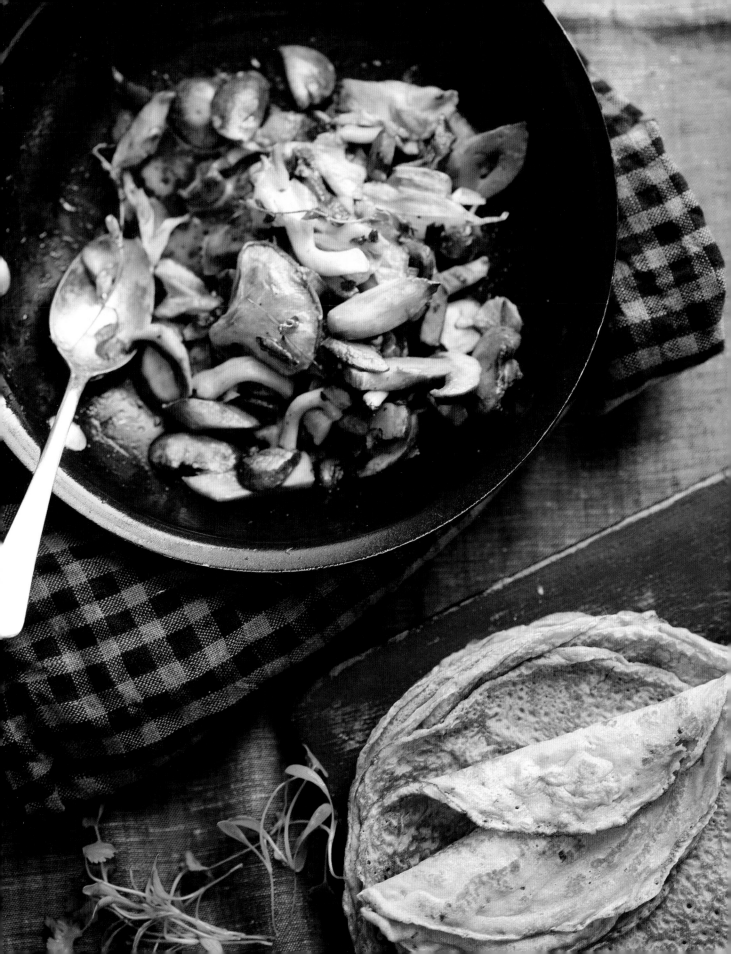

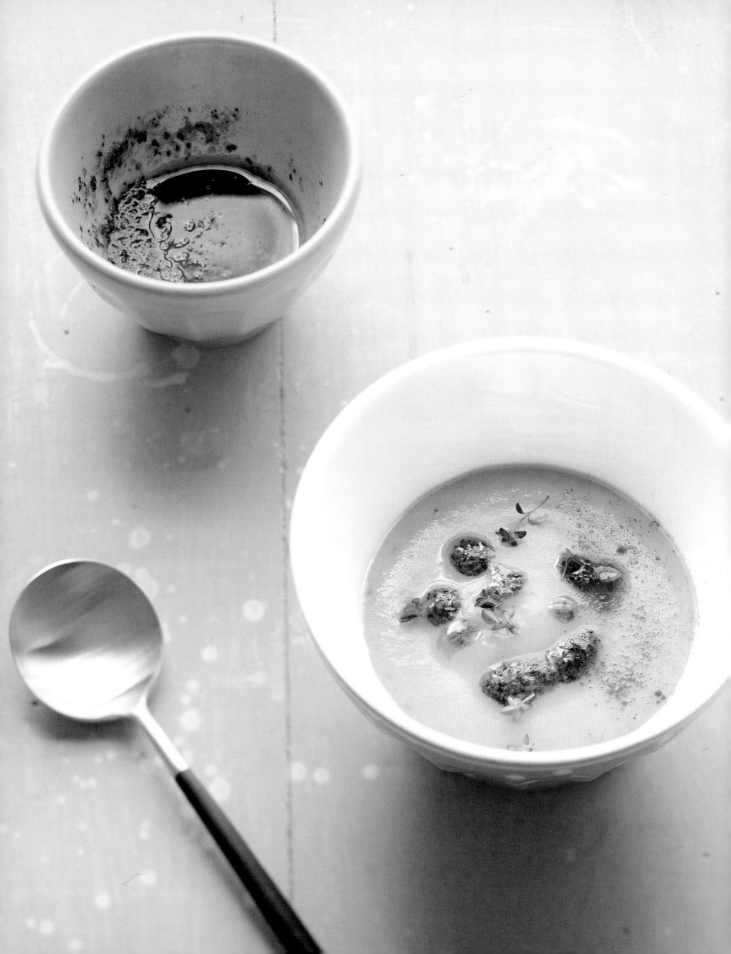

roasted cauliflower & leek soup with dandelion green & hazelnut pesto

I ALWAYS TRY TO INCORPORATE GREENS in recipes, and dandelion greens are among the most nutritious leafy greens you can find. Their bitterness works well with the sweetness of the roasted vegetables and the coconut milk. If you cannot find dandelion greens, use kale, arugula, or any other green.

SERVES 4 to 6

make the pesto

1   Place the hazelnuts in a dry skillet and toast them over medium-high heat for 5 minutes or until golden. Transfer them to a dry kitchen towel and rub them together to remove their skins.

2   Combine the garlic and hazelnuts in a food processor and process to a fine powder. Add the dandelion greens, Parmesan, and salt and continue processing. Add the olive oil in a steady stream while the machine is running until the ingredients come together into a creamy paste. The pesto may be stored in the refrigerator for up to 3 days or frozen for up to 1 month.

make the soup

1   Preheat the oven to 375°F (190°C). Toss together the cauliflower, leek, onion, garlic, olive oil, and ½ teaspoon of the salt. Transfer to a baking sheet and roast for 25 minutes or until golden.

2   Transfer the roasted vegetables to a large pot. Add the diced potato, chicken stock, coconut milk, thyme leaves, and remaining 1 teaspoon salt. Bring the liquid to a boil over medium-high heat. Reduce the heat to medium, cover, and simmer for 10 minutes or until all the vegetables are tender.

3   Puree the soup in a blender. Adjust the seasoning and serve with the Dandelion Green & Hazelnut Pesto.

DANDELION GREEN AND HAZELNUT PESTO

¼ cup (30 g) hazelnuts

1 clove garlic, minced

2 cups (40 g) dandelion greens

2 tablespoons grated Parmesan cheese

½ teaspoon salt

¼ cup (60 ml) olive oil

ROASTED CAULIFLOWER AND LEEK SOUP

1 medium cauliflower (1 pound or 450 g), cut into small florets

½ medium leek, cut into large rings

1 medium yellow onion, diced

2 cloves garlic, peeled

2 tablespoons olive oil

1½ teaspoons salt

¼ teaspoon freshly ground black pepper

1 medium russet potato, peeled and diced

3 cups (750 ml) chicken stock

½ cup (125 ml) unsweetened coconut milk

1 teaspoon fresh thyme leaves

swiss chard, pear & gruyère tart

ONE OF MY FAVORITE LUNCHES IS A savory tart accompanied by a green salad. A few years ago, I spent several weeks working on a pastry assignment in Cascais, a small seaside town outside of Lisbon, Portugal. It was a quaint beach town with cobblestone streets and outdoor cafés that catered to the many tourists who flooded the town in the summer. Tucked away on a side street was an eclectic French café that served incredible lunches. The menu, which changed daily, was mostly composed of savory tarts, tartines, and salads. It soon became my hangout spot and to this day is the inspiration for many of the savory tarts I make.

MAKES one 9-inch round tart or one 14 by 4-inch rectangular tart

PASTRY CRUST

½ cup (70 g) superfine brown rice flour, plus more for dusting

⅓ cup (45 g) quinoa flour

⅓ cup (35 g) almond flour

2 tablespoons potato starch

2 tablespoons tapioca starch

½ teaspoon salt

¼ teaspoon freshly ground black pepper

1 stick (8 tablespoons or 110 g) cold unsalted butter, cut into ½-inch cubes

6 to 8 tablespoons ice water

SWISS CHARD, PEAR, AND GRUYÈRE FILLING

2 tablespoons olive oil

1 medium leek, sliced

2 cloves garlic, minced

4 cups (175 g) chopped Swiss chard (remove tough ribs but use the tender ones)

2 tablespoons white wine

1 teaspoon salt

½ teaspoon freshly ground black pepper

Pinch of freshly grated nutmeg

2 eggs

1 tablespoon sweet rice flour or cornstarch

make the crust

1 Add the first seven ingredients to the bowl of a food processor. Pulse a couple of times to aerate. Add the cold butter to the flour mixture and pulse ten times, until the butter is cut into pea-size pieces.

2 Add 6 tablespoons ice water and pulse until the dough comes together. It will not form a ball. Check the dough to see if it holds together when pressed between your fingers. Add more water if needed.

3 Turn the dough out onto a work surface, knead it a couple of times, and press it together to form a disk. Wrap it in plastic wrap. Press it down to flatten it and refrigerate it for 30 minutes.

4 Preheat the oven to 375°F (190°C). Lightly dust your (preferably cold) work surface with superfine brown rice flour and roll out the dough to a ¼-inch thickness. If the dough cracks while rolling, pinch it back together. Fill the tart mold with the dough and press it gently into the mold. Cut off excess dough. Refrigerate the dough for 15 minutes.

5 Blind-bake the tart by covering it with a piece of parchment paper and topping the paper with pie weights or dried beans. Bake for 20 minutes. Remove the pie weights and paper and continue baking for another 10 minutes, until lightly golden. Let it cool slightly while preparing the filling. (Leave the oven on.)

prepare the filling and bake the tart

1 In a large sauté pan, heat the olive oil over medium heat. Add the leek and garlic and cook until tender, about 5 minutes.

2 Add the Swiss chard, white wine, ½ teaspoon of the salt, ¼ teaspoon of the black pepper, and nutmeg. Cook until the chard is wilted and most of the liquid has evaporated, about 5 minutes. Set aside to cool slightly.

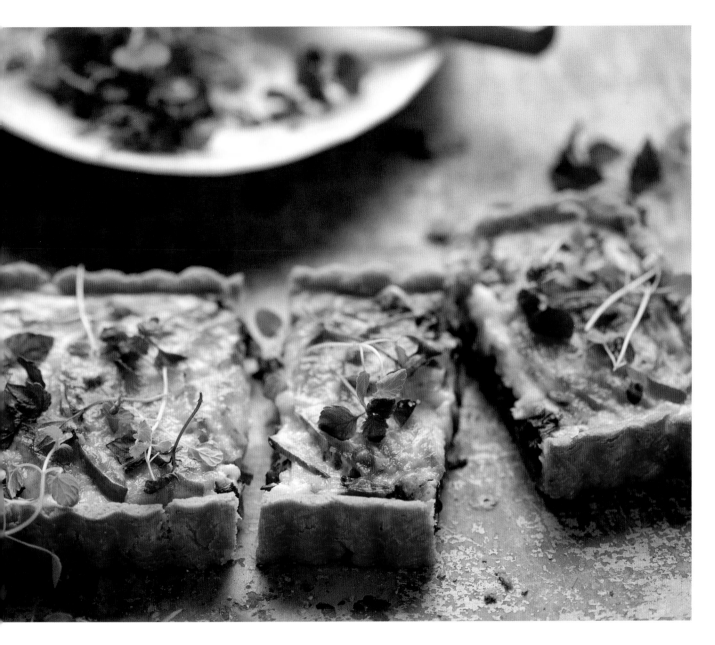

3 Whisk together the eggs, sweet rice flour, milk, coconut milk, Parmesan, 1 ounce (30 g) of the Gruyère, remaining ½ teaspoon salt, and remaining ¼ teaspoon black pepper.

4 Fill the tart crust with the Swiss chard and top with slices of pear. Lightly press the filling down and pour the custard over it. Top with the remaining 1 ounce (30 g) Gruyère.

5 Bake at 375°F (190°C) for about 25 minutes, until golden brown. Let it cool slightly before cutting. Serve the tart garnished with microgreens.

½ cup (125 ml) whole milk

½ cup (125 ml) unsweetened coconut milk

½ ounce (15 g) Parmesan cheese, finely grated

2 ounces (60 g) Gruyère cheese, grated

1 medium Bartlett or Bosc pear, thinly sliced, preferably with a mandoline

Microgreens, for garnish

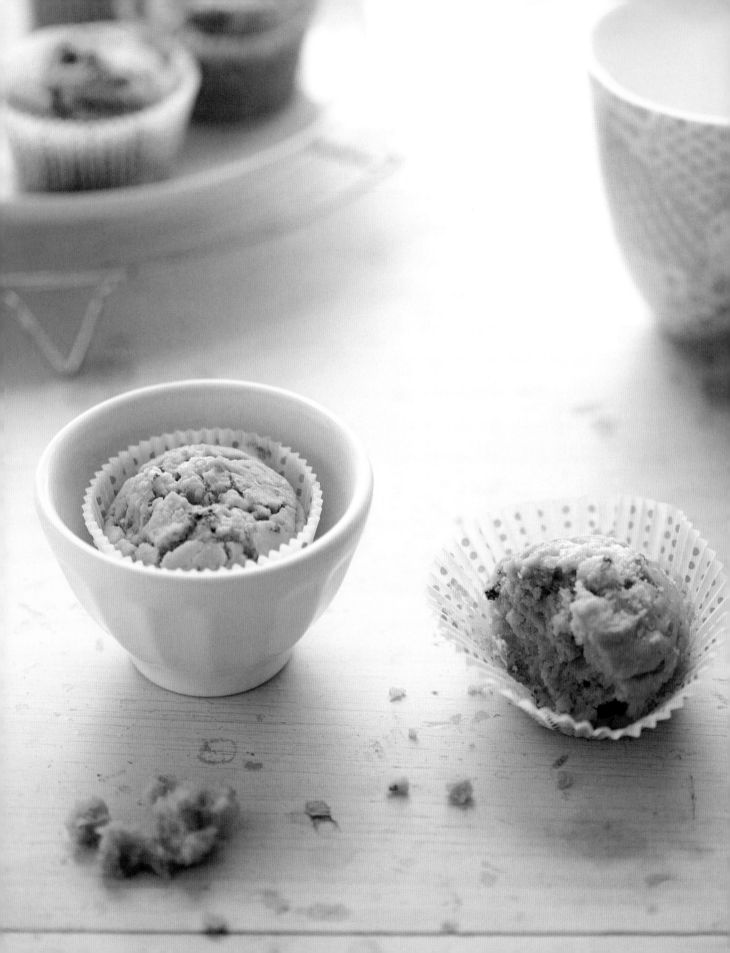

squash, apple & blue cheese muffins

SOMETIMES I LIKE TO MAKE A MEAL OF a simple soup accompanied by a piece of bread or a savory muffin. This is also how I get my children to eat most of their vegetables. I cook the vegetables into a creamy soup and I let the kids pick what kind of bread to dip into it. It never fails. With these blue cheese and squash muffins, the "bread" becomes the star of the meal.

MAKES 12 muffins

1 Preheat the oven to 375°F (190°C). Peel the squash with a vegetable peeler. Cut it in half and remove all the seeds. Cut each half into wedges. Place the wedges on a baking sheet and toss with 1 tablespoon of the olive oil and ¼ teaspoon of the salt. Bake the squash for 30 to 40 minutes or until tender. Transfer the roasted squash to a food processor or blender and puree into a smooth paste. Measure out 1 cup (250 g) of squash puree. The rest may be frozen for up to 3 months. Lower the oven temperature to 350°F (180°C).

2 In a large bowl, whisk together the superfine brown rice flour, millet flour, potato starch, baking powder, baking soda, remaining ½ teaspoon salt, sage, and thyme leaves. Add the squash puree, egg, honey, and remaining 4 tablespoons olive oil. Whisk until combined.

3 Fold in the blue cheese and grated apple, juice and all. It will be a thick batter, similar to a soft scone dough.

4 Scoop the batter into a muffin pan lined with baking cups. Bake for 18 to 20 minutes, until golden brown. Let the muffins cool in the pan for 5 minutes, and then transfer them to a cooling rack. They will keep for 3 days, or they can be frozen for up to 1 month.

TIP: Red kuri squash makes a great creamy and nutty puree, but any winter squash, such as butternut or hubbard, may be used in its place.

- 1 small red kuri squash (about 1 pound or 450 g)
- ¼ cup plus 1 tablespoon (75 ml) olive oil
- ¾ teaspoon salt
- 1 cup (140 g) superfine brown rice flour
- ½ cup (70 g) millet flour
- ¼ cup (40 g) potato starch
- 1 teaspoon baking powder
- ½ teaspoon baking soda
- 1 tablespoon finely chopped fresh sage leaves
- 1 teaspoon fresh thyme leaves
- 1 egg, lightly beaten
- ¼ cup (70 g) honey
- 2 ounces (60 g) blue cheese, crumbled
- 1 medium Gala apple, peeled, cored, and grated

amama miren's garlic soup

"MIREN, CAN YOU MAKE SOME GARLIC soup for dinner?" my grandfather Angel would ask my grandmother. I had always known he suffered from ulcers and stomach pains. He was also thin as a rail, which in retrospect makes me believe he suffered from celiac disease or was gluten intolerant at some level. That would be ironic, considering he was a pastry chef and breathed flour every day of his life. Because of his pains he wasn't able to eat much, so my grandmother took great care of him—anything he wished for, she would prepare. Garlic soup was one of his favorites.

Her recipe calls for *pimiento choricero* paste, which is the same kind used in making chorizo. Dried *choricero* peppers are reconstituted in water and their flesh is scooped out of their skin. Nowadays, this flesh can be purchased in jars in specialty shops, but if you can't find it, hot *pimentón*, *piment d'Espelette*, or paprika can be used in its place.

SERVES 4

¼ cup plus 2 tablespoons (90 ml) olive oil, plus more for garnish

4 ounces (110 g) stale gluten-free bread, cubed

6 cloves garlic, finely minced

1 tablespoon *pimiento choricero* paste or hot paprika

2 teaspoons fresh thyme leaves

6 cups (1.5 L) chicken stock

1 teaspoon salt

½ teaspoon freshly ground black pepper

4 eggs, preferably farm eggs

2 tablespoons chopped fresh parsley

1 In a large pot, heat ¼ cup of the olive oil. Add the cubed bread and toss in the olive oil. Cook until the bread starts to toast. Add the remaining 2 tablespoons olive oil, garlic, and *choricero* pepper paste. Cook for another 30 seconds or so, until the garlic is slightly cooked. You don't want to burn the garlic.

2 Add the thyme, chicken stock, salt, and pepper. Bring the liquid to a boil, reduce the heat to low, and simmer for 10 minutes.

3 Meanwhile, poach the eggs. Place 2 inches of water in a shallow pot. Bring the water to a low simmer. Do not let it boil. Break the eggs into the water. Flip the white over the yolk with a spoon and let the egg cook for a minute or until the white is cooked but the yolk remains liquidy. Remove the eggs with a slotted spoon and place them over the soup.

4 Serve with the parsley sprinkled on top and a drizzle of olive oil.

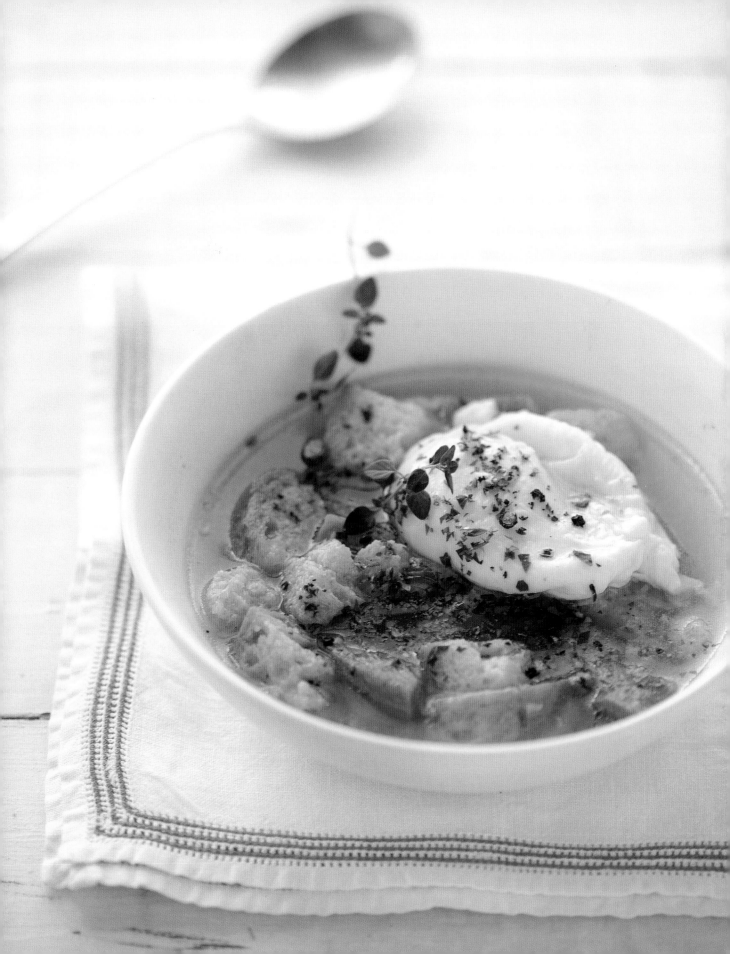

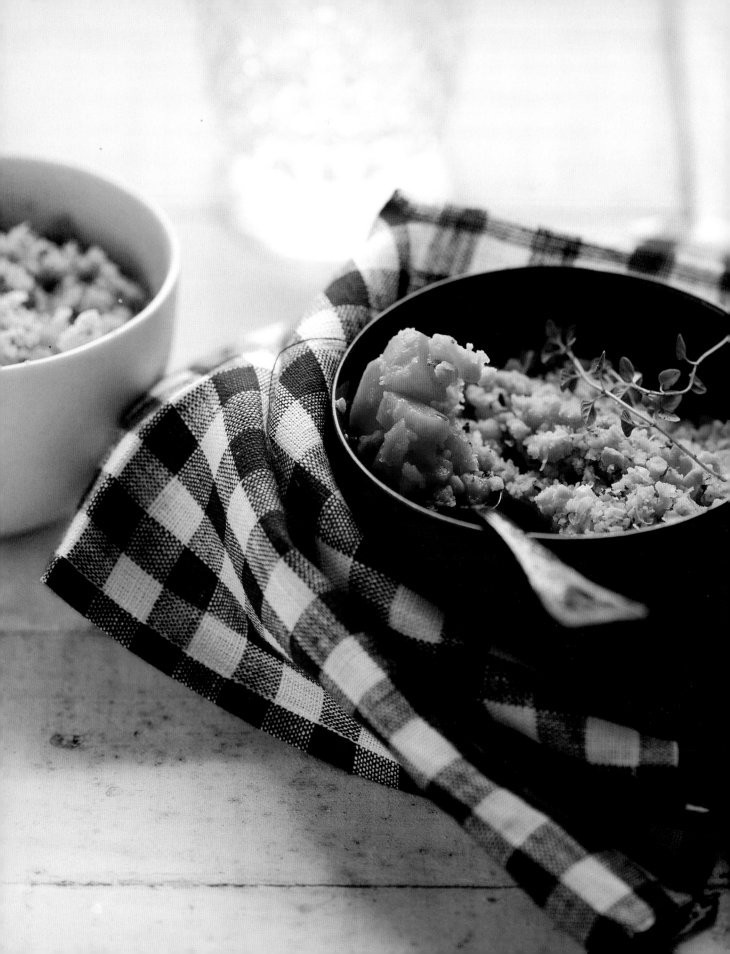

celery root, sweet potato & quinoa crumble

I WAS SIXTEEN THE FIRST TIME I celebrated an American Thanksgiving. I had never tasted a savory crumble before, so when I was served a butternut squash baked with a crumble topping, my world expanded. Today, I love making this crumble as a main vegetarian dish accompanied by a green salad.

MAKES one 8-inch square baking pan or six 8-ounce bowls

make the crumble

Whisk together the first ten ingredients in a large bowl. Add the soft butter and, using your hands, work the butter into the flour mixture until there are small pieces of butter throughout the flour. Chill the dough in the refrigerator while preparing the filling.

make the filling

1 Preheat the oven to 350°F (180°C). In a large pot, heat the olive oil over medium heat. Add the onion and cook for 3 minutes or until translucent. Add the garlic, celery root, sweet potatoes, bay leaf, parsley, salt, and pepper and cook for another 3 minutes.

2 Add the vegetable broth and bring the liquid to a boil over medium-high heat. Reduce the heat to medium-low, cover the pot, and simmer for about 10 minutes or until the vegetables are tender but not mushy. Remove the pot from the heat. Remove the bay leaf and mix in the grated cheese.

3 Transfer the filling to an oiled 8-inch square baking dish or individual bowls. Top with the crumble. Bake for 30 to 40 minutes or until the crumble is golden and the filling is bubbling.

QUINOA AND PINE NUT CRUMBLE

½ cup (70 g) superfine brown rice flour

½ cup (70 g) quinoa flour

¼ cup (40 g) pine nuts

¼ cup (25 g) quinoa flakes

1 ounce (30 g) Idiazabal or Parmesan cheese, finely grated

1 clove garlic, grated

2 tablespoons chopped fresh parsley

Leaves from 3 sprigs thyme

½ teaspoon salt

½ teaspoon freshly ground black pepper

1¼ sticks (10 tablespoons or 140 g) unsalted butter, at room temperature, cut into pieces

CELERY ROOT AND SWEET POTATO FILLING

2 tablespoons olive oil

1 small yellow onion, diced

2 cloves garlic, minced

1 medium celery root, peeled and diced

2 medium sweet potatoes, peeled and diced

1 dried bay leaf

1 tablespoon chopped fresh parsley

1¼ teaspoons salt

1 teaspoon freshly ground black pepper

1½ cups (375 ml) vegetable broth

1 ounce (30 g) Idiazabal or Parmesan cheese, finely grated

scallop, fennel, apple & hazelnut salad

THIS IS A RECIPE I HAVE COOKED for our New Year's festivities for the past couple of years. It is quick to assemble, colorful, and light. I like to serve it while the beets and scallops are still warm. The combination of crunchy hazelnuts, creamy dressing, crispy apples, and sweet scallops creates a wonderful balance of texture and flavor.

SERVES 6

8 baby golden beets or 4 large ones, stems removed

½ cup (60 g) hazelnuts

3 tablespoons olive oil

12 ounces (340 g) bay scallops

½ medium fennel bulb, thinly sliced (preferably with a mandoline)

1 Pink Lady or Gala apple, cored and thinly sliced

¼ small red onion, thinly sliced

2 cups (80 g) watercress, tough stems removed

¼ cup (60 ml) whole-milk plain yogurt

1 tablespoon freshly squeezed lemon juice

1 teaspoon Dijon mustard

2 teaspoons salt

1 teaspoon freshly ground black pepper

1 Fill a medium pot with water and bring it to a boil over high heat. Add the beets to the pot. Cover, reduce the heat to medium, and simmer for about 15 minutes for the baby beets and 30 minutes for the larger ones. The time will vary depending on the size of the beets. Insert a small knife in the center to check if they are done. Drain the beets and, when the beets are cool enough to handle, peel and slice them.

2 Meanwhile, place the hazelnuts in a dry skillet. Toast them over medium-high heat until golden and fragrant, about 5 minutes. Transfer to a dry kitchen towel and rub them together to remove their skins. Set aside to cool. When cool enough to handle, chop coarsely.

3 In a medium sauté pan, heat 2 tablespoons of the olive oil over medium-high heat and cook the scallops for 1 to 2 minutes per side, depending on their size. You want to create a little crust on each side, but do not overcook them. Set aside, keeping warm.

4 Assemble the salad by stacking the fennel, apple, red onion, watercress, sliced beets, toasted hazelnuts, and scallops on plates.

5 In a bowl, whisk together the yogurt, lemon juice, Dijon mustard, the remaining 1 tablespoon olive oil, salt, and pepper. If the dressing seems too thick, add 1 teaspoon of warm water. Drizzle the dressing over the salad and serve while the scallops are warm.

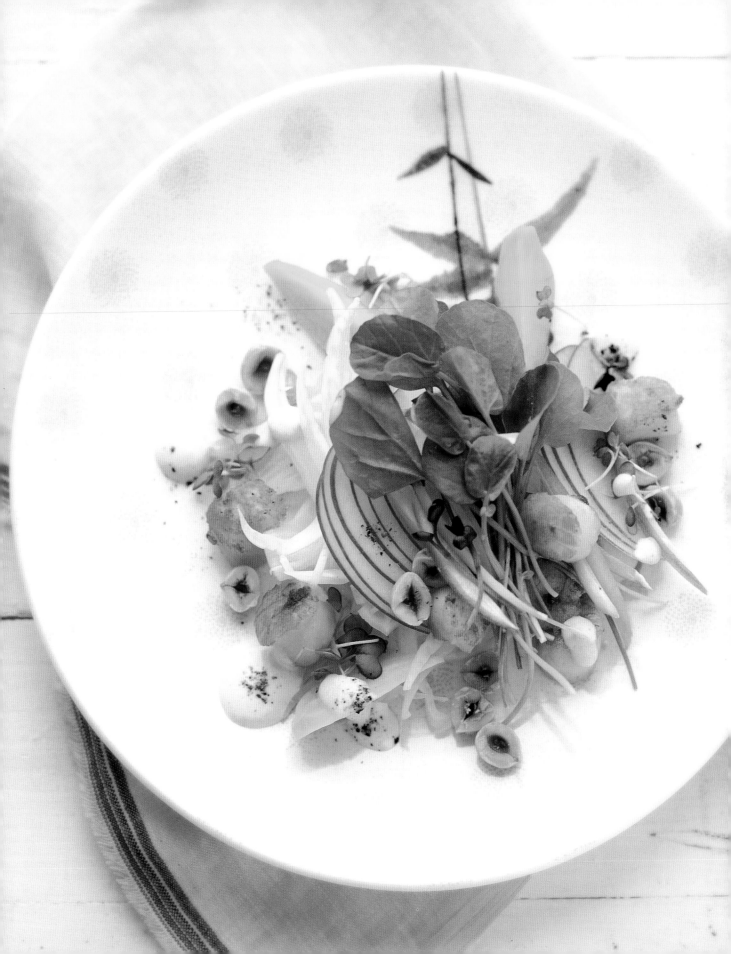

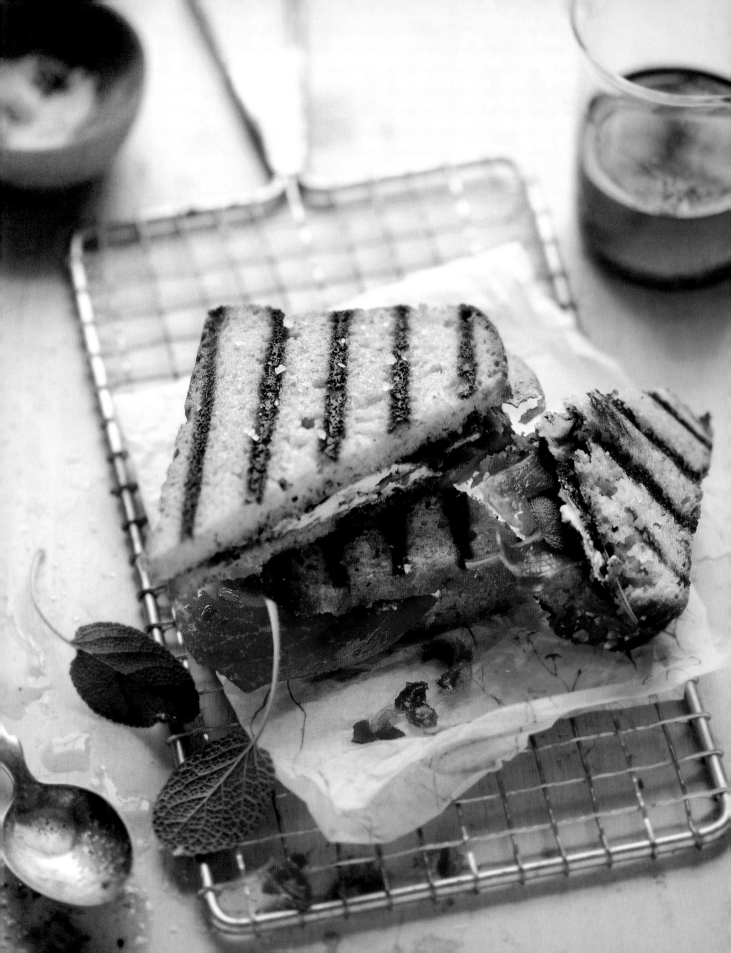

crispy serrano ham, goat cheese & pesto *bocadillos*

"**CAN I SPREAD THE GREEN STUFF ON** the bread?" asks Jon. He licks his fingers and then shrugs. *Bocadillos*, which are baguettes filled with cured meats, cheese, Spanish tortilla, or even chocolate and olive oil, are bar food—the Basque version of fast food. They are sometimes simple, sometimes layered and complex, and definitely there is an art to making them. Every day after school, Jon waits for his Idiazabal cheese and ham *bocadillo*, which I often make using the Quinoa Brioche recipe on page 125. This *bocadillo* is a bit more sophisticated, with Serrano ham, goat cheese, and pesto.

SERVES 4

make the pesto

1 Place the hazelnuts in a dry skillet. Toast them over medium-high heat until golden and fragrant. Transfer to a dry kitchen towel and rub them together to remove their skins. Set aside to cool.

2 Combine the garlic and hazelnuts in a food processor and pulse until finely chopped. Add the parsley, Parmesan, and salt and continue processing. Add the olive oil in a steady stream while the machine is running until it all comes together into a creamy paste. Store in a jar in the refrigerator.

assemble the bocadillos

1 Preheat the oven to 350°F (180°C). Lay the ham slices on a baking sheet. Bake them for about 10 minutes, until crispy.

2 Heat the 2 tablespoons olive oil in a small sauté pan over medium heat. Fry the sage leaves until crispy. Reserve.

3 Heat a griddle or panini press. Spread the pesto on top of each slice of brioche. Crumble some goat cheese on top. Place 2 slices of crispy ham per sandwich, 3 fried sage leaves, and some more goat cheese, and top with another slice of brioche, pesto side down.

4 Brush the outside of the *bocadillos* with olive oil and transfer to the griddle or panini press. Heat until the brioche is crispy and the filling is warm. Serve immediately.

PARSLEY AND HAZELNUT PESTO (MAKES ¾ CUP)

¼ cup (30 g) hazelnuts

1 clove garlic, minced

2 cups (80 g) fresh parsley, tough stems removed

2 tablespoons finely grated Parmesan cheese

½ teaspoon salt

¼ cup (60 ml) olive oil

BOCADILLOS

8 thin slices (4 ounces or 110 g) Serrano ham

2 tablespoons olive oil, plus more for brushing brioche

12 fresh sage leaves

¼ cup (60 g) Parsley and Hazelnut Pesto

8 slices Quinoa Brioche (page 125)

2 ounces (60 g) goat cheese

root vegetable & acorn squash
bravas with two aiolis

PATATAS BRAVAS ARE A FAVORITE IN *PINTXO* BARS ALL over Spain. Chunks of salty fried potatoes are served with aioli and spicy tomato sauce. This is a variation on the classic, with crispy thin-sliced root vegetable and acorn squash chips. They're perfect with some chilled Txakoli wine as a starter for any dinner party.

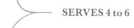

SERVES 4 to 6

AIOLI

2 cloves garlic, minced

½ teaspoon salt

2 egg yolks, at room temperature

2 teaspoons freshly squeezed lemon juice

3 tablespoons light olive oil

3 tablespoons extra-virgin olive oil

SPICY TOMATO AIOLI

½ cup (125 ml) Aioli

1 tablespoon tomato sauce

Tabasco sauce or chili oil, to taste

ROOT VEGETABLE AND ACORN SQUASH *BRAVAS*

1 small acorn squash

3 medium carrots

3 medium purple potatoes

3 medium golden beets

Vegetable oil, for frying

1 clove garlic, crushed but left whole

3 sprigs thyme

2 teaspoons sea salt

1 teaspoon freshly ground black pepper

½ ounce (15 g) Parmesan cheese, finely grated

make the aioli

1 Mix the garlic and salt in a mortar and mash with the pestle until they form a paste.

2 Combine the garlic paste, egg yolks, and lemon juice in a small blender and blend to combine.

3 While the blender is running, slowly drizzle in the light olive oil. It is very important that the oil be added slowly or else the emulsion will break. The aioli will begin to thicken. At this point, add a teaspoon of warm water. Continue by slowly adding the extra-virgin olive oil. If it becomes too thick, add another teaspoon of warm water to loosen the aioli. It will keep for up to 24 hours in the refrigerator.

TIP: If the aioli does break (it will be very runny), there is a way of fixing it. In a separate bowl, whisk another room-temperature egg yolk. Slowly add the broken aioli while constantly whisking. This should bring back the emulsion.

make the spicy tomato aioli

Whisk all the ingredients together. The mixture will keep for up to 24 hours in the refrigerator.

make the bravas

1 Thinly slice all the vegetables with a mandoline or a Y-shaped vegetable peeler. Place them in ice water for 20 minutes. Drain and pat them dry with a paper towel.

2 Meanwhile, fill a cast-iron pan with 1 inch of vegetable oil and heat it to 325°F (160°C). Add the garlic and thyme. Cook for 2 minutes or until golden. Remove them from the oil.

3 Fry the vegetables in batches and drain them on paper towels. Immediately sprinkle with the salt, pepper, and Parmesan. Serve with Aioli and Spicy Tomato Aioli.

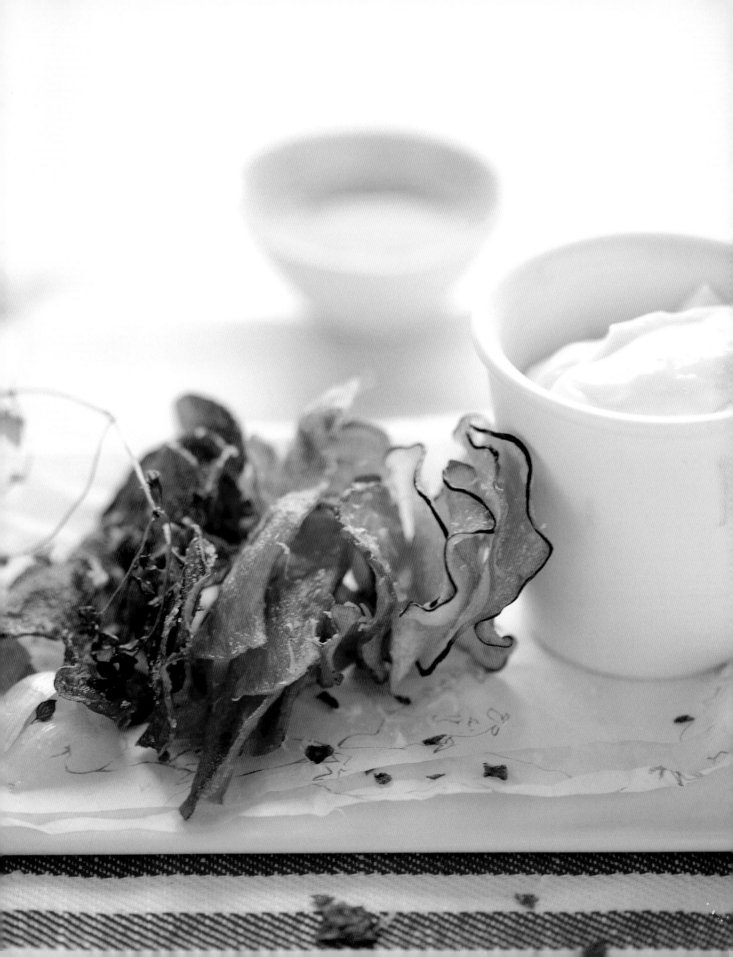

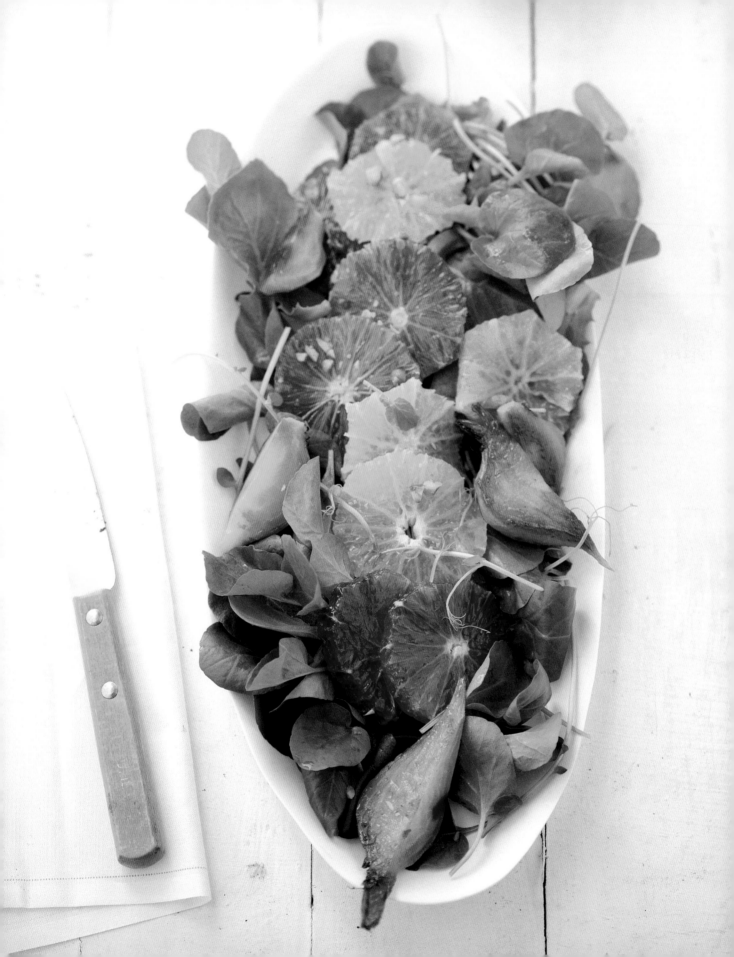

roasted beet, blood orange & mixed green salad

EVEN IN THE DEAD OF WINTER I make lots of salads with complementary textures and flavors. The acidity of the blood oranges here pairs nicely with the sweetness of the roasted beets. The pistachios add crunch. This can easily be turned into a vegetarian entrée by adding some cooked quinoa.

SERVES 4

1   Preheat the oven to 400°F (200°C). Rinse and peel the baby beets. If you are using larger beets, cut them in half or in quarters. Toss them in 2 tablespoons of the olive oil and ½ teaspoon of the salt. Place them on a baking sheet and bake them for about 40 minutes or until tender.

2   Peel the blood and navel oranges, making sure to remove the bitter white skin. Slice them thinly.

3   Place the greens on a platter and top with the orange slices, roasted beets, and pistachios.

4   Make the vinaigrette by whisking the mustard, vinegar, remaining 1 teaspoon salt, black pepper, and remaining ¼ cup (60 ml) olive oil. Drizzle the vinaigrette over the salad and serve immediately.

8 baby golden and red beets

¼ cup plus 2 tablespoons (90 ml) olive oil

1½ teaspoons salt

1 medium blood orange

1 medium navel orange

4 cups (160 g) mixed greens, such as baby romaine, spinach, watercress, or herbs

2 tablespoons chopped natural pistachios

1 tablespoon Dijon mustard

1 tablespoon champagne vinegar or apple cider vinegar

½ teaspoon freshly ground black pepper

crispy & creamy chicken, mushroom & potato bake

I WAS ELEVEN THE FIRST TIME I VISITED IRELAND. I spent a summer with the O'Sullivans, who took me in as an exchange student while I attended English classes. Every morning, Una packed my lunch in a brown bag: a chicken sandwich, an apple, and a packet of malt vinegar crisps. It seldom varied. During a lunch break at school I saw a fellow classmate pack his crisps inside his sandwich. I had never seen anything like it! "He might be on to something," I thought to myself, and he was. This dish is inspired by those flavors and textures, with a creamy chicken, mushroom, and tarragon filling and a crunchy potato, malt vinegar, and parsley topping.

SERVES 6

2 tablespoons olive oil, plus more for brushing bowls and frying

4 slices pancetta, chopped

1 medium yellow onion, diced

2 cloves garlic, minced

1 celery stalk, diced

1 pound (450 g) boneless chicken breasts or thighs, cut into bite-size pieces

1¼ teaspoons salt

1 teaspoon freshly ground black pepper

4 ounces (110 g) cremini mushrooms, sliced

1 tablespoon chopped fresh tarragon

¼ cup (60 ml) white wine

½ cup (125 ml) unsweetened coconut milk

2 medium Yukon gold potatoes, peeled

1 tablespoon malt vinegar

½ ounce (15 g) Parmesan cheese, finely grated

1 tablespoon finely chopped fresh parsley

1 Preheat the oven to 375°F (190°C). In a large sauté pan, heat 2 tablespoons of the olive oil over medium-high heat. Add the pancetta and cook until crispy. Add the onion, garlic, and celery and cook for 5 minutes.

2 Season the chicken with ½ teaspoon of the salt and ½ teaspoon of the black pepper. Add it to the pan. Cook for 5 minutes, turning once. Add the sliced mushrooms and cook for another 2 minutes. Add the tarragon, white wine, coconut milk, ½ teaspoon of the salt, and remaining ½ teaspoon black pepper. Cook for another minute.

3 Brush the inside of 6 (8-ounce) oven-safe bowls with oil. Divide the chicken mixture among the bowls and bake for 20 minutes.

4 Meanwhile, thinly slice the potatoes on a mandoline, or slice them by hand as thin as possible. Pat them dry with a paper towel. In a large sauté pan, heat ½ inch of olive oil over medium heat. Fry the potatoes in batches until crispy, making sure not to overcrowd the pan. Drain them on paper towels. Drizzle the malt vinegar and remaining ¼ teaspoon salt on top.

5 Remove the bowls from the oven and top with the crispy potatoes and Parmesan cheese. Put the bowls back in the oven for 5 minutes. Top with the parsley and serve immediately.

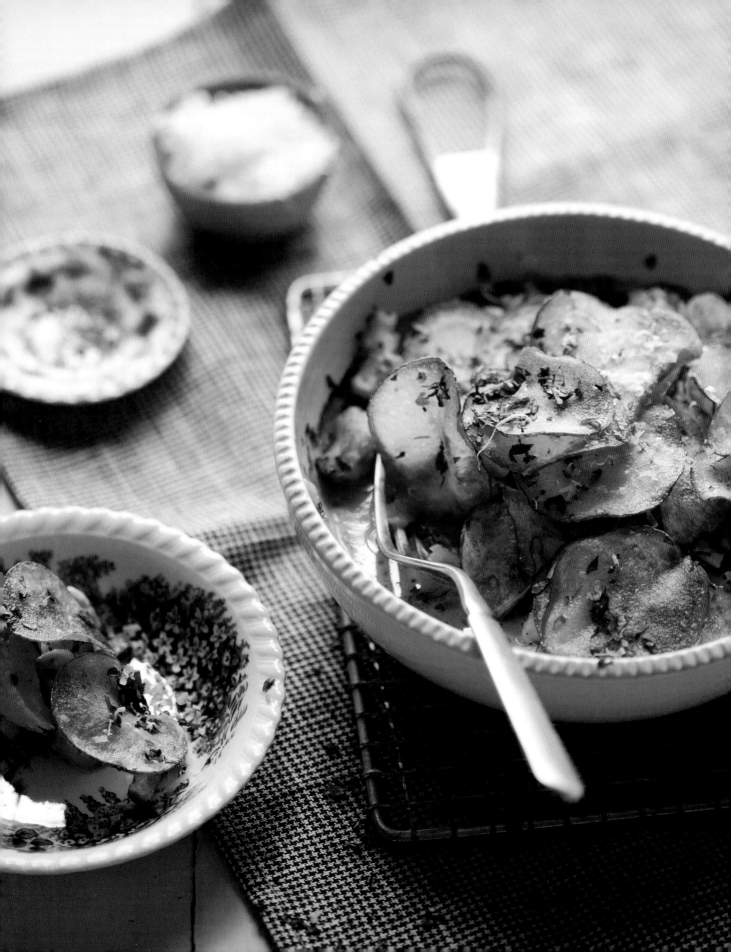

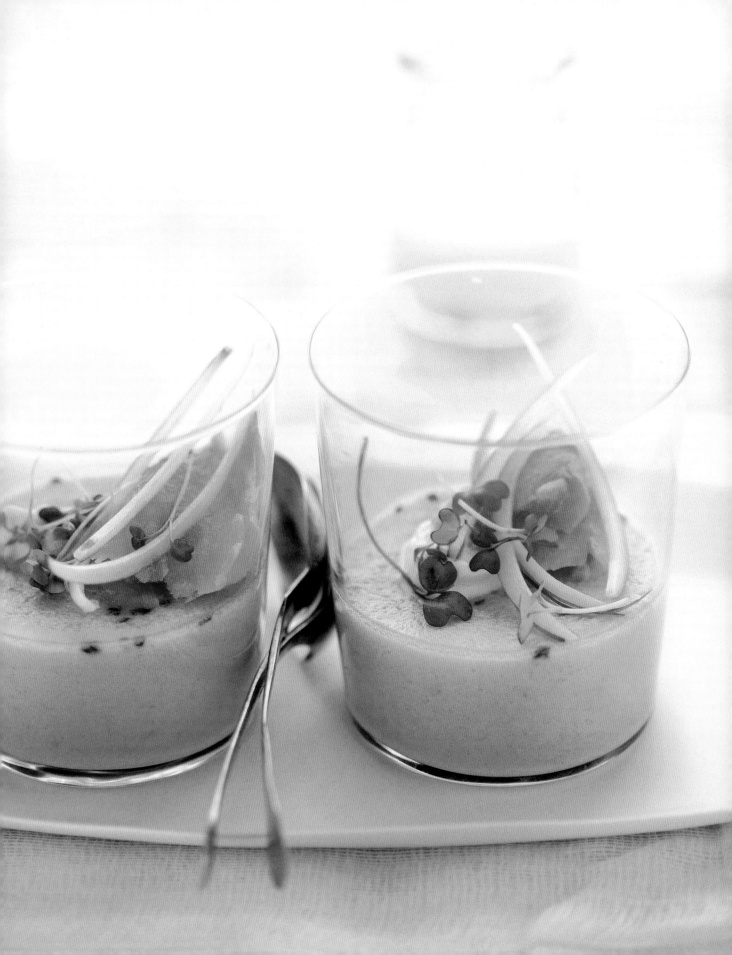

leek & chive flan with smoked salmon

THE INTENSE AROMA OF LEEKS, A STAPLE in Basque cooking, filled my childhood. My paternal grandparents grew them in their garden, and every Sunday when we visited they sent us home with bags filled with leeks, moist soil still on them. Their smell permeated my father's car all winter long. In this recipe, the leeks are first braised and later turned into a silky custard with goat cheese and coconut milk.

SERVES 4

1 Preheat the oven to 325°F (160°C). In a medium sauté pan, heat the olive oil over medium heat. Add the leeks and ¼ teaspoon of the salt. Cook them for about 5 minutes or until soft but not browned. Add the chicken stock and cook for 5 more minutes.

2 Transfer the leeks to a blender. Add the coconut milk and goat cheese and puree. Strain the mixture through a sieve.

3 In a medium bowl, whisk the eggs, the leek mixture, chives, and remaining ¼ teaspoon salt. Pour the custard into 4 (4-ounce) oven-safe glasses or ramekins. Place them in a baking dish and place on the oven rack. Pour about 1 inch of hot water into the baking dish. Bake for 20 to 25 minutes, until the custard is set. Let them cool slightly on a rack.

4 Serve lukewarm or at room temperature topped with the smoked salmon, yogurt, microgreens, and red onion.

2 tablespoons olive oil

2 medium leeks, white and tender green parts only, sliced

½ teaspoon salt

¼ cup (60 ml) chicken stock

1 cup (250 ml) unsweetened coconut milk

2 ounces (60 g) goat cheese

3 eggs

2 tablespoons finely chopped fresh chives

8 ounces (225 g) thinly sliced smoked salmon

2 tablespoons Greek-style yogurt, for garnish

Microgreens, for garnish

Thinly sliced red onion, for garnish

candy-striped beet, fennel & raclette tart with buckwheat crust

MY FRIEND LENA HYDE HAS A BEAUTIFUL garden that her two boys, Ethan and Cal, plant every year. Beets, tomatoes, green beans, peas, squash, eggplant, and all sorts of greens are among the vegetables that the boys care for so diligently throughout the year. It was a Saturday morning when my son, Jon, and I stopped by their house. I wanted to show him what Ethan and Cal were up to, because he looks up to them. The garden was overflowing with goodness. "Could you use some beets?" they asked. "Always!" I replied. Cal harvested the most beautiful candy-striped beets for us. They were sweet and earthy, and I roasted them up for this pungent tart. Thank you, Cal and Ethan!

MAKES one 9-inch round tart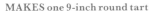

BUCKWHEAT CRUST

½ cup (70 g) superfine brown rice flour, plus more for dusting

⅓ cup (45 g) buckwheat flour

⅓ cup (40 g) cornstarch

⅓ cup (35 g) almond flour

2 teaspoons ground chia seeds

½ teaspoon salt

¼ teaspoon freshly ground black pepper

1 stick (8 tablespoons or 110 g) cold unsalted butter, cut into ½-inch cubes

6 to 8 tablespoons ice water

CANDY-STRIPED BEET, FENNEL, AND RACLETTE FILLING

3 large candy-striped, red, or golden beets, stems removed

2 tablespoons olive oil

2 medium yellow onions, thinly sliced

1 medium fennel bulb, thinly sliced

½ teaspoon salt

3 ounces (90 g) raclette or Fontina cheese, sliced into ¼-inch pieces

make the crust

1 Preheat the oven to 400°F (200°C). Combine the first seven ingredients in a food processor and pulse a couple of times to aerate. Add the cold butter and pulse ten times, until the butter is the size of peas.

2 Add 6 tablespoons ice water and pulse until the dough comes together. It does not need to form a ball. Just open the lid and press the dough between your fingers to see if it holds together. If it doesn't, add another tablespoon of water.

3 Turn the dough out onto your work surface, knead it a couple of times, and form a disk. Wrap it in plastic wrap and flatten it. Refrigerate the dough for 1 hour. (While the dough is chilling, roast the beets for the filling in the preheated oven.)

4 Dust the work surface (preferably cold, such as marble) with superfine brown rice flour. Roll the dough out to about a ⅛-inch thickness. If the dough cracks, pinch it back together. Work quickly so it doesn't get too warm. Fill a 9-inch tart mold with the dough. Press it into the mold and cut out the excess.

5 Chill the tart dough in the freezer for 10 minutes. Cover the top with a sheet of parchment paper. Place pie weights or dried beans on top and blind-bake for 20 minutes. Remove the parchment and weights and bake for another 15 minutes.

prepare the filling and bake the tart

1 While the dough is chilling, roast the beets. Wrap the beets in aluminum foil and bake them for 45 minutes to 1 hour, until you can easily

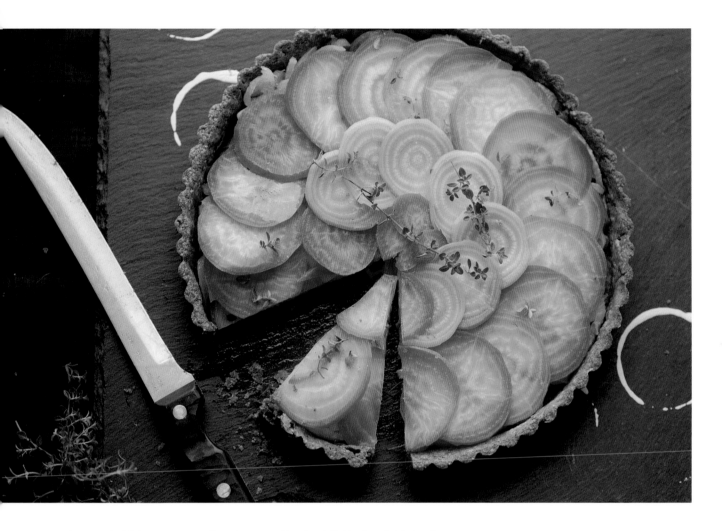

insert a knife in the center. Let them cool in the foil. Peel and thinly slice them. Reserve.

    2 Heat the olive oil in a medium sauté pan over medium-high heat. Cook the onions, fennel, and salt in it for 10 minutes or until soft, translucent, and slightly browned. Spread the mixture over the prebaked crust.

    3 Top the onion mixture with the sliced raclette and bake for 5 minutes or until the cheese is melted.

    4 Arrange the beet slices on top of the cheese and bake for 2 minutes to heat the beets through. Serve warm.

RACLETTE

Raclette is one of my favorite melting cheeses—mild, creamy, slightly nutty, and ideally suited for melting. It is made in Switzerland and parts of France from cow's milk. Raclette is also served as a meal, very much like fondue, but grilled. The cheese is melted on a special griddle and served with cured meats, vegetables, and other accompaniments.

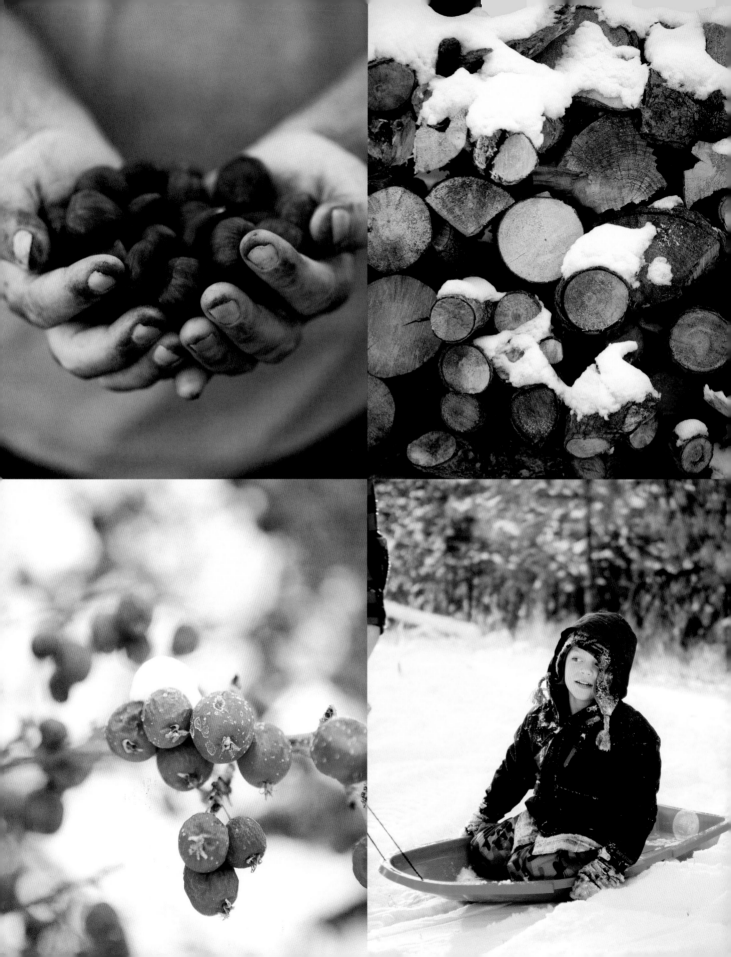

WINTER
sweet treats

Brioche • Chocolate Brioche Bread Pudding • Pistachio & Vanilla Bean Shortbread Cookies • Clementine, Green Apple & Lemon Thyme Sorbet • Hazelnut, Vanilla Bean & Cinnamon Soup Shots • Grapefruit, Champagne Sabayon, Candied Ginger & Almond Verrines • Meyer Lemon, Almond & Yogurt Custard Pots • Frozen Pistachio Nougat Mousse • Glazed Apple & Chestnut Bundt Cakes • Coconut Cream Cookies • Vanilla Bean & Cardamom Baked Arroz con Leche *• Chocolate, Hazelnut & Buckwheat Cake • Candied Sour Orange & Almond Cake • Chocolate, Banana & Hazelnut Cream Toasties*

WINTER IS THE SEASON OF chocolate, nuts, citrus, and holiday baking. I get the entire family involved in the kitchen, just as I helped out in the pastry shop growing up. Back then, when December arrived, everyone in our family knew there would be late nights and almonds to grind. Tons and tons of raw almonds arrived in grain sacks, and they needed to be blanched, peeled, and ground so we could make marzipan and *turrón* (nougat candy).

"Wait, *amatxu*," my son, Jon, asks every time he sees me pull out a bowl and the kitchen scale. "I want to help." He has been this way since I can remember, always very curious about the goings-on in the kitchen. Now, age five, he drags his blue step stool close to the kitchen counter and jumps on, ready to grab a wooden spoon. "I'm ready, *amatxu*." I carefully guide him through the steps of adding flour to a bowl and the importance of carefully weighing the ingredients. He struggles to get all the flour into the bowl, and I remind myself that it is never about the mess but about getting him involved. I remind myself over and over again.

Miren, age two, still wearing her pajamas and with her wild curls uncombed, sits on the kitchen floor playing with the flour that never made it into the bowl. She also wants to participate and stretches her arms out to let me know she wants to be up high. I hold her against my hip and help Jon scoop the Apple & Chestnut Cake batter into the Bundt pan. The kitchen smells like winter and I cannot help but smile.

brioche

FOR THE LONGEST TIME I HESITATED to refer to this recipe as a brioche. I wonder if all the master bakers I have worked with would frown upon the idea. I could say it's a yeast cake, but *brioche* sounds so much more appealing. This gluten-free version of the classic is also rich, moist, and deliciously fragrant. Warm brioche for breakfast is a favorite in our house—a treat I prepare for my family on cold winter mornings. I turn it into baked French toast, or Chocolate Brioche Bread Pudding (page 127), or I save it for sandwiches.

MAKES one 8½ by 4½-inch loaf

BASIC BRIOCHE

1 tablespoon active dry yeast

½ cup (125 ml) whole milk, heated to 115°F (46°C)

½ teaspoon natural cane sugar

1 tablespoon chia seeds

2 tablespoons boiling water

⅔ cup (90 g) superfine brown rice flour

⅔ cup (90 g) sorghum flour

½ cup (80 g) potato starch

½ cup (60 g) tapioca starch

1½ teaspoons xanthan gum

½ teaspoon salt

¼ cup (70 g) honey

2 eggs, at room temperature, plus 1 egg, lightly beaten

1 stick (8 tablespoons or 110 g) unsalted butter, at room temperature

1 tablespoon demerara sugar

1 In a small bowl, whisk together the active dry yeast, warm milk, and sugar. Let this mixture sit for about 10 minutes. It will become foamy as the yeast activates.

2 Grind the chia seeds in a coffee grinder. Stir the ground chia seeds and boiling water in a small bowl to form a thick paste. Reserve.

3 In the bowl of a stand mixer, whisk together the superfine brown rice flour, sorghum flour, potato starch, tapioca starch, xanthan gum, and salt.

4 Add the yeast mixture, chia seed paste, honey, and eggs. Mix with the dough hook on medium speed until the dough comes together.

5 Add 1 tablespoon of soft butter at a time while mixing on medium speed. Wait between each addition so that the butter becomes well incorporated into the dough. Continue mixing until all the butter has been incorporated, about 3 minutes. Turn the speed to high and mix for another 30 seconds.

6 The dough will be sticky and feel like a thick cake batter. Transfer the dough to a buttered 8½ by 4½-inch loaf pan. Smooth out the top of the dough with your wet hands. Tuck in the edges to create a slight dome on top.

7 Cover the pan with plastic wrap that has been sprayed with nonstick spray and let it ferment at room temperature for 45 minutes to 1 hour, or until the dough rises to the rim of the pan.

8 Meanwhile, preheat the oven to 350°F (180°C). Brush the top of the brioche with the lightly beaten egg and sprinkle with the demerara sugar.

9 Bake the brioche for 35 to 40 minutes, or until a toothpick inserted in the center of the bread comes out clean. Let the brioche cool in the pan for at least 15 minutes. Invert onto a wire rack and cool completely before slicing. Store at room temperature wrapped in parchment paper for up to 3 days, or freeze for up to 1 month.

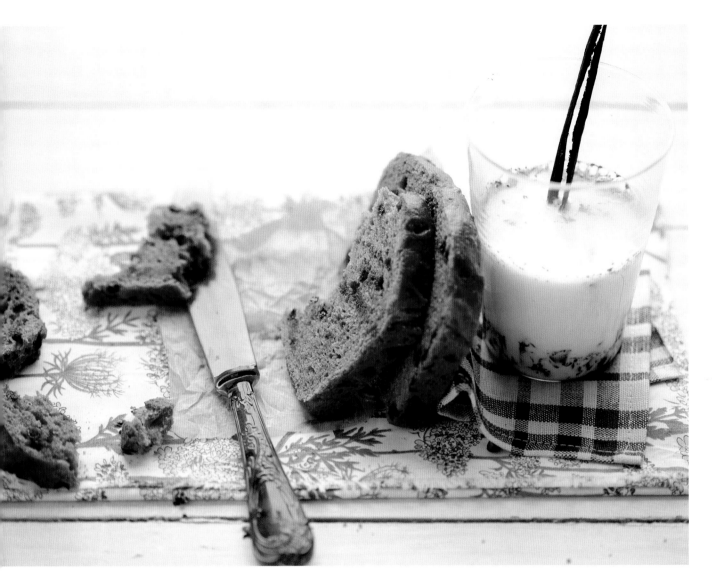

BRIOCHE VARIATIONS

CRANBERRY ORANGE BRIOCHE: Substitute millet flour for the sorghum flour. Add 2 tablespoons grated orange zest and 1 cup (150 g) dried cranberries after all the butter has been incorporated.

QUINOA BRIOCHE: For a savory variation, which I use for sandwiches and tartines, you may substitute quinoa flour for the sorghum flour. Also add ¼ teaspoon freshly ground black pepper along with the salt. Top the dough with quinoa flakes right before it goes into the oven.

CHOCOLATE BRIOCHE: For a chocolate version, add ½ cup (100 g) mini semisweet chocolate chips to the dough right after all the butter has been incorporated. Mix it for 30 seconds on high speed. The dough will take on a chocolate color and the chocolate chips will be spread evenly throughout. This variation is my personal favorite.

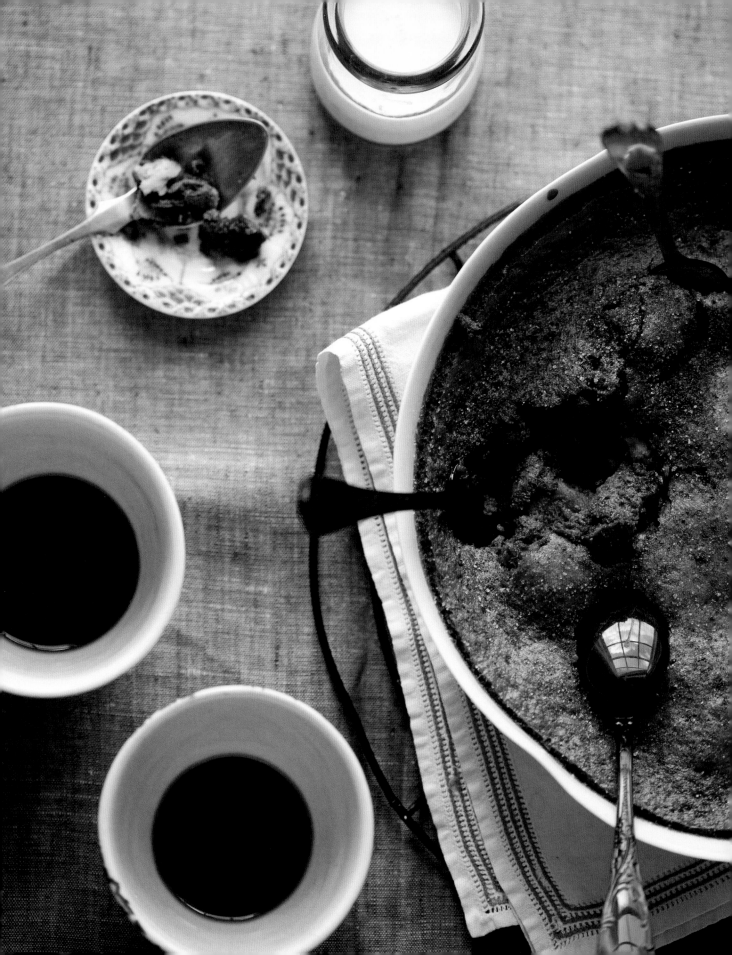

chocolate brioche bread pudding

THIS IS POSSIBLY THE BEST BREAD PUDDING I have ever made. It is based on a chocolate croissant bread pudding we made at the Ritz-Carlton Palm Beach. It is creamy and light from the whipped eggs and the cream. The combination of the warm chocolate, bread, salt, and the light custard just melts in your mouth. Serve it with thick poured cream. Heaven.

SERVES 4 to 6

1 Preheat the oven to 325°F (160°C). Place the chopped chocolate in a heatproof bowl and place it over a pot partly filled with simmering water. Melt the chocolate over this double boiler. Set it aside to cool slightly.

2 Place the eggs, egg yolk, and sugar in the bowl of a stand mixer. Whip on high speed for about 3 minutes, until the eggs are thick and form a ribbon when the beater is lifted.

3 In another bowl, whip the 1 cup heavy cream to soft peaks. Fold the heavy cream into the whipped eggs. Fold in the melted chocolate and *fleur de sel*. Make sure to scrape the bottom of the bowl well because chocolate tends to sink. Fold in the brioche cubes and chocolate chips.

4 Pour the mixture into an 8-inch cake pan. Place the cake pan on a deep rimmed baking sheet and place on the oven rack. Pour hot water into the baking sheet to a depth of about ½ inch. Bake the pudding in this water bath for 40 to 45 minutes, until the center is set and does not jiggle. Do not overbake or it will dry out. It should be light and creamy.

5 Serve with a dusting of cocoa powder and some additional whipped cream.

2 ounces (60 g) bittersweet chocolate, finely chopped

2 eggs

1 egg yolk

¼ cup (50 g) natural cane sugar

1 cup (250 ml) heavy cream, plus more for serving

¼ teaspoon *fleur de sel*

2 cups (175 g) diced Brioche (page 124)

¼ cup (50 g) mini semisweet chocolate chips

Unsweetened cocoa powder, for serving

pistachio & vanilla bean shortbread cookies

THIS SHORTBREAD GATHERS TWO OF MY favorite ingredients—pistachios and vanilla beans—in one treat. They are coated in powdered sugar while warm, which creates a slightly creamy coating. I make batch after batch of these during the holiday season. They are great to give as gifts.

MAKES about 50 cookies

1 cup (140 g) superfine brown rice flour

½ cup (80 g) potato starch

½ cup plus 2 tablespoons (70 g) gluten-free oat flour

¼ cup (30 g) tapioca starch

1 teaspoon salt

½ cup (80 g) unsalted natural pistachios

2 sticks (16 tablespoons or 225 g) unsalted butter, at room temperature

¾ cup (90 g) powdered sugar, plus more for dusting, sifted

1 vanilla bean, split lengthwise and seeds scraped

1 In a medium bowl, whisk together the superfine brown rice flour, potato starch, oat flour, tapioca starch, and salt. Measure 1 tablespoon of this flour mixture and add it to a food processor along with the pistachios. Pulse until the pistachios are ground to a fine powder.

2 Combine the soft butter, powdered sugar, and vanilla seeds in the bowl of a stand mixer fitted with the paddle attachment. Turn the mixer on low speed for a few seconds so the powdered sugar doesn't fly everywhere. Increase the speed to medium-high and cream together until light, about 2 minutes. Scrape down the sides of the bowl and the paddle.

3 Add the dry ingredients along with the ground pistachios to the mixer bowl. Mix until the dough comes together; it will be a sticky dough. Turn the dough out onto a work surface and shape it into a log that is approximately 13 inches long and 2 inches in diameter. Wrap the log in parchment and roll it, trying to make it as round as possible. Refrigerate the dough for at least 1 hour.

4 Preheat the oven to 350°F (180°C). Remove the dough from the refrigerator and unwrap it. Cut disks that are ¼ inch thick. Place them 2 inches apart on a baking sheet lined with parchment paper.

5 Bake for 10 minutes, until lightly golden on the bottom, but do not overbake, as they will become very hard. Let them cool on the baking sheet for about 10 minutes. Dust them with powdered sugar. Store tightly wrapped at room temperature for up to 3 days.

CRANBERRY & PINK PEPPERCORN SHORTBREAD COOKIES

I have a fondness for pink peppercorns in desserts. I add them to my strawberry salad in the summer or sprinkle them over vanilla ice cream. For this shortbread variation, add ½ cup (70 g) chopped dried cranberries along with 2 teaspoons ground pink peppercorns to the cookie dough in place of the chopped pistachios.

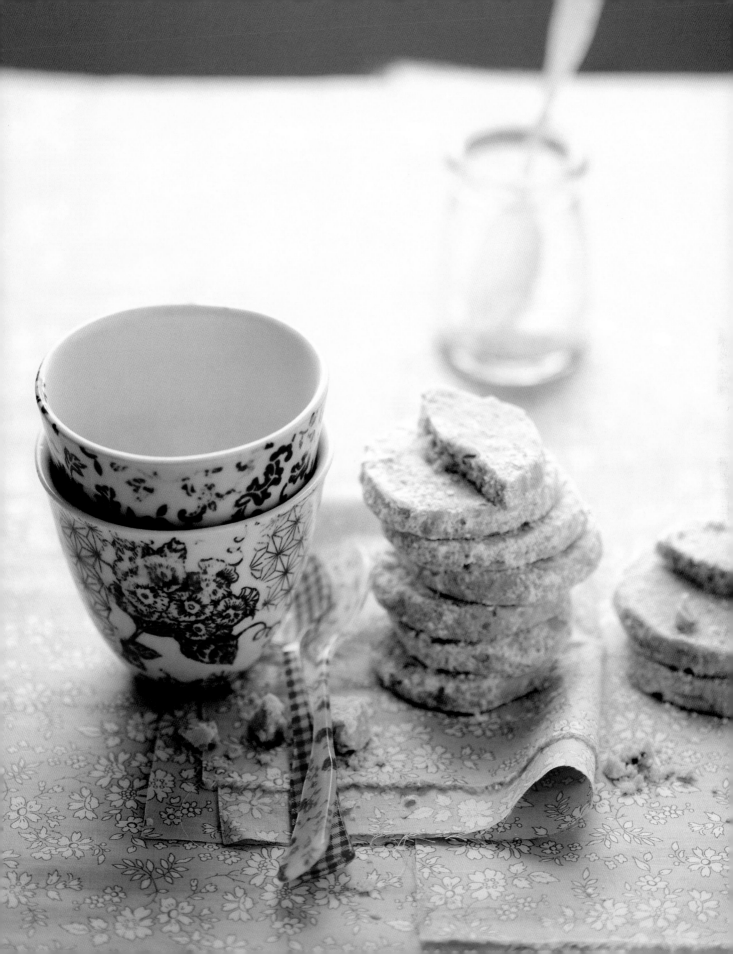

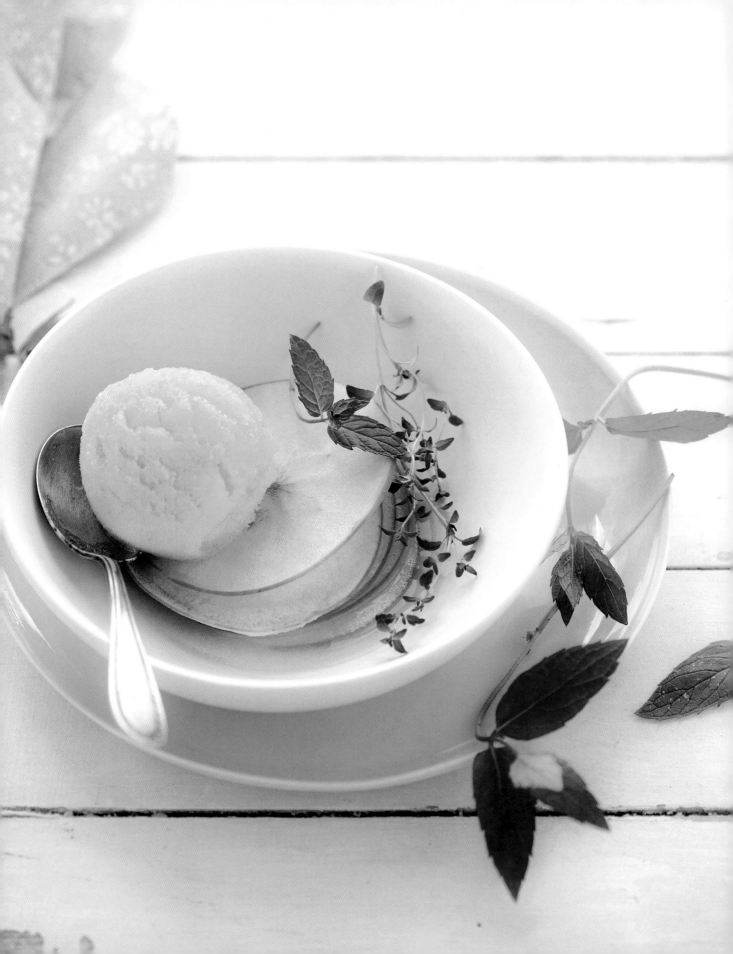

clementine, green apple & lemon thyme sorbet

CLEMENTINES, WHICH ARE ONLY AVAILABLE for a short period of time, are my winter candy. The season peaks right around the end of December, and this is when we eat them by the crate. When making this sorbet, or any fruit sorbet, taste the fruit juice first and then determine the amount of sugar needed, as the acidity and sweetness of fruit varies. It's best to start with a smaller amount and add more if needed. The green apple and lemon add tartness to the otherwise sweet clementines.

SERVES 6

1 Place ¼ cup (50 g) of the sugar, lemon zest, lemon thyme leaves, and salt in a bowl. Rub all the ingredients together between your fingers to release their natural oils.

2 In a blender, combine the clementine juice, diced apple, lemon juice, and sugar mixture. Taste to see if it has the desired sweetness; if not, add a bit more sugar. Blend on high speed until smooth. (You could also do this in a food processor, beginning with the apple and sugar mixture and then adding the juices.)

3 Transfer the fruit puree to a bowl and refrigerate for 2 hours. Churn in an ice cream machine according to the manufacturer's instructions. Transfer to a freezer-safe container and freeze for at least 4 hours.

4 Transfer the sorbet to the refrigerator for 15 minutes to soften before serving. Thinly slice the other apple. Place a few slices of apple in each bowl or glass. Scoop the sorbet on top and garnish with fresh thyme and mint.

¼ cup to ⅓ cup (50 g to 70 g) natural cane sugar

1 tablespoon finely grated lemon zest

1 teaspoon fresh lemon thyme leaves, plus more for garnish

¼ teaspoon salt

2½ cups (625 ml) freshly squeezed clementine juice, from about 2½ pounds (1.25 kg) of fruit

1 medium Granny Smith apple, peeled, cored, and diced, plus another apple for serving

2 tablespoons freshly squeezed lemon juice

Fresh mint leaves, for garnish

hazelnut, vanilla bean & cinnamon soup shots

"LET'S TAKE THE KIDS FOR A WALK and gather some hazelnuts," my mom suggested during our last visit home. I grew up in a small town surrounded by nut trees. My uncle has some beautiful walnut, hazelnut, almond, and chestnut trees around his property that I love to photograph. As kids, we would pick nuts from the ground and bring them home to eat as snacks.

This soup is a variation of the classic *intxaursaltsa* (walnut soup), which is a thick soup made with walnuts and cinnamon—a Christmas classic. I like to pour it into shot glasses and serve it with Cranberry & Pink Peppercorn Shortbread Cookies (page 128) as mini dessert starters.

SERVES 6 to 8

1 cup (120 g) hazelnuts

¼ cup (50 g) natural cane sugar

2 teaspoons finely grated lemon zest

2 cups (500 ml) whole milk

1 vanilla bean, split lengthwise and seeds scraped

1 cinnamon stick

⅛ teaspoon salt

½ cup (125 ml) heavy cream

1 Preheat the oven to 350°F (180°C). Place the hazelnuts on a baking sheet and bake them for 5 to 7 minutes or until golden and fragrant. Transfer them to a kitchen towel and rub them together to remove their skins. Let them cool. Finely chop 1 tablespoon for use as a garnish.

2 Place the skinned hazelnuts, sugar, and lemon zest in a food processor and pulse until the hazelnuts are finely ground almost into a paste.

3 Combine the milk, hazelnut mixture, vanilla bean and seeds, cinnamon stick, and salt in a medium saucepan. Bring to a simmer, reduce the heat to medium-low, and cook for about 15 minutes, while stirring, until it begins to thicken. Remove the vanilla bean and the cinnamon stick.

4 Transfer the soup to a blender and blend into a fine puree. You should have 2 cups of soup.

5 Pour the soup into a bowl and let it cool completely. The soup will thicken as it cools. Stir it before serving. You may serve it at room temperature or refrigerate and serve cold.

6 Whip the heavy cream. Pour the soup into shot glasses and top with a dollop of whipped cream and the reserved chopped hazelnuts.

REUSING VANILLA BEANS

I use vanilla beans several times. I might use them in a cake the first time around and in a custard (steeping the pods in warm milk) the second. Then I wash the pods in hot water, dry them, and place them in a jar full of sugar. I leave them there for days, weeks, and months until the sugar has been completely permeated with the vanilla. Then I grind the sugar and the vanilla beans into a powder and use them again and again.

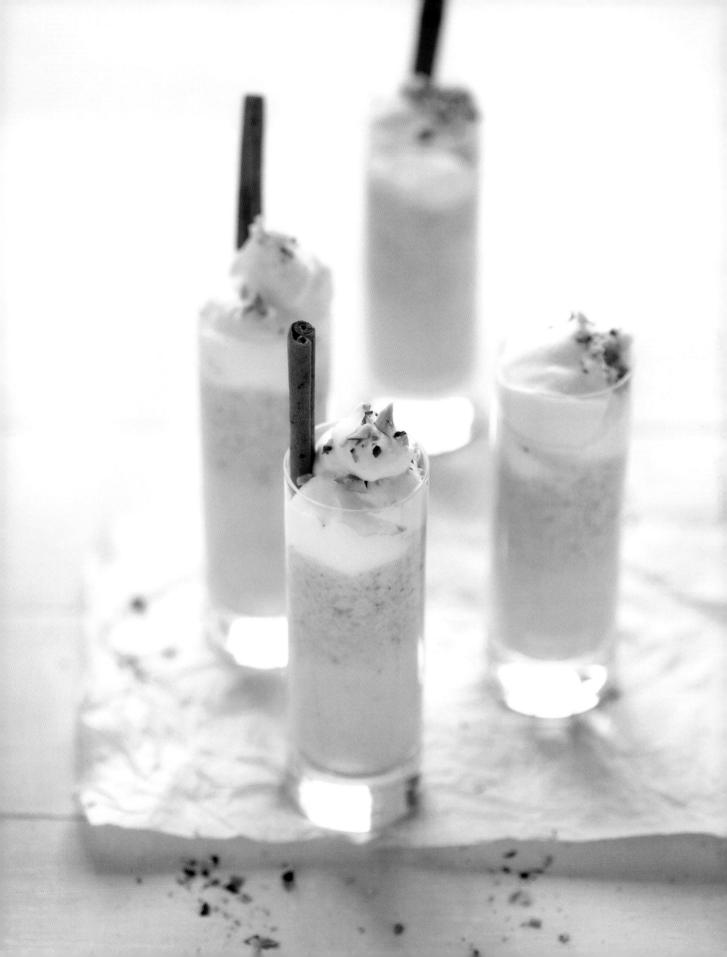

grapefruit, champagne sabayon, candied ginger & almond *verrines*

I LOVE *VERRINES*—DESSERTS THAT YOU assemble with layers of different flavors and textures in a glass. These *verrines* are fresh and light, with grapefruit segments, Champagne sabayon, and a candied ginger and almond crumble on top. For a kid-friendly and alcohol-free variation, use apple juice or apple cider instead of the Champagne.

SERVES 6

CANDIED GINGER AND ALMOND CRUMBLE

1 cup (100 g) almond flour

½ cup (100 g) natural cane sugar

½ cup (70 g) superfine brown rice flour

2 tablespoons tapioca starch

⅛ teaspoon salt

1 stick (8 tablespoons or 110 g) unsalted butter, at room temperature

¾ cup (80 g) slivered blanched almonds

2 tablespoons finely minced candied ginger

CHAMPAGNE SABAYON

6 egg yolks

½ cup (100 g) natural cane sugar

⅔ cup (165 ml) Champagne

1 cup (250 ml) heavy cream

VERRINE ASSEMBLY

3 red grapefruits

½ cup (70 g) Candied Ginger & Almond Crumble

Champagne Sabayon

Fresh mint leaves, for garnish

make the crumble

1 Preheat the oven to 350°F (180°C).

2 In a large bowl, whisk together the first five ingredients. Add the soft butter in pieces and crumble the butter into the dry ingredients with your hands.

3 Add the slivered almonds and candied ginger and toss everything together.

4 Spread the crumble on a baking sheet lined with parchment paper and freeze for 20 minutes. Scoop out half of the crumble and freeze it in an airtight container for another use (see sidebar). Bake the rest for 12 minutes, until golden brown. Let the crumble cool until you are ready to assemble the *verrines*.

make the sabayon

1 Whisk the egg yolks, sugar, and Champagne in the bowl of a stand mixer until frothy, but no need to whip it. Place the bowl over a pot partly filled with simmering water. Whisk the sabayon until it thickens. It will take about 3 minutes.

2 Immediately after, transfer the bowl to the mixer and whip the sabayon on medium-high speed until the bowl feels cool to the touch and the sabayon is pale and thick.

3 In another bowl, whip the heavy cream to soft peaks. Fold the cream into the cooled sabayon.

assemble the verrines

Peel and segment the grapefruits. Make sure to remove any of the white rind. Place 2 tablespoons of crumble on the bottom of each serving glass. Top with grapefruit segments, followed by Champagne Sabayon, and finish with some more crumble and fresh mint. Serve immediately.

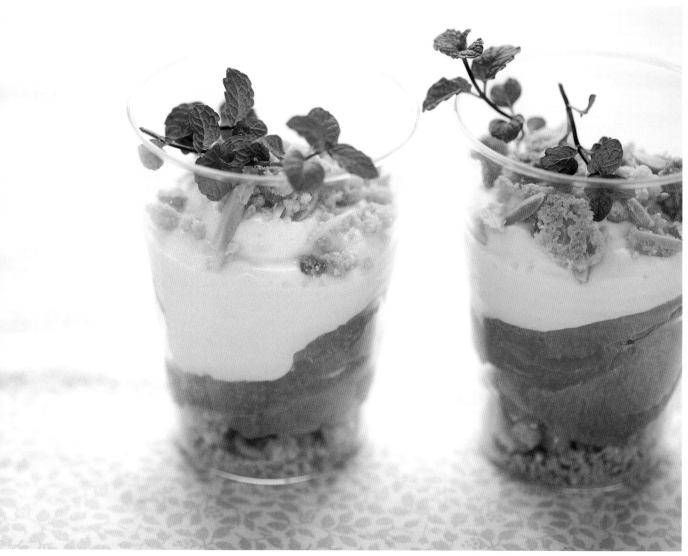

FREEZING LARGE BATCHES OF DOUGH

When I make pastry dough for tarts or crumble toppings, I tend to double the recipes and freeze what I will not be using right then. I have a freezer full of different doughs ready for when I have a last-minute get-together or I feel like having some fruit crumble in the middle of the afternoon.

Transfer the leftover crumble to an airtight container and freeze for up to 1 month. In this case, the topping does not need to be thawed out prior to using. Simply top your fruit with frozen crumble and bake.

A trick I learned in culinary school is that a tart or piecrust will use approximately 1 ounce (30 g) of dough per 1 inch (2.5 cm) of pan. For instance, if you are making a 9-inch (23 cm) pie, then you will need 9 ounces (270 g) of pie dough. Portion out your dough accordingly. Wrap tightly in plastic wrap and freeze for up to 1 month. When you are ready to use it, make sure you thaw it out in the refrigerator overnight first.

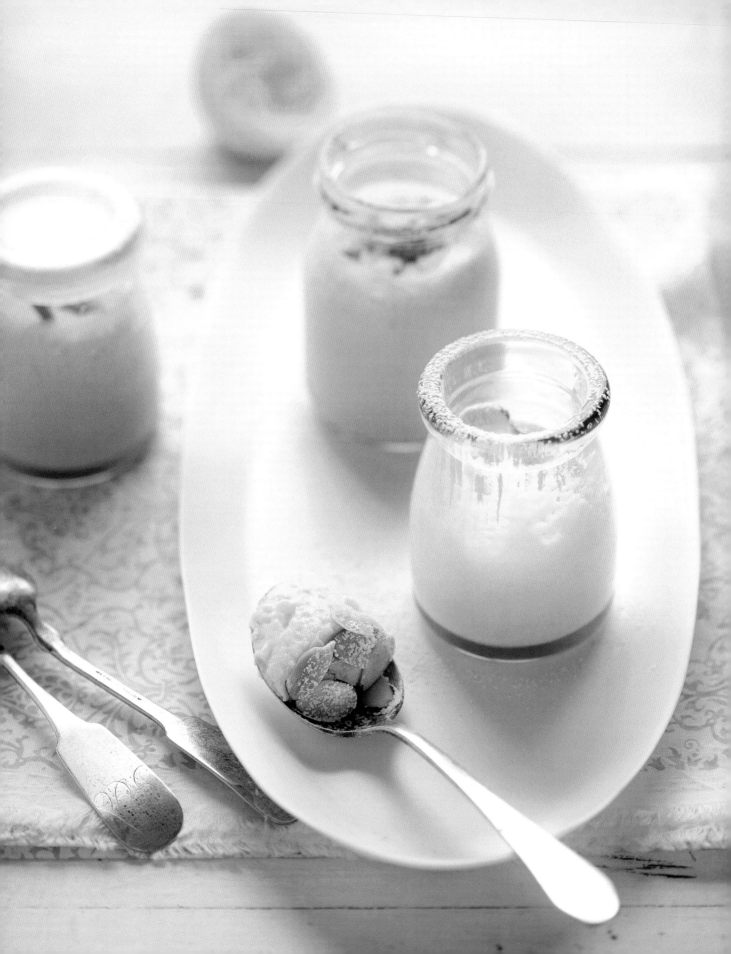

meyer lemon, almond & yogurt custard pots

I HIGHLY RECOMMEND USING FRESH FARM eggs when making custards. The intense orange yolks give this custard a bright yellow color that is rich and intense. My children love coming with me to the farm every week where we get our eggs. They run to see if any new eggs have been laid. "They are still warm!" Jon shouts as his eyes light up. "You are lucky, so lucky," I tell him.

MAKES six 4-ounce ramekins

1 Preheat the oven to 325°F (160°C). In a medium bowl, using your fingers, rub the sugar and lemon zest together. This helps release the oil in the zest. Whisk in the eggs. Add the almond flour, yogurt, coconut milk, and lemon juice. Whisk until smooth.

2 Place 6 (4-ounce) ramekins in a deep-rimmed baking pan. Pour the custard into the ramekins. Bring the baking pan to the oven and set it on the rack. Pour hot water into the baking pan, enough to come halfway up the sides of the ramekins. Bake in the water bath for 30 minutes, until set.

3 Remove the baking pan from the oven and carefully lift out the ramekins. Let them cool to room temperature on a rack and then transfer them to the refrigerator. Serve chilled with toasted almonds and powdered sugar sprinkled on top. Store in the refrigerator for up to 5 days.

⅓ cup (70 g) natural cane sugar

1 tablespoon finely grated Meyer lemon zest

4 eggs

½ cup (50 g) almond flour

1 cup (250 ml) whole-milk Greek-style yogurt

1 cup (250 ml) unsweetened coconut milk

¼ cup (60 ml) freshly squeezed Meyer lemon juice

¼ cup (30 g) toasted slivered almonds, for garnish

Powdered sugar, for garnish

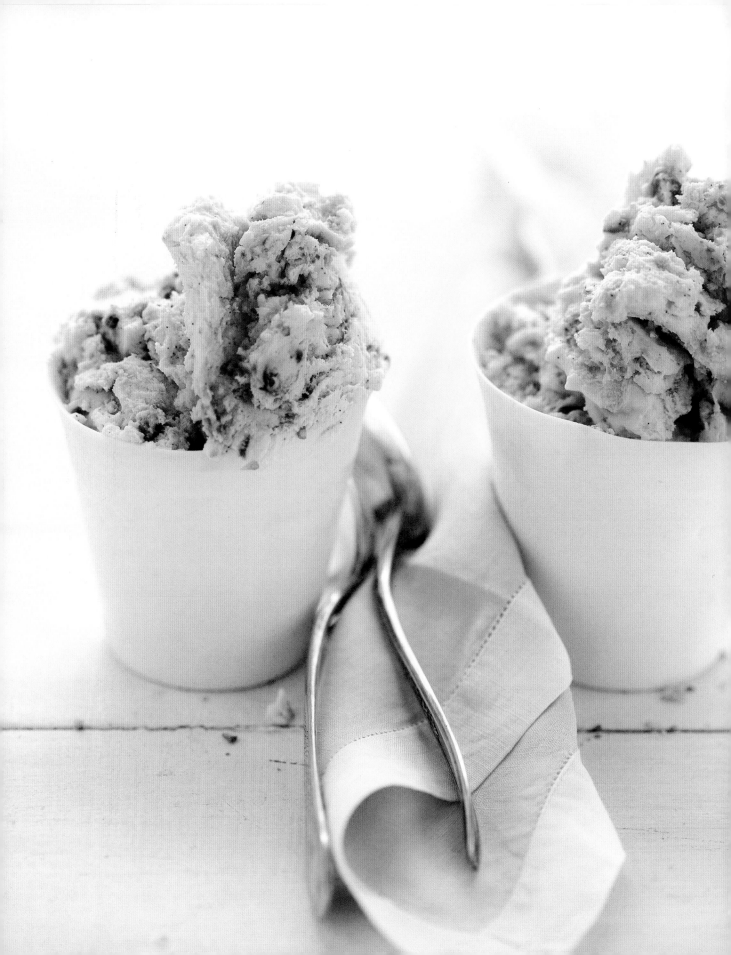

frozen pistachio nougat mousse

NOUGAT, OR *TURRÓN*, AS WE CALL IT in Spanish, is a traditional Christmastime dessert. Made with egg whites, honey, and nuts, it is the treat I looked forward to the most during the holidays when I was growing up. This is a chilled rendition of the classic treat that features pillow-like meringue made with honey and crunchy caramelized pistachios and almonds, lightened with whipped cream. Melts in your mouth.

SERVES 6 to 8

1 Sprinkle one-third of the sugar in a medium saucepan. Heat over medium-high heat until the sugar begins to melt. Sprinkle in another one-third and let this melt as well. Add the rest of the sugar and continue cooking until the color is a medium amber. Swirl the pan so that all the sugar caramelizes evenly.

2 Stir in the pistachios and almonds and immediately pour the caramel onto a baking sheet lined with a silicone mat or lightly greased parchment paper. Let it cool completely, and then chop it coarsely.

3 In a bowl of a stand mixer, whip the heavy cream and vanilla seeds to soft peaks. Reserve in the refrigerator until ready to use.

4 Place the egg whites in another bowl on the stand mixer and whip them on high speed until very light and tripled in volume. In the meantime, place the honey in a microwave-safe bowl and heat for 30 seconds or until it comes to a simmer. Gradually, on low speed, pour the honey into the whipped whites. Turn the speed to high and finish whipping to firm peaks and until the bowl feels cool to the touch.

5 Gently fold the meringue and the caramelized nut pieces into the reserved cream. Pour into a freezer-safe container and freeze until solid. Remove from the freezer 5 minutes before serving.

1 cup (200 g) natural cane sugar

⅓ cup (55 g) unsalted natural pistachios

2 tablespoons slivered blanched almonds

1 cup (250 ml) heavy cream

1 vanilla bean, split lengthwise and seeds scraped

3 egg whites, preferably from farm eggs

¼ cup (70 g) honey

glazed apple & chestnut bundt cakes

BROWN BUTTER, CHESTNUT FLOUR, and hazelnut flour make these cakes nutty and rich. Glazed while warm, they make a gooey and sticky dessert, perfect for any holiday table or a weekend treat.

MAKES twelve 4-ounce mini-Bundt cakes

APPLE AND CHESTNUT CAKES

1¼ sticks (10 tablespoons or 140 g) unsalted butter

½ cup (70 g) superfine brown rice flour

½ cup (50 g) chestnut flour

½ cup (50 g) hazelnut flour

2 tablespoons tapioca starch

1½ teaspoons baking powder

¼ teaspoon salt

3 eggs

¾ cup (150 g) light brown sugar

½ vanilla bean, split lengthwise and seeds scraped

2 Granny Smith apples, peeled, cored, and grated

APPLE GLAZE

⅔ cup (80 g) powdered sugar, sifted

½ stick (4 tablespoons or 55 g) unsalted butter, melted

1 tablespoon apple juice

make the cakes

1   Preheat the oven to 350°F (180°C). Place the butter in a small saucepan and cook it over medium heat until the milk solids start to brown on the bottom of the pan. It will smell like roasting nuts. Strain it into a bowl and let it cool.

2   In a large bowl, whisk together the superfine brown rice flour, chestnut flour, hazelnut flour, tapioca starch, baking powder, and salt.

3   In a separate bowl, whisk together the eggs, brown sugar, vanilla seeds, grated apple, and brown butter. Add this mixture to the dry ingredients and mix until incorporated. Spoon the batter into 12 greased mini Bundt molds.

4   Bake for about 20 minutes or until a toothpick inserted in the center comes out clean. Let them cool in the molds for 5 to 10 minutes, and then transfer them to a cooling rack.

TIP: If chestnut flour is not available, make your own (see sidebar), or substitute ⅓ cup (45 g) of buckwheat flour.

make the glaze and finish the cakes

Whisk all the ingredients together until a thin glaze forms. Glaze the cakes while they are still warm.

HOW TO MAKE YOUR OWN CHESTNUT FLOUR

Start with 1 pound (450 g) of chestnuts. Make two crisscross cuts on the skin of each nut. Roast the whole chestnuts at 400°F (200°C) for 15 minutes. When they are cool enough to handle, peel the skin off. Spread the skinned chestnuts on a baking sheet and leave them to dry in the oven with the pilot light on (but the oven turned off) overnight or for up to 20 hours if possible. (If you have an electric oven, simply turn the oven light on and leave the chestnuts in there to dry overnight. The heat from the oven light should be enough.) Pulverize the dry chestnuts in a food processor or a high-powered blender. Sift and discard the large pieces. The flour can be stored for up to 6 months in the freezer.

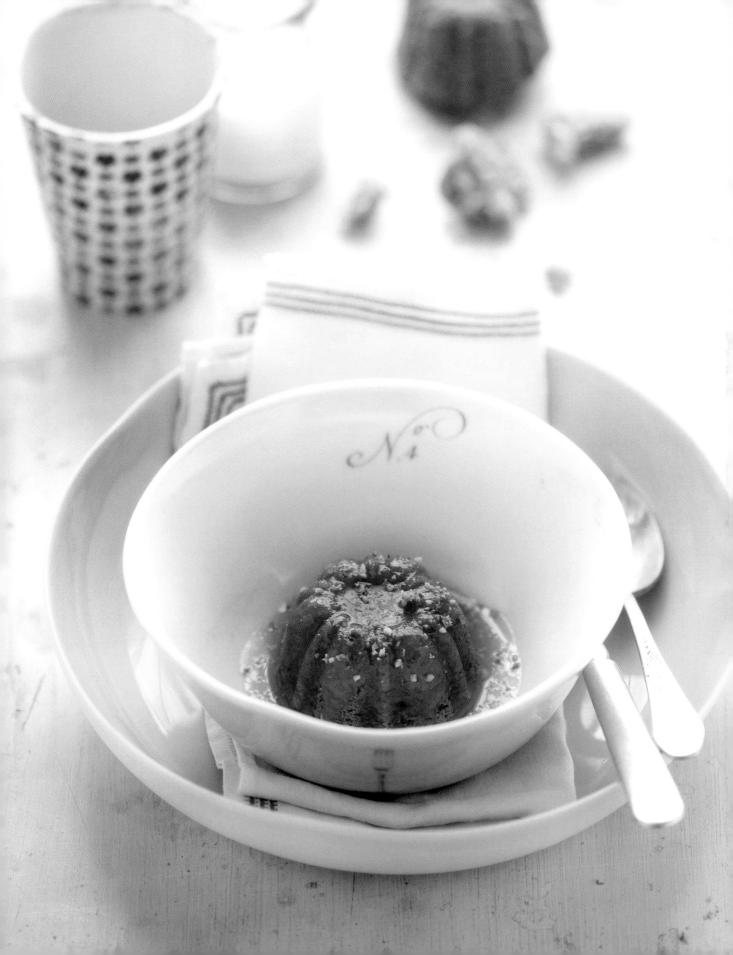

coconut cream cookies

I HAVE ALWAYS HAD A SOFT SPOT FOR shortbread cookies filled with a creamy center. I like to give them out as holiday gifts. The dough for these cookies can be stiff to pipe, so it is best to fill the pastry bag with small amounts, keeping your hand and grip close to the tip. This will allow you to apply more pressure and pipe more easily.

MAKES 20 sandwich cookies

COCONUT COOKIES

1 stick (8 tablespoons or 110 g) unsalted butter, at room temperature

½ cup (100 g) natural cane sugar

3 egg yolks, at room temperature

½ teaspoon finely grated lemon zest

¼ teaspoon coconut extract

¾ cup (105 g) superfine brown rice flour

¼ cup plus 2 tablespoons (50 g) coconut flour

2 tablespoons tapioca starch

¼ teaspoon salt

⅓ cup (80 ml) unsweetened coconut milk

COCONUT BUTTERCREAM FILLING

2 egg whites

½ cup (100 g) natural cane sugar

1½ sticks (12 tablespoons or 170 g) unsalted butter, at room temperature

½ teaspoon coconut extract

⅛ teaspoon salt

make the cookies

1 Preheat the oven to 350°F (180°C). In a stand mixer using the paddle attachment, mix the butter and sugar together on medium speed until light, about 2 minutes. Scrape the sides of the bowl. Add the egg yolks, lemon zest, and coconut extract and mix until combined.

2 In a separate bowl, whisk together the superfine brown rice flour, coconut flour, tapioca starch, and salt. Add the dry ingredients to the mixer bowl and mix. Add the coconut milk and mix until thoroughly combined.

3 Transfer about one-third of the dough to a pastry bag fitted with a star tip (#4). Press the dough down toward the tip of the bag. Pipe 1-inch rosettes onto two baking sheets lined with silicone mats, spacing them 2 inches apart. The dough will be stiff, so you must apply pressure. If you are having difficulty, grab the bag close to the tip, which will allow you to apply more pressure. Finish piping all the dough, adding more batter to the bag in batches as you use it. Alternatively, you could scoop the dough using a 1-inch mini ice cream scoop. In this case, slightly flatten the tops with your fingers.

4 Bake them for 12 to 15 minutes, until lightly golden on the bottom. Let them cool on the pan for 5 minutes before trying to remove them. Cool them completely before filling them.

prepare the filling

1 Whisk the egg whites and sugar in the bowl of a stand mixer. Place the bowl over a pan filled partway with simmering water. Whisk the egg whites and sugar over the heat for about 5 minutes, until the egg whites feel hot to the touch.

2 Transfer the bowl to a stand mixer and whip the meringue on high speed until thick and the bowl feels cool to the touch.

3 Turn the speed to medium and add 1 tablespoon of soft butter at a time. When all the butter has been incorporated, turn the mixer to high

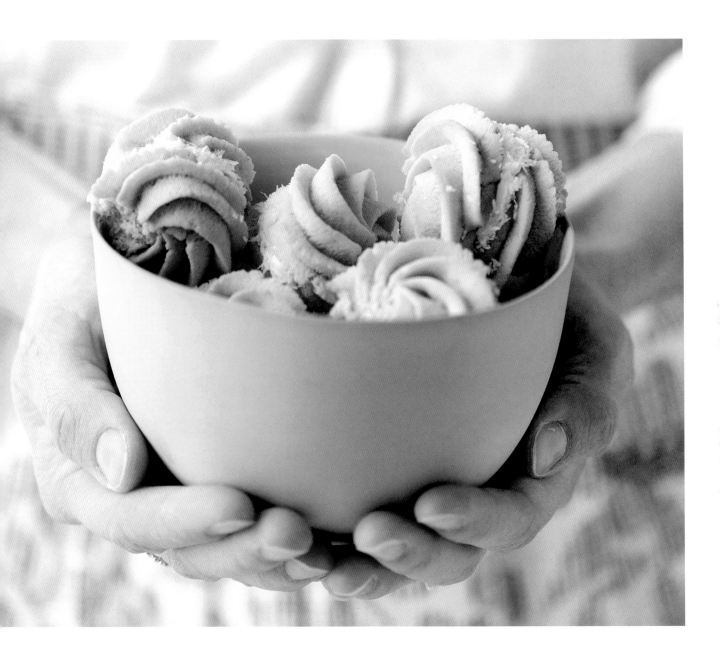

and whip for 1 minute, until it comes together as a smooth buttercream. Add the coconut extract and salt.

4 Place the buttercream in a pastry bag fitted with a plain tip (#4) and pipe a dab of cream on the underside of half of the cookies. Top with another cookie, flat side down, and lightly press them together. You can freeze the leftover buttercream for up to 1 month.

5 The filled cookies may be stored at room temperature for up to 4 hours; after that refrigerate them for up to 2 days. After refrigeration, let them come to room temperature before serving.

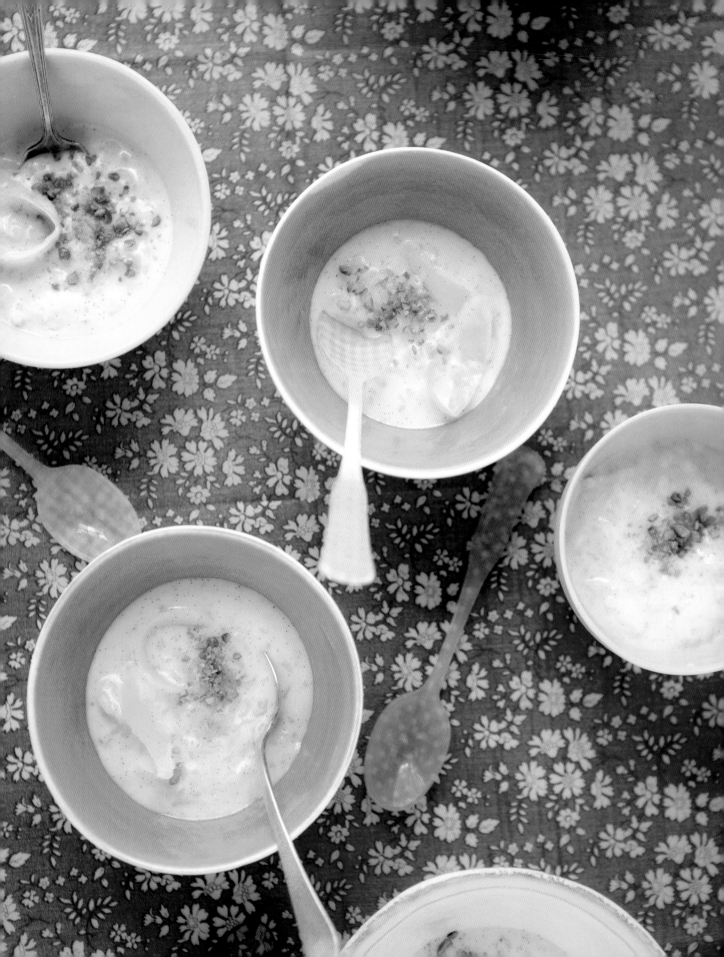

vanilla bean & cardamom
baked *arroz con leche*

I HAVE LONG CHRONICLED MY LOVE FOR *arroz con leche,* or rice pudding, in my blog. In fact, I named the blog Cannelle et Vanille after the smells of cinnamon and vanilla simmering on the stove. It is the dessert my grandmother used to make with the raw milk that was delivered to our pastry shop daily from the dairy farm up the road, and it is the dessert I make for my family when we crave comfort. The traditional recipe can be time-consuming, as it requires constant supervision and stirring. This version is less demanding because it is slowly baked in the oven, but it is equally creamy and delicious.

Cardamom and lemon zest give it a little something extra.

SERVES 4

1   Preheat the oven to 325°F (160°C). Combine all the ingredients in a 2-quart baking dish or one large enough to hold all the liquid. Cover with parchment paper and then aluminum foil.

2   Bake for 1 hour. Remove the foil and parchment, stir, and bake for an additional 15 to 30 minutes or until thick and creamy. This will depend on the size of dish you are using, but remember that the *arroz con leche* will thicken as it sits. Serve at room temperature or chilled.

4 cups (1 L) whole milk

½ cup (100 g) Arborio rice

¼ cup (50 g) natural cane sugar

1 vanilla bean, split lengthwise and seeds scraped

1 cinnamon stick

4 cardamom pods, cracked

Zest of ½ lemon

⅛ teaspoon salt

chocolate, hazelnut & buckwheat cake

"DO YOU ALWAYS HAVE DESSERT WITH your meal?" asked my friend Nadia. "Well, yes—it almost feels like I have to." Whether it is a piece of dark chocolate or a cookie, I always look forward to ending a meal with something sweet. This light and moist chocolate cake is one of my favorites to have after a nice soup or a piece of vegetable tart. It is quite easy to make and fairly healthy, so I never feel guilty eating it. And my kids love licking the bowl. I actually like the cake better the next day.

MAKES one 8-inch cake

¼ cup (30 g) hazelnuts

6 ounces (170 g) bittersweet chocolate, finely chopped

½ cup (125 ml) coconut oil

4 eggs, separated

½ cup (100 g) coconut palm sugar

⅓ cup (80 ml) whole-milk plain yogurt

1 teaspoon vanilla extract

¾ cup (75 g) hazelnut flour

¼ cup (35 g) buckwheat flour

½ teaspoon salt

1 Preheat the oven to 350°F (180°C) and set the oven rack in the middle. Place the hazelnuts on a baking sheet and roast them for 5 to 7 minutes, until fragrant. Using a dry kitchen towel, rub the hazelnuts together to remove their skins. Cool, then coarsely chop them.

2 In a medium bowl, combine the chopped chocolate and coconut oil. Place the bowl over a pot filled partway with simmering water and melt the contents over the water bath. Let it cool slightly.

3 Whisk together the egg yolks and ¼ cup (50 g) of the sugar in a large bowl. Add the yogurt, vanilla extract, melted chocolate mixture, hazelnut flour, buckwheat flour, and salt. Whisk to combine.

4 In a separate bowl, whip the egg whites until they form semi-stiff peaks. Slowly sprinkle in the remaining ¼ cup sugar while continuously whipping. Whip to stiff peaks. Fold one-third of the meringue into the yolk-chocolate base to lighten it. Fold in the rest of the meringue, folding gently to keep as much air as possible in the mixture. Fold in the chopped hazelnuts.

5 Line the bottom of an 8-inch round cake pan with a circle of parchment paper. Spray the pan with nonstick spray or brush with melted butter. Pour the batter into the pan and bake for 30 to 35 minutes or until the center is set and a toothpick inserted in the center comes out clean. Be careful not to overbake it or the chocolate will burn. Let it rest in the pan until it cools slightly, and then invert it onto a cooling rack.

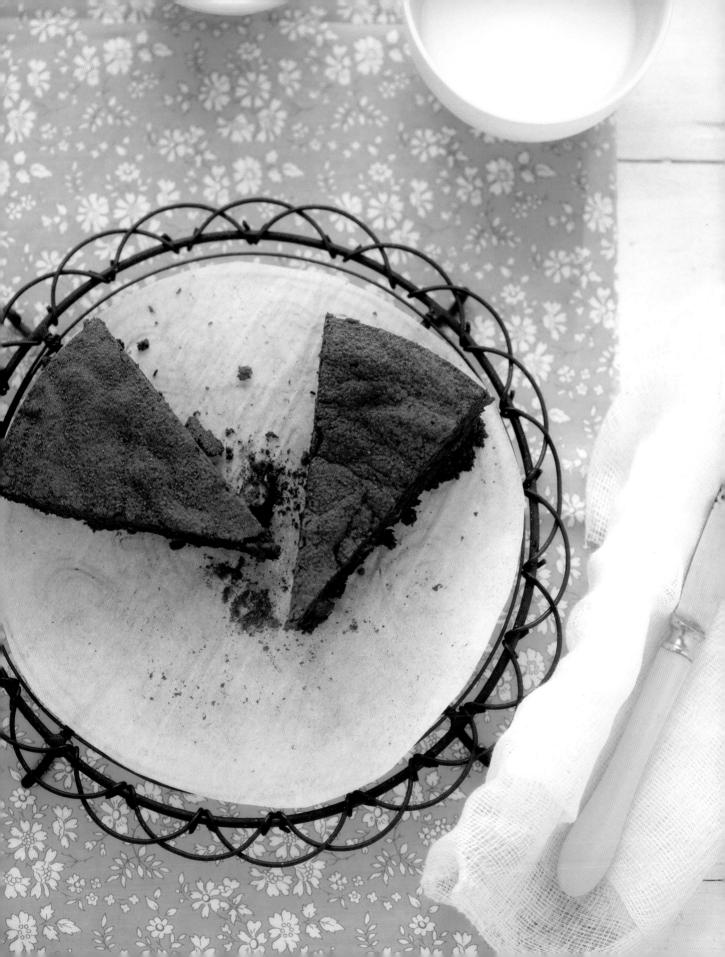

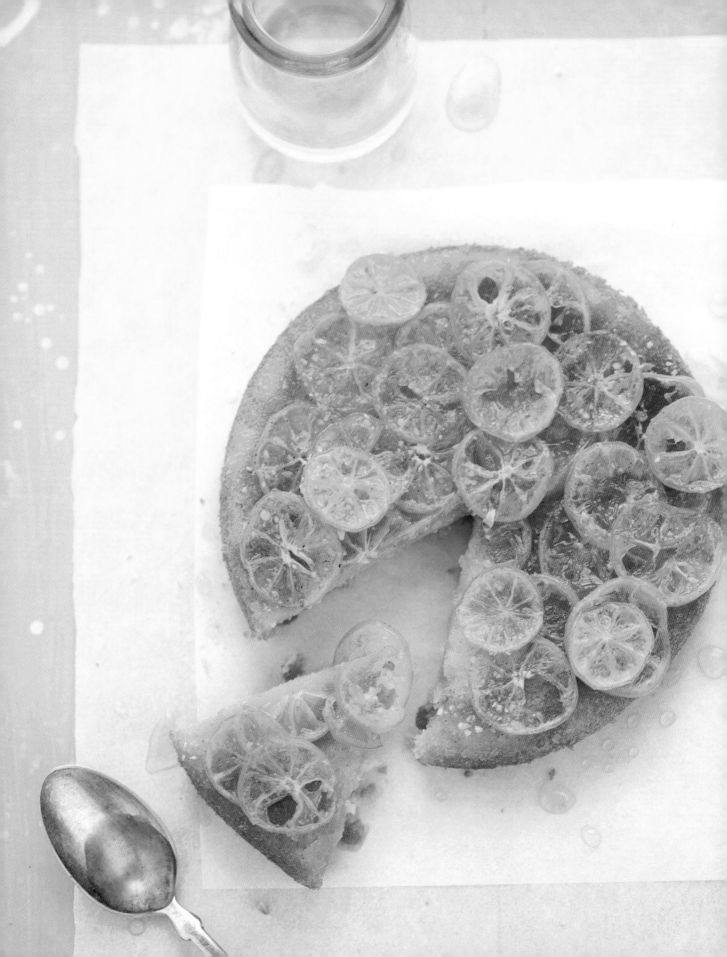

candied sour orange
& almond cake

"WOULD YOU LIKE SOME OF THESE?" Lena texted me this tantalizing query along with a photo of the tiniest sour oranges I have ever seen. "Certainly! I'll make you a cake with them," I replied. I love it when friends know you well enough that they can anticipate your excitement over a simple bag of sour oranges.

In my recipe the sour oranges are lightly candied in vanilla syrup, which makes a nice sweet-and-sour contrast. They are also wonderful served over vanilla bean ice cream. If sour oranges are not available in your area, try using kumquats. Unsprayed, thin-skinned oranges are ideal for this recipe.

MAKES **one 9-inch cake**

1 Preheat the oven to 350°F (180°C). Combine the sugar and ½ cup (125 ml) water in a medium saucepan. Add the vanilla bean and seeds to the pan. Bring it to a boil, lower the heat, and simmer until the sugar has dissolved. Add the thin slices of sour orange and cook them for 10 minutes, until translucent. Do not boil the syrup; just gently simmer it. Remove from the heat and keep the candied oranges in the syrup.

2 Combine the almond paste, 1 of the eggs, orange zest, and lemon zest in the bowl of a stand mixer. Using the paddle attachment, mix on medium-high speed until a thick and smooth paste forms. There might be some small lumps left, which is fine. Add the remaining 3 eggs. Switch to a whip attachment and whip the mixture for 5 minutes on high speed, until thick and pale in color.

3 Add the millet flour, baking powder, salt, and melted butter. Whip on high speed for another 30 seconds, until all the ingredients are incorporated.

4 Line the bottom of a 9-inch round cake pan with a circle of parchment paper. Grease the paper and pan and pour in the batter. Bake for 30 minutes. When a toothpick inserted in the center of the cake comes out clean, it is done. Let the cake cool in the pan for 20 minutes. Invert it onto a cooling rack.

5 Serve the cake with the candied sour oranges on top as well as some of the vanilla syrup.

1 cup (200 g) natural cane sugar

1 vanilla bean, split lengthwise and seeds scraped

1 pound (450 g) small sour oranges, seeded and thinly sliced (do not peel them)

⅔ cup (200 g) gluten-free almond paste

4 eggs

Zest of 1 orange

Zest of 1 lemon

¼ cup (30 g) millet flour

½ teaspoon baking powder

¼ teaspoon salt

¾ stick (6 tablespoons or 85 g) unsalted butter, melted and cooled

chocolate, banana
& hazelnut cream toasties

MY CHILDREN CAN NEVER GET ENOUGH of this Chocolate & Banana Bread recipe. It is loaded with whole grains and stays moist for days thanks to the olive oil and ripe bananas. On cold afternoons, when we bundle up with blankets and crave something special and very chocolaty, I add the ganache filling and make toasties. They are not only delicious but also nutritious.

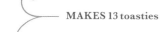

MAKES 13 toasties

CHOCOLATE AND BANANA BREAD (MAKES ONE 8½ BY 4½-INCH LOAF)

3 ripe bananas

1 cup (140 g) superfine brown rice flour

¼ cup (35 g) buckwheat flour

¼ cup (25 g) hazelnut flour

2 tablespoons tapioca starch

1 tablespoon unsweetened Dutch-process or black cocoa powder

½ teaspoon salt

½ teaspoon baking soda

3 eggs

1 cup (200 g) natural cane sugar

½ cup (125 ml) olive oil

2 teaspoons vanilla extract

CHOCOLATE AND HAZELNUT GANACHE (MAKES 1½ CUPS)

1 cup (250 ml) unsweetened coconut milk

2 tablespoons hazelnut butter

10 ounces (290 g) bittersweet chocolate, finely chopped

2 teaspoons vanilla extract

½ teaspoon *fleur de sel*

make the bread

1 Preheat the oven to 375°F (190°C). Puree the bananas in a blender or food processor. You should have approximately 1¼ cups (250 g) banana puree.

2 In a large bowl, whisk together the superfine brown rice flour, buckwheat flour, hazelnut flour, tapioca starch, cocoa powder, salt, and baking soda.

3 In a separate bowl, whisk together the eggs, sugar, banana puree, olive oil, and vanilla extract. Add the wet ingredients to the dry and whisk until smooth.

4 Pour the batter into a greased 8½ by 4½-inch loaf pan. Bake for 50 minutes to 1 hour or until a toothpick inserted in the center comes out clean. Let the bread cool in the pan for 15 minutes. Invert it onto a cooling rack and cool completely. It may be stored for 5 days in the refrigerator, wrapped tightly.

make the ganache

1 In a small saucepan, combine the coconut milk and hazelnut butter. Bring to a simmer over medium-high heat.

2 Place the finely chopped chocolate in a medium bowl. Add the simmering coconut milk and stir until the chocolate is melted and smooth. Add the vanilla extract and *fleur de sel*. Stir to combine, but do not whisk too much, as the ganache can separate and lose its smoothness.

3 The ganache will harden as it cools. To bring it back to a spreadable consistency, place the ganache in a bowl over a pot partway filled with simmering water. Stir it and let the heat soften it. It will keep in the refrigerator for up to 1 week.

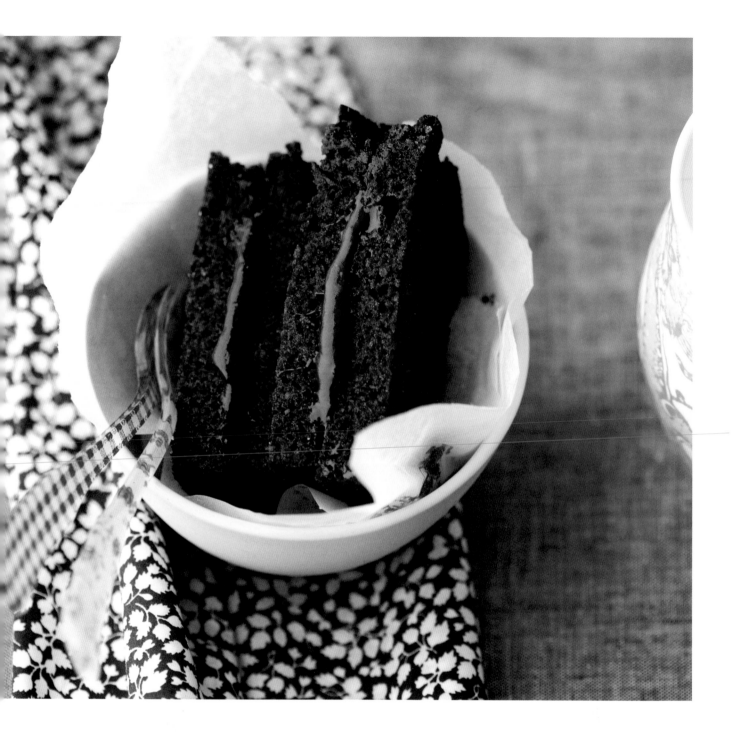

assemble the toasties

Cut the Chocolate & Banana Bread into ¼-inch-thick slices. Spread 2 tablespoons of Chocolate & Hazelnut Ganache on one slice and top it with another. Toast it on a griddle or panini press until crispy on the outside and melted on the inside. Serve warm.

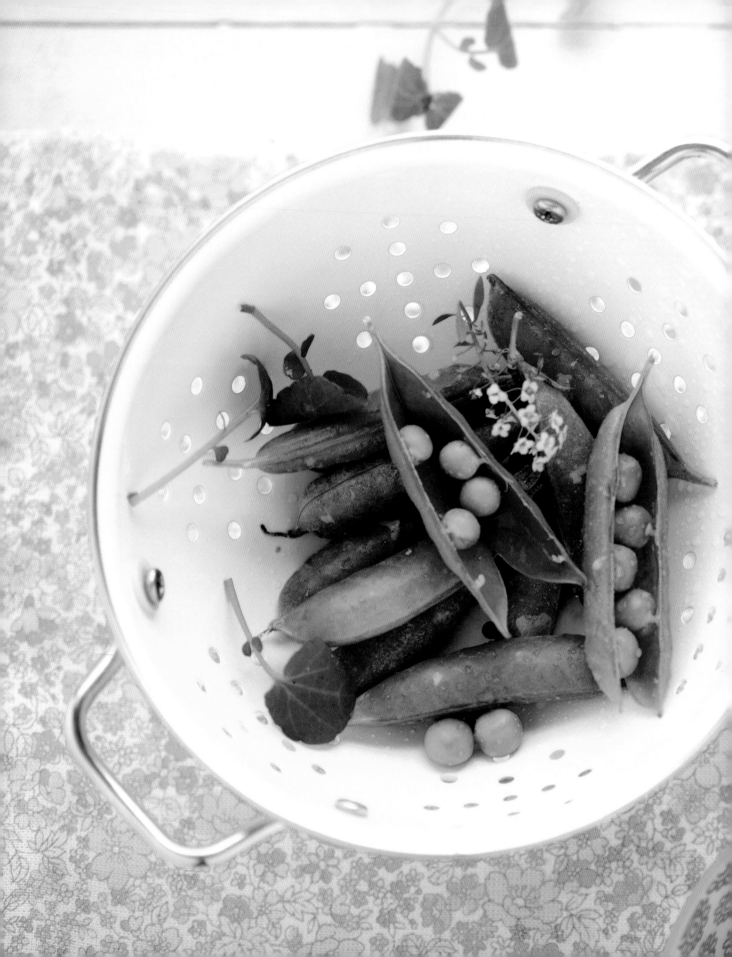

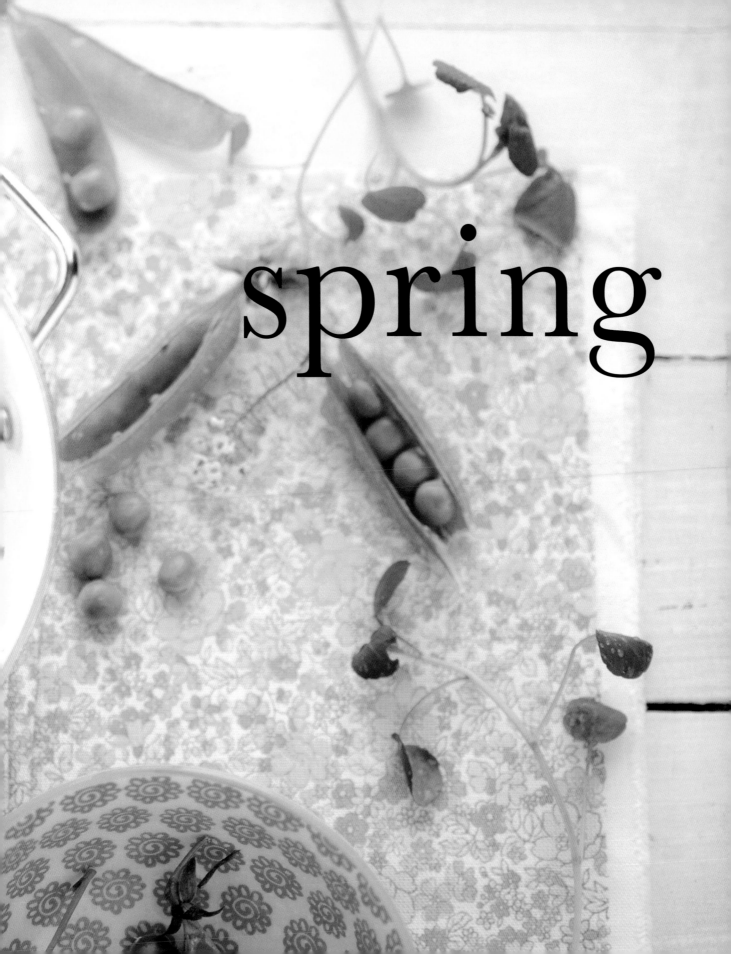

spring

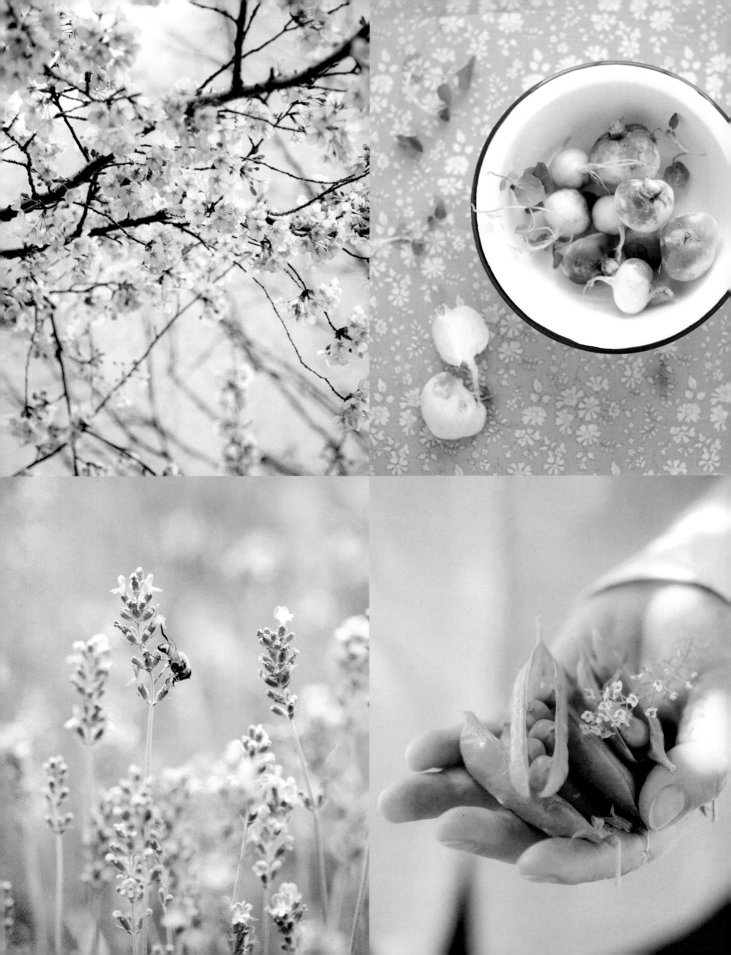

SPRING
small plates

Ricotta & Quinoa Gnocchi with Pea Shoot & Almond Pesto • Asparagus, Arugula & Avocado Soup with Crab • Shrimp & Grapefruit Risotto • Zucchini, Quinoa & Goat Cheese Tart • Potato, Salmon & Pea Fritters with Pea Shoot Mayonnaise • Crushed Bean & Prosciutto Tartines • Tuna, Grapefruit & Avocado Salad with Spicy Garlic Vinaigrette • Clams, Peas & Potatoes en Papillote • Spring Quinoa Salad • Chamomile-Poached Salmon with Cucumber & Fennel Slaw • Salty Herb, Walnut & Corn Crackers • Creamy Fennel & Spinach Soup • Herbed Lamb Meatballs in Coconut Milk • Chicken, Sugar Snap Pea & Rice Soup • Watercress Pudding with Soft-Boiled Quail Eggs, Asparagus & Watermelon Radish

IN SPRING 2010 I WAS DIAGNOSED with gluten intolerance. I had spent the winter weak and bedridden, debilitated by vertigo. Both my mind and my body needed a fresh start. I never thought I would be so enthusiastic about hearing the words *gluten intolerant* come out of my doctor's mouth. I thought of how perfect the timing was, and that, just like spring, a lighter version of myself was about to emerge.

My parents flew in from the Basque Country to help me through this healing process. We took trips to the farmers' markets, where week after week new produce appeared. Bright, crispy English peas for soups and risottos, their shoots turned into pesto; tender asparagus; and all sorts of fresh herbs ignited my appetite for fresh cooking once again. Having my mom next to me was a reminder of what Basque cooking is all about—finding the best produce available and preparing it simply. She and I spoke of the garden my grandmother's family kept in the small town of Lezama. It touched me to hear how my mother's childhood memories were tied to gardens, trees, and afternoons playing in the kitchen, just as mine were. I found this time of cooking and bonding very therapeutic.

That spring was good to me. A strong sense of cooking for nourishment directed our lives. The children sensed it. "Now that you are healthy, I want to go have a picnic," Jon asserted. It was the perfect idea. That weekend we packed my white bicycle basket with slices of Zucchini, Quinoa & Goat Cheese Tart (page 162), a thermos of Asparagus, Arugula & Avocado Soup with Crab (page 159), and a loaf of Brioche (page 124). We didn't go far; the park behind our home was good enough for them. After this we made a habit of weekly picnics—our baskets filled with an assortment of small bites to share over stories of cherry blossoms and wild strawberries.

ricotta & quinoa gnocchi with pea shoot & almond pesto

PEA SHOOTS ALWAYS REMIND ME OF spring gardens. The delicate and tender leaves are great in many preparations, such as salads, quick sautés with garlic, or in frittatas. Here I turned them into a bright green pesto that goes perfectly with the ricotta gnocchi.

My children love helping shape the little pillows of pasta every time I make this recipe. They take turns. Miren holds the gnocchi board and Jon rolls the dough; then they switch. I tell them stories about the days I made gnocchi for a living and Jon says to me, "You are a great chef."

In autumn, I make a variation of this recipe with roasted winter squash or red kuri squash, which is dry and creamy, with a lovely chestnut-like flavor.

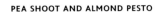

SERVES 4

PEA SHOOT AND ALMOND PESTO

1 clove garlic, minced

⅓ cup (40 g) slivered almonds

2 cups (60 g) pea shoots, tough stalks removed and chopped

1 ounce (30 g) Parmesan cheese, finely grated

½ teaspoon salt

½ teaspoon freshly ground black pepper

½ cup (125 ml) olive oil

RICOTTA AND QUINOA GNOCCHI

8 ounces (225 g) whole-milk ricotta cheese

2 egg yolks

½ cup (70 g) superfine brown rice flour, plus more for dusting

¼ cup (40 g) potato starch

¼ cup (35 g) millet flour

1 teaspoon salt

⅛ teaspoon freshly grated nutmeg

make the pesto

Place the garlic and almonds in the bowl of a food processor and pulse until the almonds are finely chopped. Add the pea shoots and process into a paste. Add the Parmesan, salt, and pepper. Pulse one more time. Add the olive oil in a light stream while the processor is on and process until a smooth paste forms. Scrape down the sides and mix well.

TIP: If pea shoots are not available, watercress or spinach would be a great substitute. The pesto can be made in advance. It will keep in the refrigerator for up to 5 days or frozen for up to 1 month.

make the gnocchi

1 Stir all the ingredients together in a large bowl. The dough must be a little sticky but still hold together. If it's too wet, add a little bit more flour, but be careful not to add too much or the dough will be dry and heavy.

2 Dust the work surface with superfine brown rice flour. Knead the dough until it's smooth. Form it into a ball and cut it into four pieces.

3 Roll each piece into a log that is about ½ inch in diameter. Dust the blade of the knife with flour and cut the log into ½-inch-long pieces. Roll these pieces over a gnocchi board or a fork to create the signature indentations. Place them on a baking sheet dusted with superfine brown rice flour. Repeat with the rest of the dough.

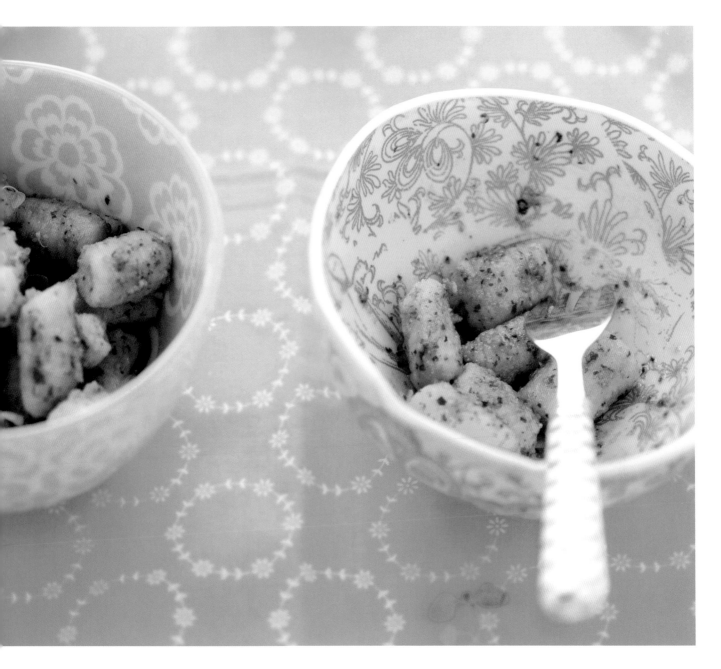

4   Refrigerate the gnocchi for 15 minutes to set. They can also be
frozen at this point by placing the baking sheet in the freezer and, once
frozen solid, transferring them into a freezer bag.

5   In the meantime, fill a large pot with water and bring it to a boil.
Salt the water generously. Cook the gnocchi in batches. When they rise
to the surface, they are cooked. It should take between 2 and 3 minutes.
Remove the gnocchi with a slotted spoon as they finish cooking. Toss them
with the Pea Shoot & Almond Pesto and serve immediately.

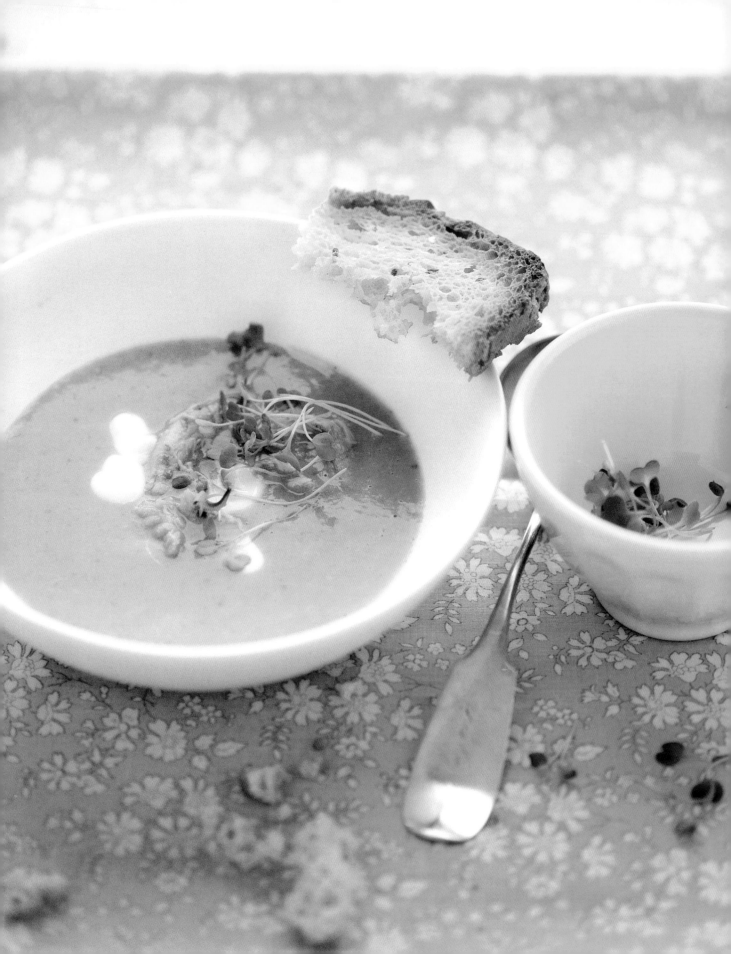

asparagus, arugula & avocado soup with crab

THIS SOUP IS GREAT FOR SPRING. It is light and creamy from the avocados, with peppery arugula and slightly sweet crabmeat. It can be served warm or chilled for an outdoor party.

SERVES 4 to 6

1 Heat the oil in a large pot over medium heat. Add the shallot, garlic, asparagus, and ¼ teaspoon of the salt. Cook the vegetables for 3 minutes or until tender but not browned.

2 Add the vegetable stock. Bring it to a boil, turn the heat to low, and simmer for 4 minutes or until the asparagus is tender.

3 Add the arugula and cook for 1 additional minute. Remove the pot from the heat. Add the diced avocado and remaining ½ teaspoon salt. Puree the soup in a blender and then strain it into a clean bowl. Adjust the seasoning if needed.

4 Serve the soup warm or chilled, topped with the crabmeat and garnished with the yogurt and greens, if desired. Store leftovers in the refrigerator for up to 3 days.

2 tablespoons olive oil

1 shallot, minced

2 cloves garlic, minced

1 pound (450 g) green asparagus, tough bottoms trimmed and diced

¾ teaspoon salt

3 cups (750 ml) vegetable stock

2 cups (60 g) tightly packed arugula

1 avocado, pitted and peeled

4 ounces (110 g) crabmeat (I used canned claw meat)

2 tablespoons whole-milk plain yogurt, for serving

Arugula microgreens, for garnish, optional

shrimp & grapefruit risotto

RISOTTO, OR *ARROZ CALDOSO*, AS WE CALL IT, is a favorite in our house. I cook different variations of it for my family at least once a week. Sometimes I add cheese, sometimes we do without it. Sometimes it's baked, sometimes stirred. In this recipe, the grapefruit adds a touch of fruity freshness—unexpected but delicious.

Many people are afraid to buy fish and shellfish that still have their heads on, but if you are lucky enough to be able to find them, please go for it. There is remarkable flavor in the head, and it makes wonderful stock.

SERVES 4

12 ounces (340 g) medium pink shrimp, shells on

5 cups (1.25 L) vegetable stock

1¼ teaspoons salt

3 tablespoons olive oil

½ small red onion, diced

1½ cups (290 g) Arborio rice

½ cup (125 ml) white wine

1 red grapefruit, segmented and juiced by squeezing with your hands

1 teaspoon finely grated red grapefruit zest

2 tablespoons finely chopped fresh parsley

1 tablespoon fresh thyme leaves

1 ounce (30 g) Parmesan cheese, finely grated

1   Peel the shrimp and reserve the shells. In a small pot, bring the vegetable stock to a boil. Add the shells and ½ teaspoon of the salt to the stock and simmer for 5 minutes. Skim the foam and impurities from the surface of the stock. Strain it into a clean pot and keep it on the stove over low heat. Discard the shells.

2   In a large pot, heat 1 tablespoon of the olive oil over medium-high heat. Season the shrimp with ½ teaspoon of the salt and cook the shrimp, flipping once, just until they turn pink, about 1 minute. Transfer the shrimp to a plate and keep them covered until ready to use.

3   Add the remaining 2 tablespoons olive oil to the pot and turn the heat to medium. Add the diced onion and remaining ¼ teaspoon salt and cook for 5 minutes or until softened. Add the rice and cook it for 2 minutes, stirring constantly, until all the grains are well coated with the oil. Add the white wine and let it cook for a minute or two.

4   Add ½ cup (125 ml) shrimp stock and stir. Continue cooking the rice, stirring constantly. When the stock has been absorbed, add another ½ cup (125 ml) and continue, stirring, until the rice is cooked al dente, 16 to 18 minutes.

5   Add the grapefruit juice, segments, and zest. Cook for another 2 minutes. Add the parsley, thyme, Parmesan cheese, and cooked shrimp. Stir until the shrimp is heated through, then serve immediately.

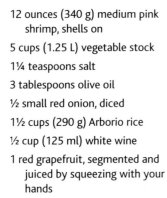

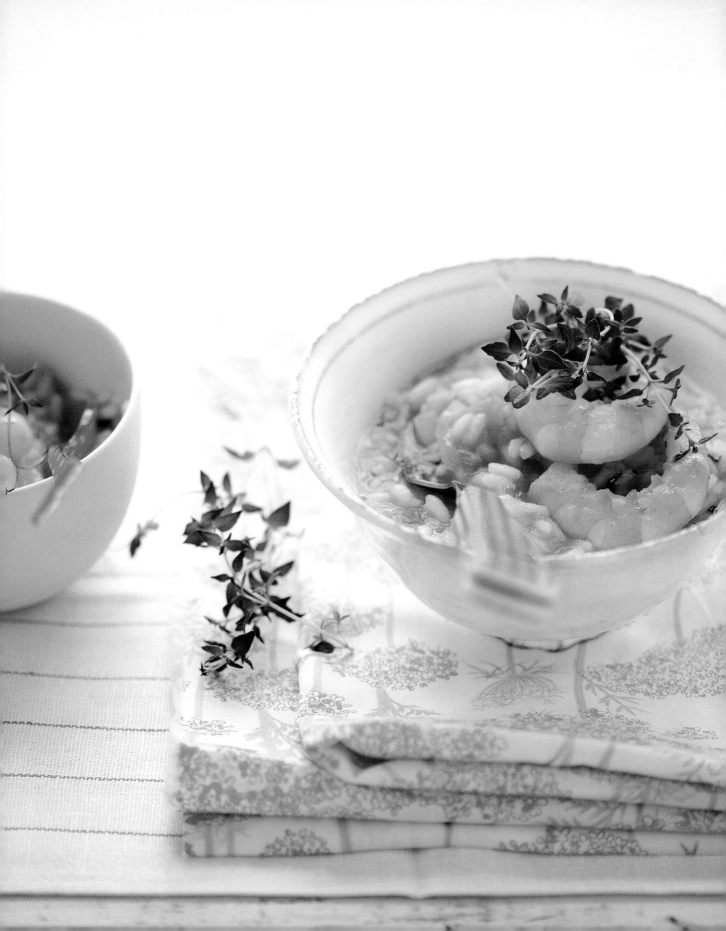

zucchini, quinoa & goat cheese tart

THIS TART IS A MAIN COURSE IN ITSELF. Quinoa flour in the crust and cooked quinoa in the filling add lots of protein, magnesium, iron, and a distinct nutty flavor. You may substitute cooked rice, which will result in a milder-tasting tart.

MAKES one 9-inch square or round tart

QUINOA AND OLIVE OIL CRUST

½ cup (70 g) superfine brown rice flour, plus more for dusting

½ cup (70 g) quinoa flour

⅓ cup (35 g) almond flour

¼ cup (30 g) amaranth flour

1 teaspoon salt

1 teaspoon fresh thyme leaves

¼ cup (60 ml) olive oil

ZUCCHINI, QUINOA, AND GOAT CHEESE FILLING

¼ cup (50 g) quinoa, rinsed

1½ teaspoons salt, plus more for quinoa

2 medium zucchini, grated

2 tablespoons olive oil

6 spring onions or 2 medium leeks, diced

3 eggs

2 ounces (60 g) crème fraîche or heavy cream

½ teaspoon finely grated lemon zest

¼ teaspoon freshly ground black pepper

2 ounces (60 g) goat cheese, crumbled

Watercress, for garnish

make the crust

1   Combine the first six ingredients in a food processor. Pulse a couple of times to aerate the ingredients.

2   Add the olive oil and ½ cup (125 ml) cold water. Pulse until the dough comes together.

3   Transfer the dough to a work surface, knead it a couple of times, and press it into a disk. Wrap in plastic wrap and refrigerate it for 30 minutes.

4   Dust a work surface with superfine brown rice flour and roll the dough to a ⅛-inch thickness. Roll the dough carefully around the rolling pin and place it over a 9-inch square or round tart mold. Fill the mold. Pinch the cracked pieces together and trim the edges. Transfer the tart mold to the refrigerator and chill for 30 minutes.

5   Preheat the oven to 375°F (190°C). Place the tart on a baking sheet and cover it with a piece of parchment paper. Add pie weights or dry beans and blind-bake for 20 minutes. Remove the beans and the parchment and bake for another 10 minutes. Let the crust cool while preparing the filling (leave the oven on).

prepare the filling and bake the tart

1   Reduce the oven heat to 350°F (180°C). In a small saucepan, combine the quinoa, ½ cup (125 ml) water, and a pinch of salt. Bring to a boil, reduce the heat to low, cover, and cook for 15 minutes.

2   Place the grated zucchini in a bowl and add ½ teaspoon of the salt. Transfer to a colander set on top of a bowl and let macerate for 15 minutes. This will release some of the moisture from the zucchini. Discard the water collected in the bowl.

3   In a large sauté pan, heat the olive oil over medium heat. Add the drained zucchini and spring onions. Cook for about 5 minutes, until they soften. Add the cooked quinoa and stir. Remove from the heat and set aside.

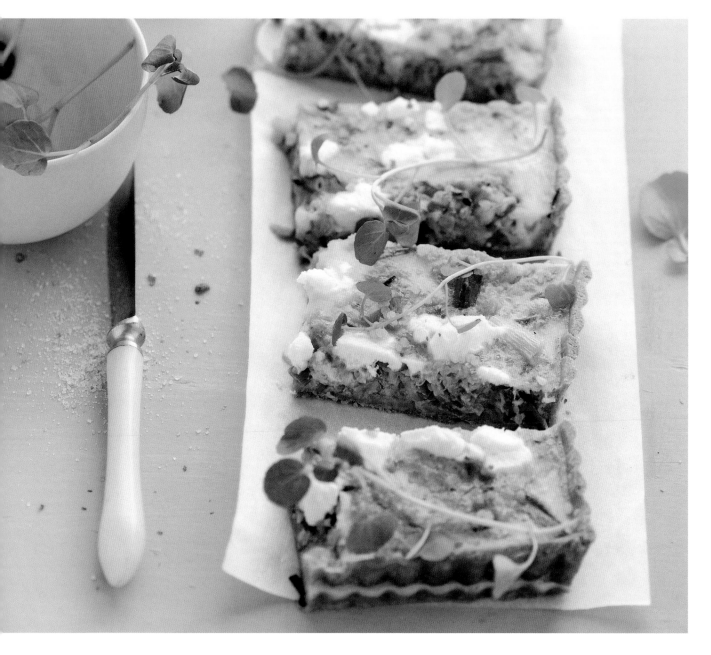

4 In a large bowl, whisk together the eggs, crème fraîche, remaining 1 teaspoon salt, lemon zest, and pepper.

5 Spread the zucchini mixture over the tart crust. Pour the custard over the vegetables. Top with the crumbled goat cheese.

6 Bake for 25 to 30 minutes, until the custard sets. Let the tart cool for 15 minutes before cutting. Serve warm or at room temperature garnished with the watercress. The tart can be stored in the refrigerator for up to 3 days or frozen for up to 1 month.

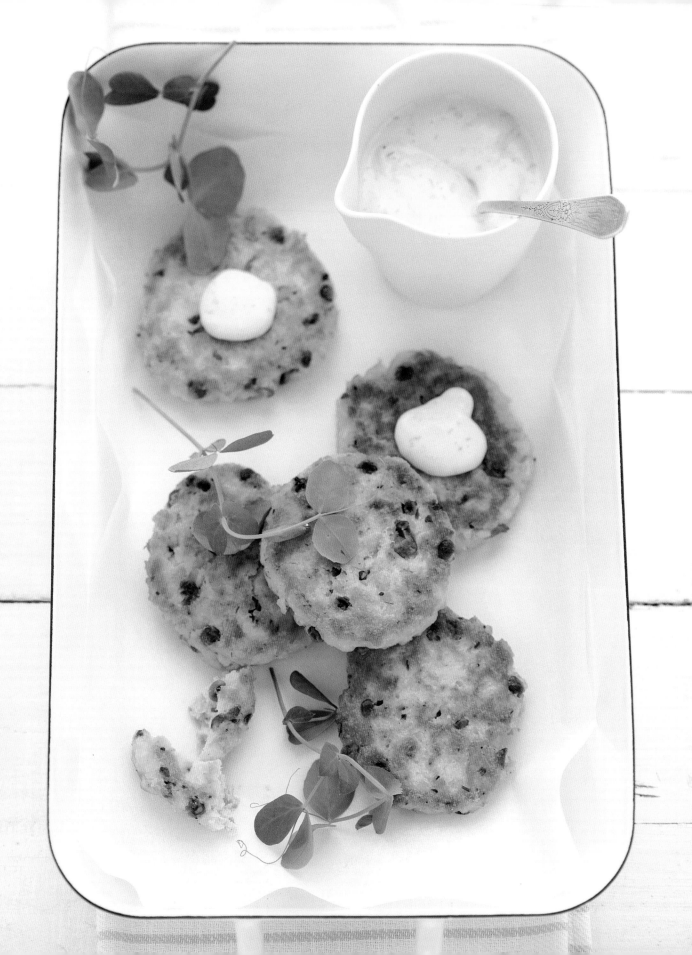

potato, salmon & pea fritters with pea shoot mayonnaise

THESE FRITTERS ARE INSPIRED BY one of my all-time favorite recipes, cod brandade: salted cod poached in milk and mixed into fluffy mashed potatoes. This version includes mashed potatoes, crushed English peas, and salmon poached in a mixture of coconut milk, thyme, and garlic. It is served with pea shoot mayonnaise, but if shoots are not available, you may use spinach or watercress.

SERVES 4 to 6

make the mayonnaise

In a blender, combine the egg, Dijon mustard, lemon juice, salt, and pea shoots. Slowly, with the blender running, drizzle in the olive oil, followed by the grapeseed oil. It will create an emulsion. Chill the mayonnaise until ready to use. Use the mayonnaise within 1 day.

make the fritters

1   Place the potatoes in a medium saucepan. Cover them with water and bring to a boil. Cover the saucepan, turn the heat to medium-low, and cook for 9 minutes or until you can easily insert the tip of a knife in the center. Drain the water and let the potatoes cool in the pan.

2   Meanwhile, place the coconut milk, vegetable broth, garlic, and thyme in a medium saucepan. Bring it to a boil. Turn the heat off and let it steep for 10 minutes. Bring back to a simmer. Add the salmon, cover the pan, and cook over low heat (do not let it boil), flipping halfway through, until the salmon is cooked through, 6 to 8 minutes. Remove the salmon from the poaching liquid and remove the skin. Discard the poaching liquid. Transfer the salmon to a small bowl and flake with a fork.

3   In a small saucepan, bring 1 cup (250 ml) water to a boil. Add the peas and blanch them for 1 minute. Drain and submerge them in ice water to stop the cooking process. Drain them once they are cool.

4   In a medium bowl, mash the potatoes and blanched peas with a fork. Add the salmon, eggs, salt, pepper, and parsley and mix to combine.

5   Heat the olive oil in a large nonstick skillet over medium heat. Remove ⅓-cup portions of the salmon mixture and form them into patties. Cook the patties in batches, flipping halfway through, until golden brown, 2 to 3 minutes per side. Add an additional 1 tablespoon of olive oil if needed for cooking. Serve with the Pea Shoot Mayonnaise.

PEA SHOOT MAYONNAISE
(MAKES 1 CUP)

1 egg

½ teaspoon Dijon mustard

1 teaspoon freshly squeezed lemon juice

¼ teaspoon salt

¼ cup pea shoots, stems removed

2 tablespoons olive oil

½ cup (125 ml) grapeseed oil

POTATO, SALMON, AND PEA FRITTERS
(MAKES 12 CAKES)

2 medium russet potatoes (1½ pounds or 680 g), peeled and cut into 2-inch pieces

⅔ cup (165 ml) unsweetened coconut milk

⅓ cup (80 ml) vegetable broth

2 cloves garlic, crushed but left whole

2 sprigs thyme

8 ounces (225 g) salmon

½ cup (60 g) English peas

2 eggs, lightly beaten

1 teaspoon salt

½ teaspoon freshly ground black pepper

1 tablespoon finely chopped fresh parsley

3 tablespoons olive oil, plus more if needed

crushed bean & prosciutto tartines

WHEN I WAS FIRST DIAGNOSED WITH gluten intolerance and temporarily gave up grains, snacks were the hardest thing to come up with. This bean spread served with raw vegetables became a staple. I carried it with me everywhere packed in small containers to keep my blood sugar stable. Now, I spread it on toasted Quinoa Brioche (page 125) as a tartine and serve it with soup or a salad to make a complete meal.

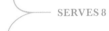

SERVES 8

¾ cup (450 g) green flageolet beans or cannellini beans

1 teaspoon salt

2 tablespoons diced scallions, plus more for garnish

¼ cup (10 g) watercress, plus more for garnish

½ cup (125 ml) olive oil

8 slices Quinoa Brioche (page 125), toasted

2 ounces (60 g) radishes, thinly sliced

8 thin slices (4 ounces or 115 g) sliced prosciutto

1 Place the beans in a medium pot. Add enough water to cover the beans plus 2 inches more. Soak the beans overnight. The following day, drain the beans. Transfer them to a clean pot and cover them with water. Bring the water to a boil, reduce the heat to low, and let the beans cook until tender, 1½ to 2 hours. Season with ½ teaspoon of the salt.

2 Drain the cooked beans and transfer them to a food processor. Add the scallions, watercress, and remaining ½ teaspoon salt. Add the olive oil while pulsing. Process until it becomes a chunky paste, but do not turn it into a puree.

3 Top the toasted Quinoa Brioche slices with the bean spread, sliced radishes, and prosciutto. Garnish with scallions and watercress.

TIP: Use canned cannellini beans as a shortcut. This makes a superfast appetizer for impromptu get-togethers.

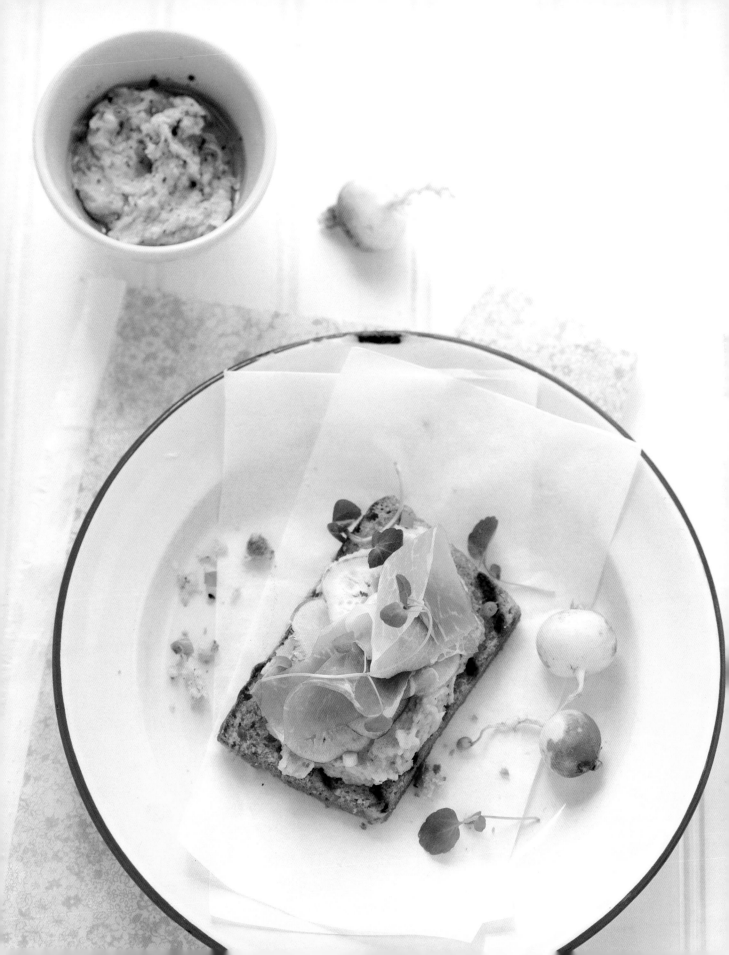

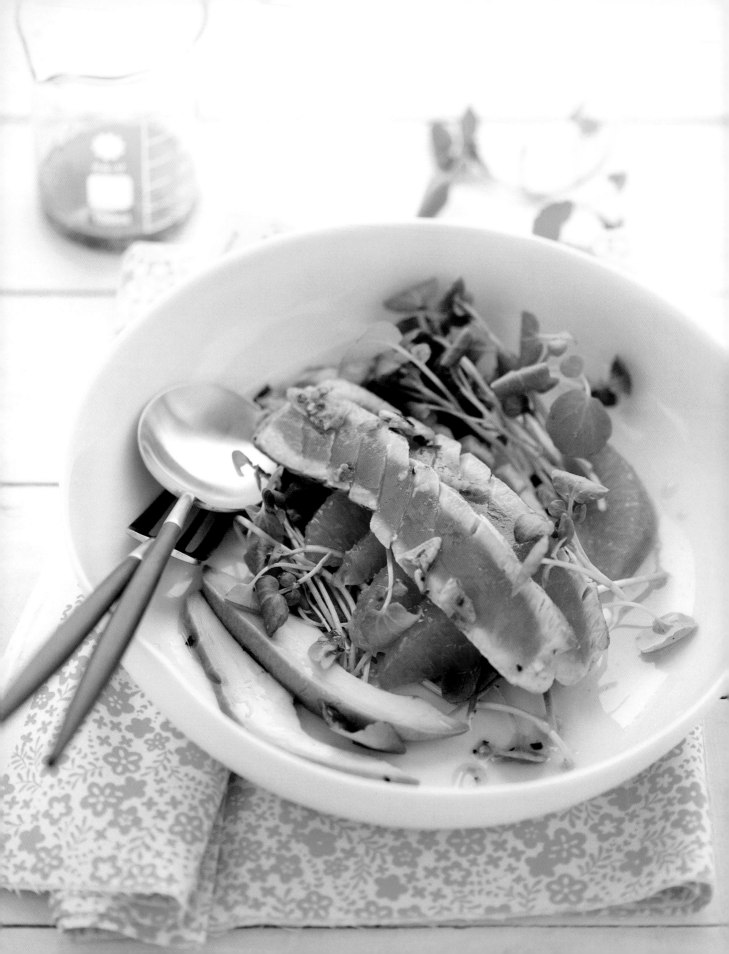

tuna, grapefruit & avocado salad
with spicy garlic vinaigrette

"ARE YOU SURE YOU WILL BE OKAY?" Mom asked. It was a Saturday morning and I was determined to cook lunch. I was twelve, and it was the first time I was cooking a meal for the entire family. I laid out all the ingredients to make *patatas en salsa verde*—potatoes, garlic, peas, and olive oil. I even cleaned and gutted the small hake Mom bought at the market. I felt empowered by her trust and all this food laid out in front of me. To this day, I love gutting and preparing fish.

This is one of my mom's favorite salads. It's sweet, sour, and a little spicy.

SERVES 4

1   Heat a medium skillet over medium-high heat and add 1 tablespoon of the olive oil. Season the tuna with ¼ teaspoon each of salt and pepper. Sear each side for 1 minute and remove the tuna from the pan. Transfer the tuna to a cutting board and slice thinly against the grain.

2   In the same pan, heat the remaining 2 tablespoons olive oil. Add the red pepper flakes and garlic and cook until the garlic starts to get a bit toasted, but do not let it burn. Immediately add the grapefruit juice. It will splatter, so be careful not to get burned. Pour the vinaigrette into a bowl, add the remaining ½ teaspoon salt, and mix to combine.

3   In a large bowl, toss together the watercress, grapefruit segments, avocado, sliced tuna, and the vinaigrette. Serve immediately.

3 tablespoons olive oil

1 (12-ounce or 340 g) tuna steak

¾ teaspoon salt

¼ teaspoon freshly ground black pepper

½ to 1 teaspoon red pepper flakes, depending on how spicy you like it

2 cloves garlic, thinly sliced

1 tablespoon freshly squeezed grapefruit juice

2 cups (80 g) watercress

1 red grapefruit, peeled and cut into segments

1 avocado, pitted, peeled, and sliced

BONITO TUNA

Bonito del Norte, also known as skipjack tuna, is a source of pride and sometimes conflict for the Basques. Fishing for bonito is a tradition that goes back centuries, and many of my friends who lived in coastal towns, like Bermeo and Lekeitio, come from a long line of fishermen. The high-quality tuna is line-caught in the Bay of Biscay and then hand-packed by local artisans. Every year, my parents drove to Bermeo to buy bonito right off the boat to later preserve in olive oil. We ate it in salads or on simple toasted bread. Bonito tuna is smaller in size than other tuna species, usually not reaching more than 30 pounds (15 kg). Its flesh is white in color and very soft in texture.

clams, peas & potatoes
en papillote

THIS IS A VERSION OF A TRADITIONAL Basque recipe, *almejas en salsa verde*, which is a simple dish of clams cooked in olive oil, garlic, lots of parsley, and a touch of red pepper flakes. Here, the clams are cooked in parchment instead of the traditional clay pot. Served with bread, it is one of my favorite light lunches.

SERVES 4

¾ cup (75 g) English peas

2 tablespoons olive oil, plus more for brushing

2 medium Yukon gold potatoes, peeled and thinly sliced

2 pounds (1 kg) littleneck clams

¼ cup (15 g) chopped fresh parsley

4 sprigs thyme

1 teaspoon red pepper flakes

Zest of 1 lemon

¼ stick (2 tablespoons or 30 g) unsalted butter, cut into pieces

¼ cup (60 ml) white wine

2 cloves garlic, very thinly sliced

1   Preheat the oven to 400°F (200°C). In a small saucepan, bring 1½ cups (375 ml) water to a boil. Add the peas and blanch them for 1 minute. Drain and submerge them in ice water to stop the cooking process. Drain.

2   Cut 4 pieces of parchment paper to approximately 13 by 9 inches. Fold each sheet of parchment in half and lay them on a work surface. Brush a little bit of olive oil on the center of each of the folded halves; this is where the potatoes will go.

3   Using a mandoline, very thinly slice the potatoes. Arrange the potatoes on top of the olive oil on all the pieces of parchment. Place the clams and peas on top. Sprinkle with the parsley, thyme, red pepper flakes, lemon zest, and butter. Pour the wine over the top, distributing evenly on the parchment. Fold the edges and seal the packets. Tighten with paper clips if necessary. Place the packets on two baking sheets.

4   Bake for 20 minutes or until the clams open. You will be able to feel through the paper that they have opened.

5   About 2 minutes before the clams are done cooking, combine the 2 tablespoons of olive oil and garlic in a small sauté pan and cook over low heat until the garlic is fragrant. Remove the packets from the oven, open them, and drizzle the garlic and olive oil on top of the clams. Serve immediately.

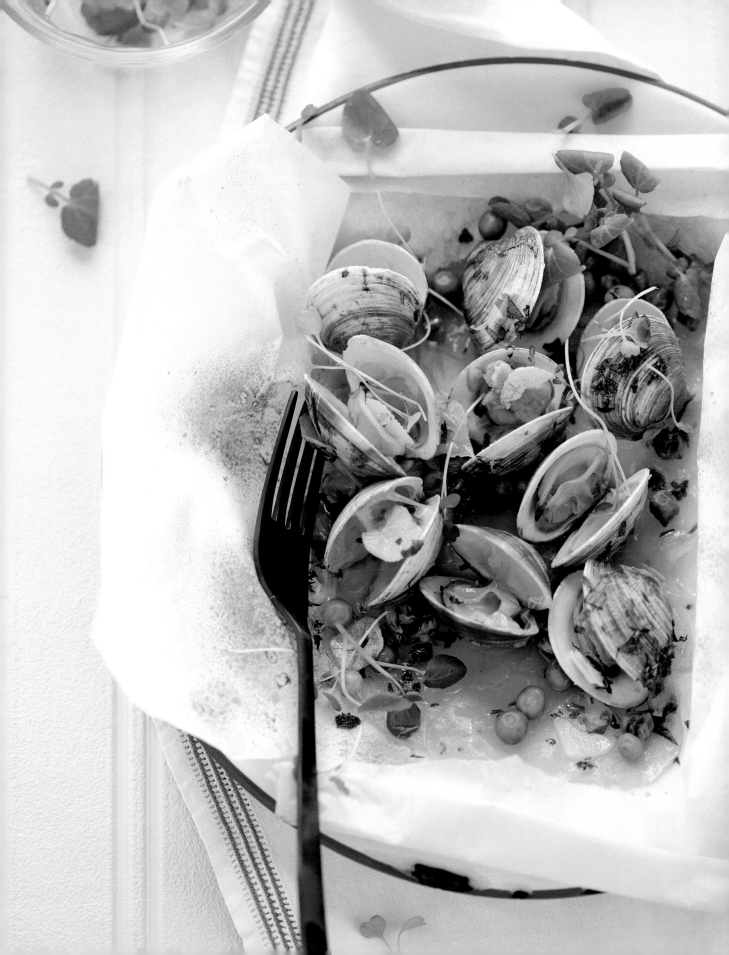

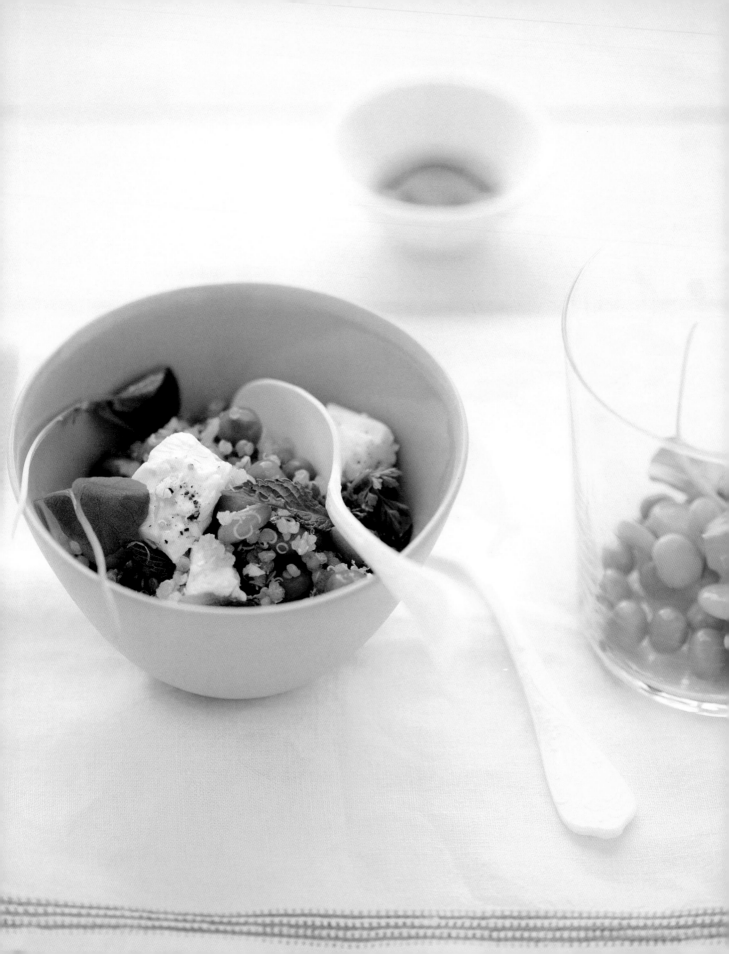

spring quinoa salad

QUINOA SALADS ARE ALWAYS FULL OF nutrients and high in protein. They are one of my go-to, quick-lunch fixes. It takes no longer than 20 minutes to cook this complete meal. The touch of mint and lemon, along with the crumbled feta, makes this one of my favorite spring dishes.

SERVES 4 to 6

1 In a medium saucepan, bring the chicken stock and ½ teaspoon of the salt to a boil. Add the quinoa, lower the heat to a simmer, cover the pan, and cook for 15 minutes. The quinoa will absorb all the water. Transfer to a large bowl to cool, about 15 minutes.

2 Meanwhile, in a medium saucepan, bring about 3 cups (750 ml) water and the remaining 2 teaspoons salt to a boil. Blanch the peas and lima beans in the water for about 1 minute. Drain the water and immediately submerge the peas and lima beans in a bowl of ice water. This will stop the cooking process and keep their color.

3 Add the blanched peas, lima beans, and the rest of the ingredients to the bowl with the quinoa. Toss and serve at room temperature or chilled.

- 2 cups (500 ml) chicken stock or water
- 2½ teaspoons salt
- 1 cup (175 g) quinoa, rinsed
- ¾ cup (160 g) English peas
- ¾ cup (160 g) baby lima beans
- 2 ounces (60 g) feta cheese, crumbled
- ¼ cup (15 g) fresh mint leaves
- ½ cup (20 g) watercress
- 2 teaspoons finely grated lemon zest
- ¼ cup (60 ml) olive oil
- ½ teaspoon freshly ground black pepper

QUINOA VARIETIES

After I was diagnosed with gluten intolerance, my doctor asked me to give up grains for a few months to see if that would help my digestive system heal and reduce inflammation. It was probably harder to do than giving up gluten or dairy altogether. But during this process, I learned that quinoa is safe, as it is technically the starchy fruit seed of an herb, or a *pseudo-grain*, as it is sometimes called. It is mainly grown in Peru and Bolivia, where they supposedly store seeds from more than 1,800 varieties of quinoa, but three are widely available in most shops.

IVORY QUINOA: This is the most commonly found variety. It is pale ivory in color and has the mildest flavor of the three. It cooks faster and has a softer texture. It is great for salads, fillings, soups, and desserts.

RED QUINOA: It contains slightly more protein, calcium, iron, phosphorus, and riboflavin than ivory quinoa. It takes a bit longer to cook and has a crunchier texture and a slightly nuttier flavor. It is great for salads, as it holds its texture better than ivory quinoa.

BLACK QUINOA: It is earthier and sweeter than white quinoa. It also takes a bit longer to cook, and it retains its striking black color after it is cooked. This variety is also perfect for salads.

chamomile-poached salmon
with cucumber & fennel slaw

GENTLY POACHING FISH REALLY PRESERVES its tenderness and flakiness.
Have fun experimenting with different poaching liquids. I particularly love this one,
made with chamomile tea and aromatics.

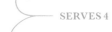

SERVES 4

CUCUMBER AND FENNEL SLAW

1 medium seedless cucumber,
   thinly sliced

1 medium fennel bulb, thinly sliced

1 medium shallot, minced

2 tablespoons fresh cilantro or
   chervil leaves

1 teaspoon salt

½ teaspoon freshly ground black
   pepper

½ teaspoon Dijon mustard

1 teaspoon freshly squeezed
   lemon juice

2 tablespoons olive oil

1 teaspoon ground pink
   peppercorns

CHAMOMILE-POACHED SALMON

1 shallot, halved

1 medium carrot, peeled and diced

4 strips lemon zest

¾ teaspoon salt

1 teaspoon fennel seeds

1 tablespoon loose dried
   chamomile leaves or
   4 chamomile tea bags

4 (6-ounce or 170 g) pieces salmon

make the slaw

Toss all the ingredients together in a bowl and let them macerate while
preparing the salmon.

poach the salmon

1　In a medium saucepan, combine 6 cups (1.5 L) water, the shallot,
carrot, lemon zest, ½ teaspoon of the salt, and the fennel seeds. Bring the
liquid to a boil, reduce the heat to low, and simmer for 15 minutes. Add
the chamomile. Turn off the heat and let steep for 15 minutes. Strain the
liquid into a large deep skillet.

2　Bring the liquid back to a low simmer over medium-high heat.
Remove the pan from the heat. Season the salmon with the remaining
¼ teaspoon salt. Lay the pieces of salmon in the pan with the hot broth.
Cover the pan and let the salmon cook for about 10 minutes, depending
on the thickness. Remove a piece and check for doneness. The center
should be cooked but not dry.

3　Remove the salmon from the poaching liquid and serve with the
Cucumber & Fennel Slaw.

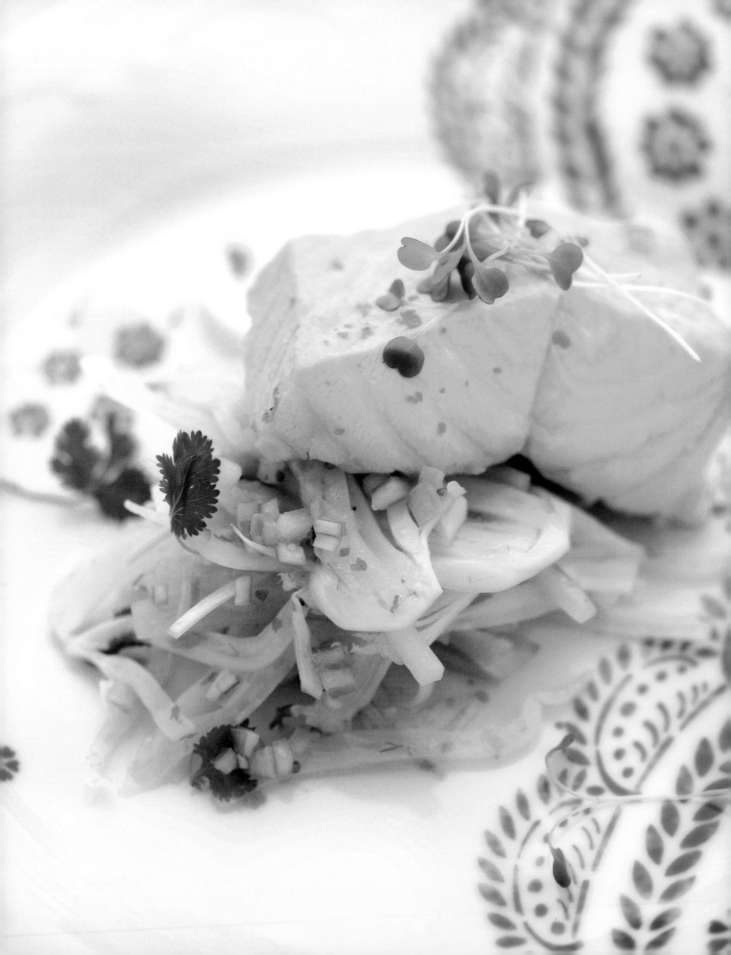

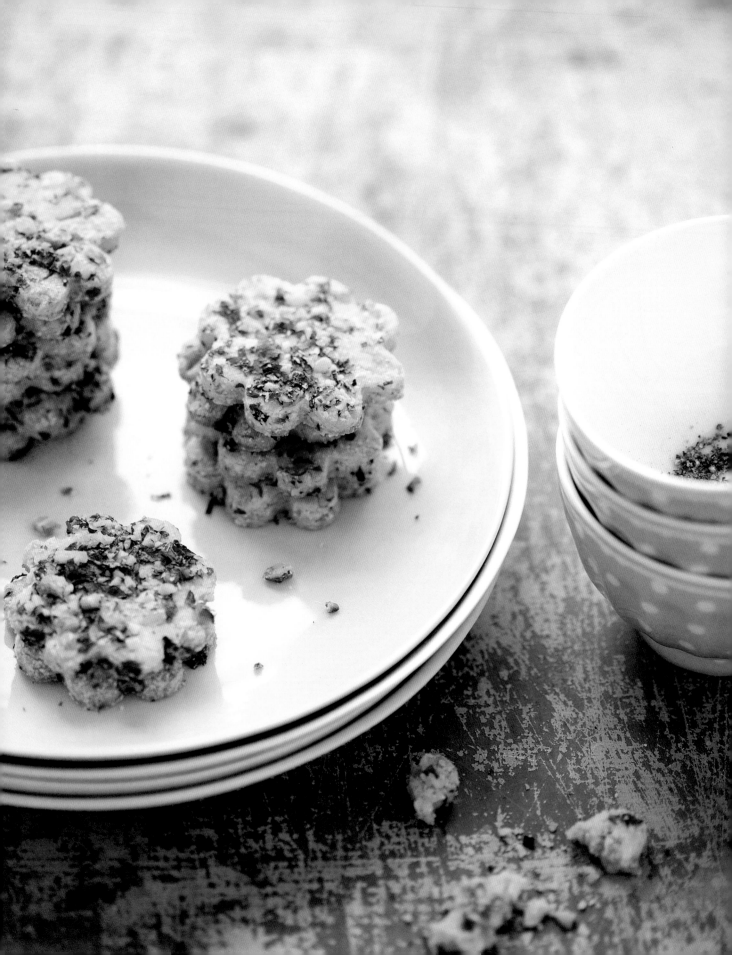

salty herb, walnut & corn crackers

THIS IS A BASIC SAVORY CRACKER RECIPE that can be adapted in many ways. Substitute quinoa flour for the corn flour and add ¼ cup of crispy sautéed prosciutto to the dough for a heartier variation. You can also cut the crackers into larger circles and top them with goat cheese, smoked salmon, and chives.

MAKES 20 crackers

1 In a medium bowl, whisk together the first six ingredients. Add the soft butter and mix it into the flour with your fingers. It will be a crumbly mixture. Add the egg and mix. Knead it a couple of times and form into a disk. Wrap with plastic wrap, flatten it, and refrigerate for 1 hour.

2 Preheat the oven to 400°F (200°C). Spread the chopped walnuts and parsley on a work surface. Place the dough on top and, with a lightly dusted rolling pin, roll out to a ¼-inch thickness. Refrigerate until firm, about 15 minutes. Cut with a 2-inch round or fluted cookie cutter. Place the crackers on a baking sheet lined with parchment paper.

3 Brush the tops with the olive oil and bake for 13 to 15 minutes, until lightly golden. Cool on the baking sheet for 10 minutes before transferring to a wire rack to cool completely.

½ cup (70 g) superfine brown rice flour

⅓ cup (45 g) gluten-free corn flour (not cornmeal)

3 tablespoons gluten-free oat flour

2 tablespoons tapioca starch

1 teaspoon salt

½ teaspoon freshly ground black pepper

½ stick (4 tablespoons or 55 g) unsalted butter, at room temperature, cut into pieces

1 egg, lightly beaten

¼ cup (30 g) walnuts, finely chopped

⅓ cup (20 g) finely chopped fresh parsley

2 tablespoons olive oil

creamy fennel & spinach soup

"PUT YOUR WELLIES ON AND LET'S GO GET some potatoes for lunch," said *amama* Dolores while holding on to a long branch that served as a makeshift cane. Even at ninety years old, she was still going down to the garden every day to harvest vegetables for lunch. She leaned down with the wooden cane in her left hand and picked potatoes with her right. "They only need a light scrubbing and they will be ready for soup." She was right. New potatoes in the spring are tender like butter. Serve this soup with the Salty Herb, Walnut & Corn Crackers (page 177).

SERVES 4 to 6

2 tablespoons olive oil

1 large shallot, diced

1 medium fennel bulb, diced

½ teaspoon salt

¼ teaspoon freshly ground black pepper

3 small Yukon gold potatoes, diced

¼ teaspoon ground coriander

¼ teaspoon ground fennel

2½ cups (625 ml) chicken stock

½ cup (30 g) spinach leaves

2 ounces (60 g) mascarpone cheese

Olive oil, for drizzling

1 In a medium saucepan, heat the olive oil over medium heat. Add the shallot, fennel, salt, and black pepper. Cook for 5 minutes, until tender but not caramelized.

2 Add the potatoes, ground coriander, ground fennel, and chicken stock. Bring the liquid to a boil, reduce the heat to low, cover, and simmer for 15 minutes, until the vegetables are soft.

3 Add the spinach and cook for another minute. Turn off the heat and add the mascarpone. Transfer to a blender and puree. Adjust the seasoning if needed. Serve with a drizzle of olive oil.

TIP: New potatoes have such thin skin that they really do not need to be peeled. Because of their high moisture content, they are best boiled and in soups. If you cannot find them, use regular golden potatoes, but peel them.

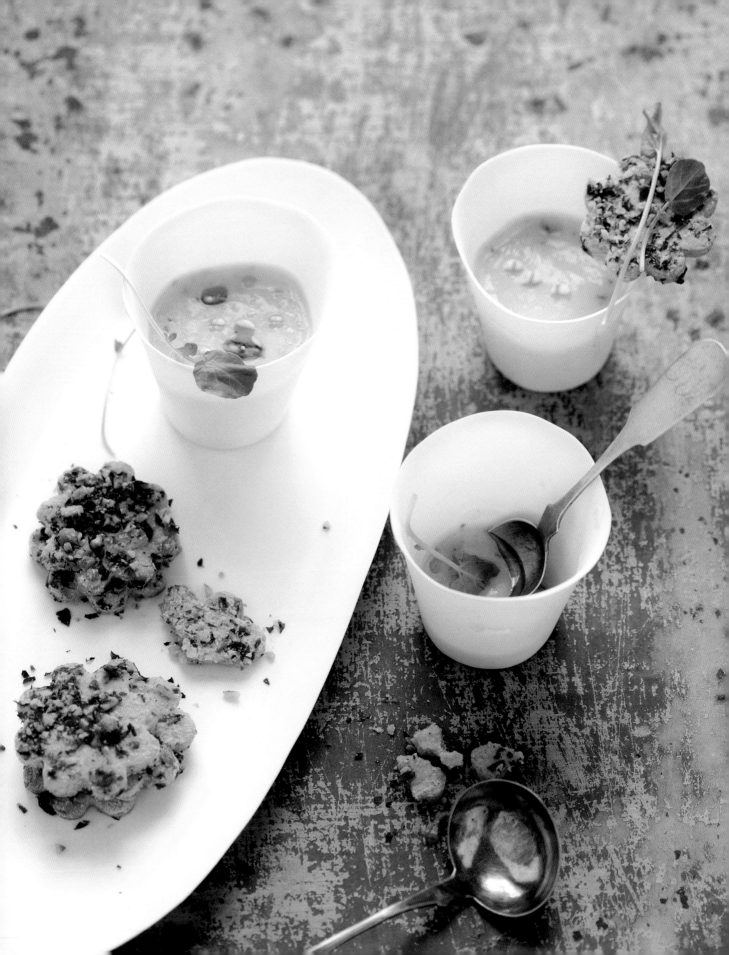

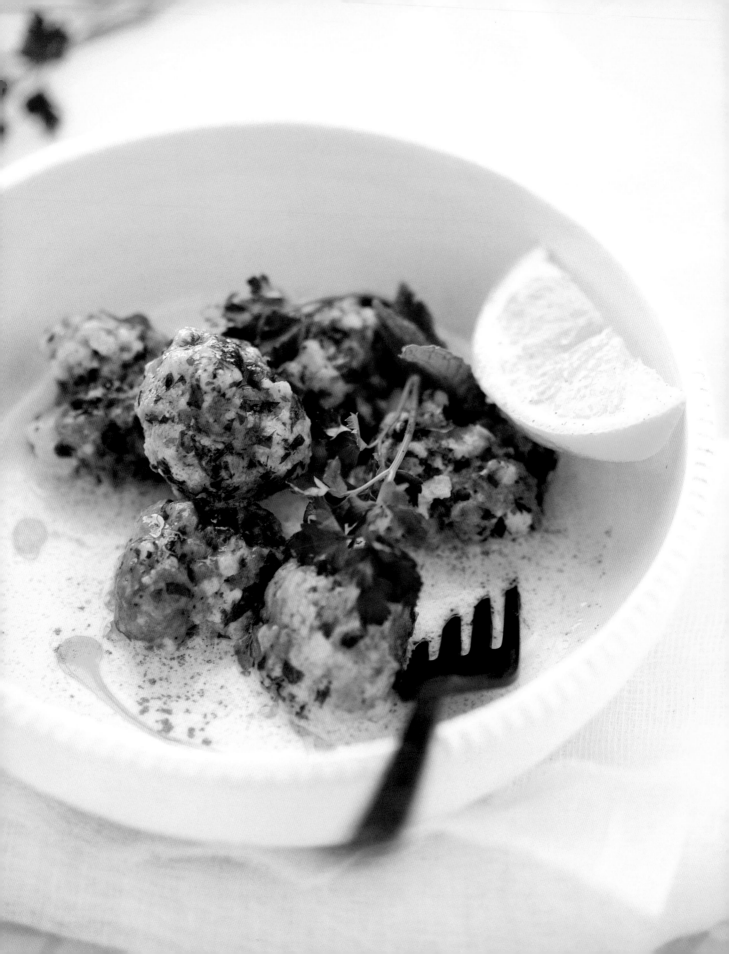

herbed lamb meatballs in coconut milk

PINTXO **BARS IN THE BASQUE COUNTRY** have an endless assortment of little bite-size nibbles on display. But I always tell people who visit for the first time to look for the blackboard that lists the day's *raciones*, or small plates. Traditionally they are served in small clay pots, and most of the time they are sauce-based dishes. It could be an oxtail stew, mussels in a spicy broth, or calamari cooked in their own ink. It's important to ask for extra bread for dipping in that leftover sauce. Meatballs were always my favorite. In this recipe, they are cooked in a coconut milk broth and flavored with lots of fresh herbs.

SERVES 4 to 6

1   In a medium bowl, combine the lamb, bread, garlic, egg, parsley, mint, oregano, ½ teaspoon of the salt, paprika, and black pepper. Mix with your hands. Do not overwork the meat or it will become tough when cooked. Make 1-inch meatballs and set them on a tray.

2   In a large shallow pan, bring the coconut milk and remaining ½ teaspoon salt to a low simmer over medium heat. Add the meatballs, reduce the heat to low, cover, and simmer for 20 minutes.

3   Add the yogurt and lemon juice and gently stir it into the sauce to thicken it. Serve warm.

TIP: You may substitute ground chicken or turkey for the ground lamb.

1 pound (450 g) ground lamb

2 slices (45 g) gluten-free bread, crumbled

1 clove garlic, grated

1 egg, lightly beaten

2 tablespoons finely chopped fresh parsley

2 tablespoons finely chopped fresh mint

1 tablespoon finely chopped fresh oregano leaves

1 teaspoon salt

½ teaspoon hot paprika

¼ teaspoon freshly ground black pepper

1½ cups (375 ml) unsweetened coconut milk

½ cup (125 ml) whole-milk plain yogurt

1 tablespoon freshly squeezed lemon juice

chicken, sugar snap pea & rice soup

THIS IS A VERY SIMPLE BUT FLAVORFUL broth. The trick is to use really fresh herbs and chicken with the bone in and skin on. You could skip the first stage of making the broth and use store-bought chicken stock to cut down the cooking time, but make sure to add the herbs for freshness.

SERVES 4

2 chicken breasts, with skin on and bones in (you could also use dark meat, such as thighs)

2 baby spring leeks or 1 medium leek, cut into strips

1 medium carrot, peeled

2 cloves garlic, crushed but left whole

1 bunch parsley

1 bunch chervil

2 sprigs thyme

2 teaspoons salt

1 teaspoon freshly ground black pepper

¼ cup (50 g) Arborio rice

1 cup (40 g) sugar snap peas

Olive oil, for drizzling

1 In a medium pot, combine the first nine ingredients (use only half the leeks) along with 2 quarts (2 L) water. Bring the liquid to a boil over medium-high heat. Skim the impurities and foam that rise to the top. Reduce the heat to low, cover, and simmer for 1 hour. Do not stir during this time.

2 Remove the chicken from the broth. Strain the broth into a clean medium pot. Discard the vegetables and aromatics.

3 Bring the broth back to a boil over medium-high heat. Add the rice, cover the pot, and reduce the heat to low. Cook for 10 minutes.

4 In the meantime, shred the reserved chicken. After 10 minutes of cooking the rice, add the remaining leeks, the snap peas, and shredded chicken to the broth. Cover and cook for an additional 5 minutes. Adjust the seasoning if needed and serve with a drizzle of olive oil.

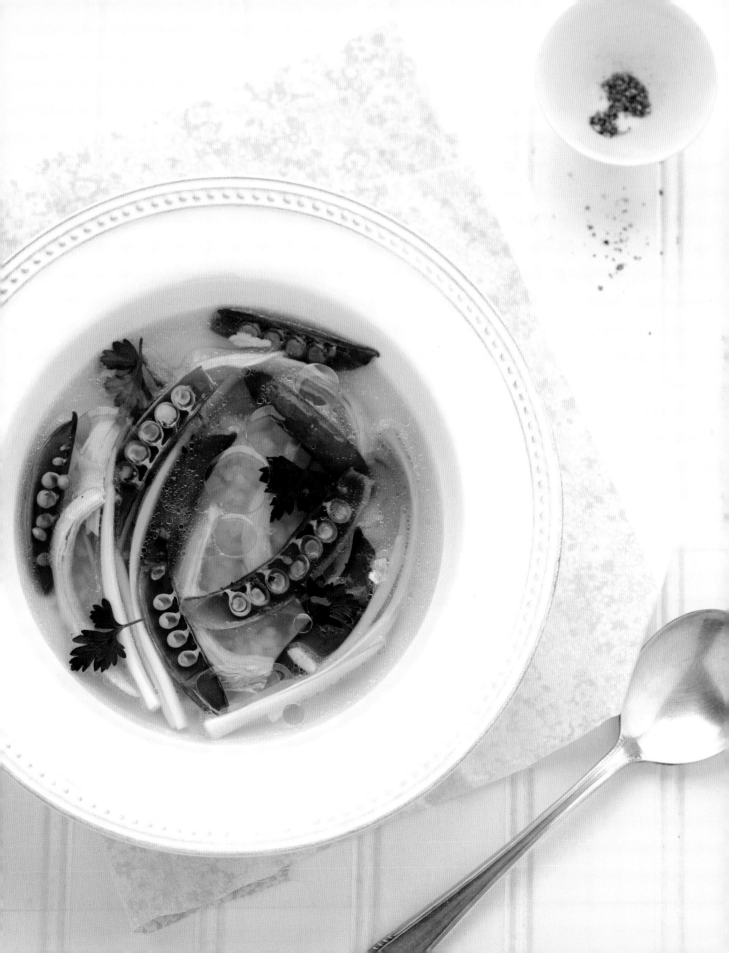

watercress pudding with soft-boiled quail eggs, asparagus & watermelon radish

ON LAZY WEEKEND MORNINGS, we sit around, play with the kids, maybe have a bowl of fresh fruit, and then we cook brunch. It feels luxurious and worth the wait. Waffles and eggs are everyone's favorites, but sometimes I need something a little bit more sophisticated—delicate soft-boiled quail eggs with creamy watercress custard. The watermelon radish and asparagus add an extra layer of texture and crunch.

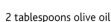

SERVES 6

2 tablespoons olive oil

2 cloves garlic, crushed but left whole

2 cups (80 g) watercress

1 teaspoon celery salt

½ teaspoon freshly ground black pepper

½ teaspoon freshly grated nutmeg

1 cup (250 ml) unsweetened coconut milk

1 cup (250 ml) heavy cream

4 eggs

6 quail eggs

3 ounces (90 g) asparagus tips

1 watermelon radish, thinly sliced

¼ teaspoon salt

1 Preheat the oven to 325°F (160°C). In a medium sauté pan, heat 1 tablespoon of the olive oil over medium heat. Add the garlic and cook for 1 minute or until it starts to turn golden. Remove the garlic from the oil. Add the watercress, celery salt, black pepper, and nutmeg. Cook the watercress for 1 minute or until wilted. Remove from the heat.

2 Place the wilted watercress in a blender along with the coconut milk and heavy cream. Blend to a fine puree. Add the 4 regular eggs and blend.

3 Divide the custard among 6 (6-ounce) ramekins. Place the ramekins in a deep baking dish. Bring the dish to the oven and place on the rack. Pour hot water into the baking dish, enough to go halfway up the sides of the ramekins.

4 Bake the custards in the water bath for 30 to 35 minutes or until the center is set.

5 In the meantime, bring 3 cups water to a boil in a medium saucepan. Make a swirling motion with a spoon in the boiling water. Gently add the quail eggs and continue to spin them around for a few seconds. This will ensure the yolks are perfectly set in the center of the egg. Cook for 1 minute and then transfer the eggs to a bowl of ice water to cool. Gently peel the shells and cut the eggs in half. You should have a runny yolk right in the center of each egg.

6 Blanch the asparagus tips in salted boiling water for 1 minute and then shock them in ice water. This will help preserve the green color.

7 Toss the asparagus tips and sliced watermelon radish with the salt and remaining 1 tablespoon olive oil. Serve the warm watercress custards with the quail eggs, asparagus, and watermelon radish.

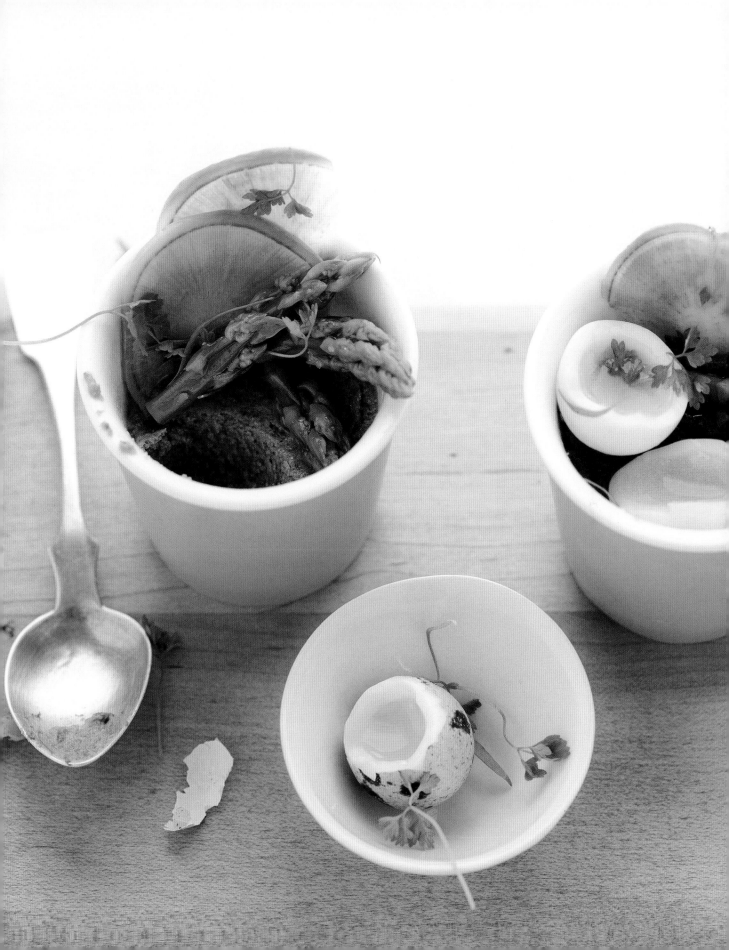

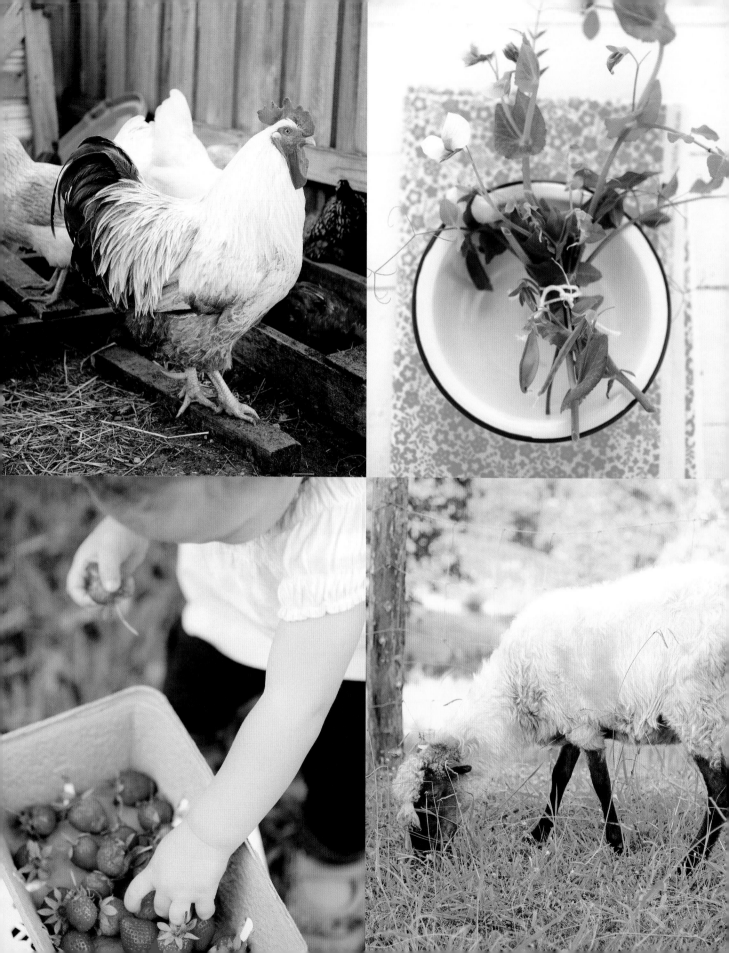

SPRING
sweet treats

THERE IS A NATURAL ORDER to the way the dreary winter weather unfolds and the brightness and freshness of spring sets in. Cherry trees line the calm street we walk every morning on our way to school. Sometime around mid-April, these trees go into full bloom, with white and pink blossoms that turn the landscape into a beautiful spectrum of pastels.

"Strawberries will soon follow!" I tell my son, Jon. The cherry blossoms are the first sign of great things to come, starting with the giant wooden crates filled with ripe strawberries that we end up bringing home. We don't even refrigerate them. Never make it that far. Simply macerated strawberries with a touch of sugar and orange juice make the perfect after-lunch dessert. And then there is the canning. My mom always saves the lightly bruised ones to make her favorite jam. She likes it light, not too sweet, not too thick.

"Who are they trying to fool with those strawberry stands on the side of the road?" I asked my husband, Chad, during our first winter in Florida. It was sometime in January, and impromptu farm stands were suddenly crowding every corner. I couldn't believe it. We quickly learned the benefits of living in a warm climate. "Strawberries in January? It must be so."

Late May and June are the months of cherries, followed by the first apricots as spring turns into summer. This is the season of tarts, clafoutis, and the first homemade ice cream.

lemon, buttermilk &
olive oil madeleines

"AMATXU, **CAN YOU MAKE SOME OF** those bumpy cakes?" asks Jon, mimicking a dunking motion. He has watched my dad dunk madeleines in his *café con leche* many times before. In our family, dipping cookies, cake, or bread in milk is not something reserved for children alone. We all take great pleasure in it, especially with our afternoon coffee and tea.

MAKES 36 madeleines

¾ stick (6 tablespoons or 80 g) unsalted butter

1 cup (200 g) natural cane sugar

Finely grated zest of 3 lemons

3 eggs

¾ cup (105 g) superfine brown rice flour

⅓ cup (45 g) millet flour

¼ cup (30 g) tapioca starch

1 tablespoon flaxseed meal

1 teaspoon baking powder

½ teaspoon salt

¼ cup (60 ml) full-fat buttermilk

½ cup (125 ml) olive oil

1 In a small saucepan, melt the butter. Let it cool completely.

2 Combine the sugar and lemon zest in the bowl of a stand mixer. Rub the zest and the sugar together between your fingers. This will release the oil in the zest. Add the eggs and whip on high speed for 5 minutes, until light and thick.

3 In a separate bowl, whisk together the superfine brown rice flour, millet flour, tapioca starch, flaxseed meal, baking powder, and salt. Add the dry ingredients to the whipped egg mixture while mixing on low speed.

4 Add the buttermilk, olive oil, and melted butter on low speed. Turn the mixer back to high and whip for another 30 seconds, until all the ingredients are well incorporated.

5 Cover the bowl with plastic wrap and refrigerate for 2 hours. If you wish, you may keep the batter in the refrigerator for up to 2 days and bake small batches of madeleines as you need.

6 Preheat the oven to 425°F (220°C). If using a plain aluminum pan, make sure to grease the pan. If you have a pastry bag, fit it with a plain pastry tip that is ½-inch wide and then scrape the batter into it. Pipe the batter into the mold. Otherwise, spoon the batter into the mold.

7 Bake the madeleines for 8 minutes. Do not open the oven door during baking. Turn the temperature down to 350°F (180°C) and bake for another 5 minutes or until golden. Let them cool in the mold for 5 minutes. Transfer the madeleines to a plate.

TIP: If you do not have flaxseed meal on hand, simply increase the amount of superfine brown rice flour by 1 tablespoon.

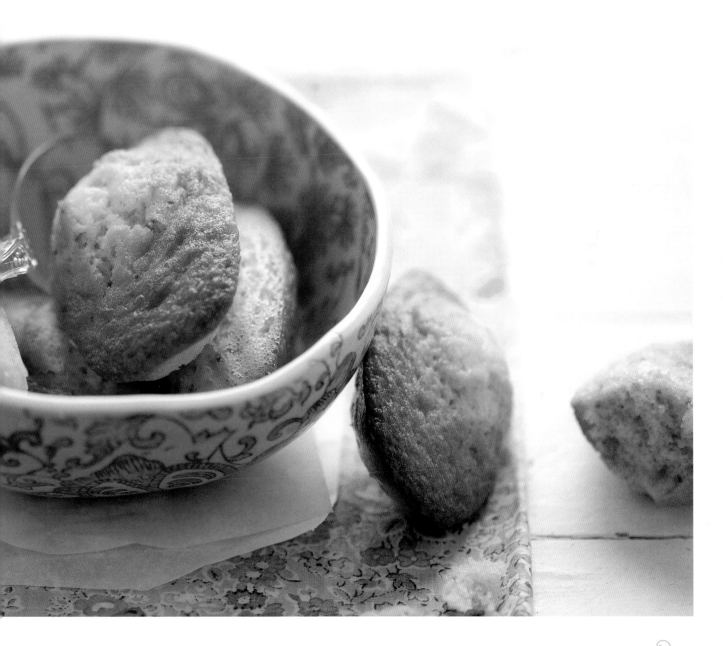

MOLDS FOR MADELEINES

There are many options for madeleine molds: nonstick, aluminum, and silicone. I have a set of each and more, as I love to experiment with different molds. Metal molds in general yield darker cake exteriors, and the same applies to madeleines.

It is all a matter of personal preference. I like the tender texture and light color that result from using silicone molds. But you may prefer the darker color that metal yields.

rhubarb, ladyfinger & crème fraîche trifle

BAKING LADYFINGERS IS ONE OF the pleasures of life—the gentle folding of whipped egg whites and the infinite rows of symmetrically piped batter give me a sense of purpose. I love having ladyfingers handy in the freezer for those times I want to make a last-minute tiramisu or a trifle.

This recipe makes more ladyfingers than you will need for the trifle, but leftovers freeze well. Stack them on top of each other in an airtight container and freeze for up to 1 month.

You can also make this recipe without the ground chia seeds, but they do add a bit more structure to the batter.

SERVES 4

LADYFINGERS (MAKES ABOUT 35 LADYFINGERS)

4 eggs, separated

⅓ cup (70 g) natural cane sugar

2 teaspoons finely grated lemon zest

½ cup (60 g) powdered sugar, plus more for dusting, sifted

½ cup (70 g) superfine brown rice flour

¼ cup (30 g) cornstarch

2 teaspoons ground chia seeds

make the ladyfingers

1   Preheat the oven to 375°F (190°C). Line two baking sheets with parchment paper.

2   Combine the egg yolks, sugar, and lemon zest in the bowl of a stand mixer. Whisk immediately with the whip attachment. Do not let the sugar sit on top of the egg yolks without whisking or it will "burn" and create a skin. Whip the mixture on high speed until very thick and very pale, about 7 minutes. Transfer the whipped yolks to a large bowl.

3   Thoroughly wash the mixer bowl and the whip attachment in warm, soapy water. If there is any fat residue left behind, the egg whites will not whip properly. Dry the bowl and attachment thoroughly.

4   Add the egg whites to the clean bowl. Whip them on high speed until light and soft peaks start to form. Slowly add the sifted powdered sugar, in four batches, and continue to whip until stiff peaks form.

5   Add one-third of the meringue to the yolk mixture and fold. Add the rest of the meringue and fold gently so as not to deflate the mixture.

6   Sift the superfine brown rice flour, cornstarch, and ground chia seeds together into a bowl. Add the dry ingredients to the egg mixture. Fold carefully, so as not to deflate the batter, until no more flour particles are visible. It will be a thick batter and should hold its shape when piped. If it's runny, it means you did not whip your egg yolks or egg whites fully, or that you folded the batter too much.

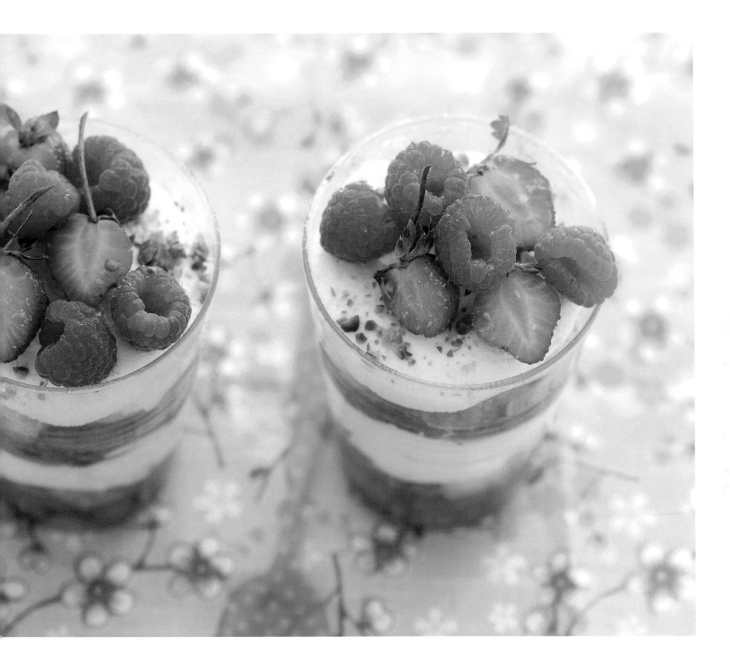

7   Transfer the batter to a pastry bag fitted with a #6 or #7 plain tip.
Pipe three rows of 2½-inch ladyfingers onto the parchment paper, leaving
1 inch in between. Dust the tops with a little bit of sifted powdered sugar.

8   Bake for 13 to 14 minutes, until golden. Do not open the oven
door during the first 8 minutes. Let the baked ladyfingers cool completely
on the pan. Carefully peel the parchment paper from the back of the
ladyfingers and set aside.

recipe continues

RHUBARB COMPOTE (MAKES 1½ CUPS)

1 pound (450 g) rhubarb, cut into
2-inch pieces

3 tablespoons freshly squeezed
orange juice

2 tablespoons honey

1 teaspoon freshly grated
orange zest

CRÈME FRAÎCHE

12 ounces (340 g) crème fraîche
or heavy cream

1 tablespoon superfine sugar

1 teaspoon orange flower water,
optional

TRIFLE ASSEMBLY

12 Ladyfingers

1 cup (120 g) sliced strawberries
and whole raspberries

make the compote

Place all the ingredients in a medium saucepan and cook over medium heat for 5 minutes or until the rhubarb is tender but not mushy. Let the compote cool completely.

make the crème fraîche

Place all the ingredients in a bowl. If you are using crème fraîche, lightly whisk by hand until soft peaks form, which will not take very long. Do not overmix it or it will turn to butter very quickly. If you are using heavy cream, whip it on high speed in a stand mixer until soft peaks form.

assemble the trifle

Spoon half of the Rhubarb Compote evenly among 4 glasses. Top each with 1½ Ladyfingers, breaking them as needed to fit. Top with half of the Crème Fraîche. Repeat with another layer of Rhubarb Compote, Ladyfingers, and Crème Fraîche. Top with the fresh berries.

HOMEMADE CRÈME FRAÎCHE

This is not the traditional way of making crème fraîche; the original is made with unpasteurized cream and bacteria that are naturally present in the air. Just as with sourdough bread, cheese, or wine, true crème fraîche made in one location will differ from that made in another location due to the presence of different bacteria. This is what I love about it: the uniqueness and the surprise.

Most people don't have access to unpasteurized milk, so I have come up with a recipe that is easy to make and still wonderfully creamy and delicious. You will get the best results if you do not use ultra-

pasteurized heavy cream. Here is how I make my crème fraîche at home:

Combine 2 cups (500 ml) heavy cream and 2 tablespoons full-fat buttermilk in a small saucepan. Heat the mixture over medium heat until an instant-read thermometer reads 80°F (27°C). Pour the mixture into a clean glass jar and partially cover it with a lid. Let the mixture stand at room temperature for 6 to 24 hours, or until slightly thickened. Stir, and then refrigerate it for at least 24 hours before using. The crème fraîche will thicken in the refrigerator and will keep for 10 days.

macarons

I LOVE TO WALK INTO FINE PASTRY SHOPS and just stare and feel inspired. I was eighteen the first time I visited Paris, and I fell in love with the macaron towers that decorated many pastry shops. In Barcelona, I love visiting Pasteleria Escribà and Bubo, where the flavor combinations wow me every time.

This recipe is an adaptation of a recipe from master pastry chef Sébastien Cannone, which I have been using for years. It always works for me. The macarons have a thin, crispy shell with a chewy interior.

MAKES about 48 macarons

1   Take the aged egg whites out of the refrigerator and leave them at room temperature for at least 1 hour before beginning. Then weigh 5 ounces (140 g) of the egg whites. If you are only a few grams short, do not panic. The recipe will work.

2   Line four baking sheets with silicone mats or parchment paper. In a large bowl, sift together the almond flour, powdered sugar, and salt. If you are using powdered food coloring, sift it with the dry ingredients. Remember that the intensity of the color will diminish once the meringue is added, so plan for that. If you are using liquid food coloring, save this for step 4.

3   If you are using the egg white powder, place it in a small bowl, add 1 tablespoon egg whites, and whisk to combine. Add this mixture to the rest of the egg whites.

4   Place the egg whites in the bowl of a stand mixer and start whipping on medium speed. Whipping them slowly creates a more stable meringue structure. After a couple of minutes, the egg whites will begin to foam. When they are almost fully whipped, slowly add the natural cane sugar, 1 tablespoon at a time. Continue to whip. When all the sugar has been added, turn the speed to high and let it finish whipping to firm peaks. Add your liquid food coloring at this point, but only 2 or 3 drops, or the batter will be too wet and will crack.

5   Add all of the dry ingredients to the meringue at once. Fold them together until a shiny magma-like mass forms. Do not be afraid to fold at the beginning, but as the batter starts to become shiny, watch it to see how it flows. Place 1 teaspoon of the batter on a silicone mat. Watch it for

5 egg whites, aged (see Mastering Macarons, page 196)

1¾ cups (175 g) sifted almond flour

2 cups (240 g) powdered sugar, sifted

½ teaspoon salt

Food coloring (powder or liquid, optional)

1½ teaspoons egg white powder, optional (see Mastering Macarons, page 196)

¼ cup plus 2 tablespoons (80 g) natural cane sugar

Filling or buttercream of your choice, such as Basic Swiss Buttercream Filling (page 197)

recipe continues

30 seconds. If it leaves a point on the top, then it needs more folding. You want a batter that flows enough that it leaves no point but does not spread too much. If it spreads too much, it will not develop the desired "feet."

6   Transfer the batter to a pastry bag fitted with a plain pastry tip that is ½ inch wide. Pipe 1-inch circles onto the baking sheets, spacing the macarons 1 to 2 inches apart. Pipe all the batter. Let the macarons sit at room temperature for 30 to 45 minutes, depending on the humidity in the air. After this time, the tops should develop a thin skin and your finger should not stick to the top.

7   Preheat the oven to 350°F (180°C). Place one baking sheet in the center rack of the oven. Reduce the heat to 300°F (150°C). Bake for 8 minutes, rotate the baking sheet, and bake for an additional 5 minutes. Ovens may vary, so to check for doneness, gently jiggle a macaron between your fingers. It will stick to the silicone mat, but the center will feel set and not runny. Remove the baking sheet from the oven and let the macarons cool completely before attempting to lift them.

8   Increase the oven temperature to 350°F (180°C) once again and repeat the process with the rest of the baking sheets.

9   Once completely cooled, turn half of the macarons upside down. Fit a pastry bag with a plain pastry tip that is ½ inch wide. Fill the bag with the filling or buttercream of your choice. Pipe a bit of filling on each upside-down macaron and top with another one, flat side down. Gently press them together.

10   Filled macarons are best kept at room temperature. Storing them in the refrigerator will make them soggy. They may also be frozen after being filled, but once they thaw, they must be eaten immediately. Unfilled macarons are best stored at room temperature, wrapped, for up to 1 day. They may also be frozen, tightly wrapped, for up to 1 month.

macaron variations

PISTACHIO MACARONS: Use 1 cup (100 g) unsalted natural pistachios and ¾ cup (80 g) almond flour. In a food processor, pulse the pistachios, almond flour, and powdered sugar together until a fine powder forms. Follow the basic recipe and add 2 drops of gel food coloring to the meringue (optional). For the filling, whisk together 1 cup of mascarpone cheese and 2 teaspoons finely grated lemon zest.

CHOCOLATE MACARONS: Add 2 tablespoons sifted really dark unsweetened Dutch-process cocoa powder to the dry ingredients. Fill with espresso-flavored buttercream by adding 2 teaspoons instant espresso powder to 1 cup of the basic buttercream.

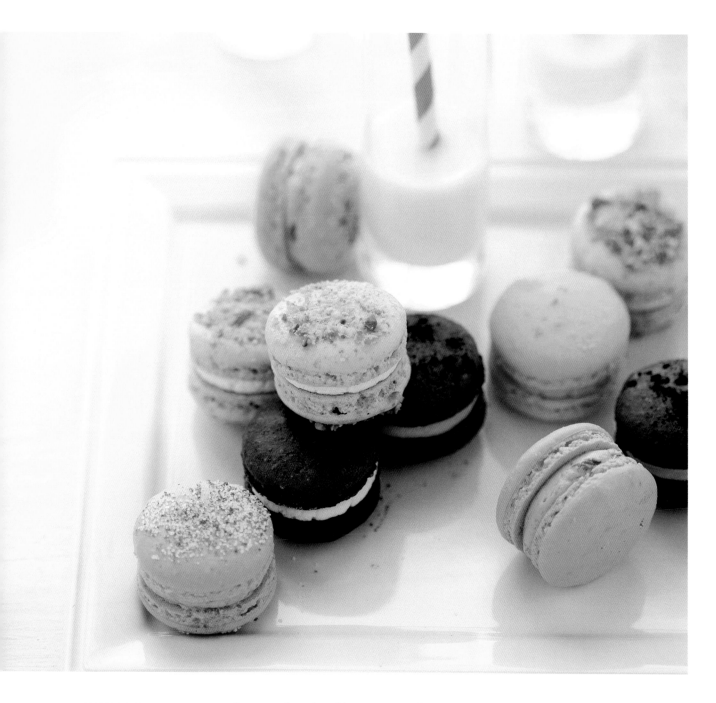

VANILLA SALT MACARONS: Increase the salt to ¾ teaspoon and use vanilla sugar in place of the granulated sugar. Fill with vanilla buttercream.

RASPBERRY MACARONS: Add 2 teaspoons freeze-dried raspberry powder and 2 drops red food coloring (optional) to the batter. For the filling, whisk together 1 cup of the basic buttercream with 1 tablespoon crushed fresh raspberries.

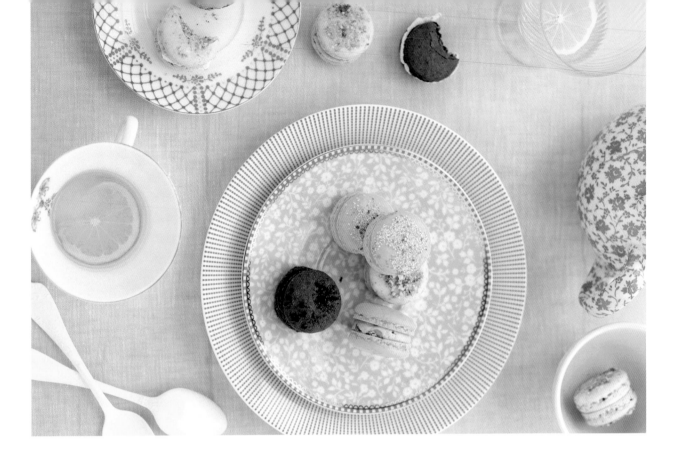

MASTERING MACARONS

Macarons are not difficult to make, but there are a few points to keep in mind:

1 I recommend weighing the ingredients, as measuring in cups is not very accurate.

2 The egg whites must be aged, which means you must separate the whites from the yolks at least 2 days in advance. Store the egg whites uncovered in the refrigerator. This allows some of the water in the whites to evaporate, increasing their solids content. Aging also turns the egg whites acidic, which helps create more volume while whipping.

3 Humidity in the air plays a big role, so it is important to use egg white powder (not meringue powder) in high-humidity locations. When there is too much moisture in the batter, the macarons tend to crack while baking. I also recommend drying the almond flour and powdered sugar when humidity is an issue. Evenly spread the almond flour and powdered sugar on a baking sheet and leave them in the oven overnight with the pilot light on (and the oven turned off). If you have an electric oven, leave them in the oven overnight with the door closed and the oven light on.

4 For intense color, it is best to use powdered food coloring. I prefer natural colors in liquid form, but this means that only a couple of drops can be added without affecting the dough. My macarons tend to be light in color as a result.

5 All ovens are different, so you really must experiment with the temperature. Preheat the oven to 350°F (180°C), then lower it to 300°F (150°C) once the macarons are in. Bake only one baking sheet at a time and place it in the center of the oven.

6 Silicone mats are my preference, but parchment paper will also work. Make sure to use baking sheets that are flat, not warped, or else the macarons will lose their shape before they are fully baked.

basic swiss buttercream filling

YOU MAY FREEZE THIS BUTTERCREAM IN AN AIRTIGHT container for up to 3 months. To thaw, simply leave it at room temperature overnight.

MAKES about 3 cups

1 Whisk the egg whites, sugar, and salt in the bowl of a stand mixer. Place the bowl over a pan filled partway with simmering water. Continue whisking until the sugar has dissolved and the mixture feels hot to the touch. Bring the bowl back to the mixer and, with the whip attachment, whip until a stiff meringue forms and the bottom of the bowl feels cool.

2 While whipping on low to medium speed, start adding the butter 1 tablespoon at a time. Add all the butter in this manner. It might look curdled, but do not worry; it will come together. Turn the speed to high and mix until the buttercream comes together.

3 Add the flavorings and fold to combine.

3 egg whites

¾ cup plus 2 tablespoons (180 g) natural cane sugar

¼ teaspoon salt

2½ sticks (20 tablespoons or 280 g) unsalted butter, at room temperature

Flavorings, such as vanilla extract, lemon zest, espresso powder, and so on, optional

chocolate frangipane & raspberry tarts

THIS IS AN INTENSELY DARK AND RICH TART with a creamy chocolate, almond, and raspberry filling that melts in your mouth. It is beautiful topped with the fresh raspberries.

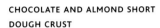

MAKES five 4½-inch tarts

CHOCOLATE AND ALMOND SHORT DOUGH CRUST

1 stick (8 tablespoons or 110 g) unsalted butter, at room temperature

⅓ cup (70 g) natural cane sugar

½ vanilla bean, split lengthwise and seeds scraped

1 egg, at room temperature

¾ cup (105 g) superfine brown rice flour, plus more for dusting

¼ cup (35 g) buckwheat flour

¼ cup (25 g) almond flour

3 tablespoons potato starch

3 tablespoons unsweetened Dutch-process cocoa powder

¼ teaspoon salt

CHOCOLATE FRANGIPANE AND RASPBERRY FILLING

4 ounces (110 g) bittersweet chocolate, finely chopped

¼ cup (60 ml) whole milk

⅔ cup (200 g) gluten-free almond paste

⅓ cup (35 g) almond flour

2 eggs, at room temperature

¼ teaspoon baking powder

¼ teaspoon salt

1 pound (450 g) raspberries

Powdered sugar, for dusting

make the crust

1   In the bowl of a stand mixer, mix the butter, sugar, and vanilla seeds with the paddle attachment on medium speed until light, about 2 minutes. Add the egg and mix until combined. Scrape down the sides and bottom of the bowl.

2   In a small bowl, whisk together all the dry ingredients. Add them to the butter mixture and mix until the dough comes together; it will be a very soft dough. Turn it out onto a work surface, and form it into a disk. Wrap it in plastic wrap, flatten it, and refrigerate for 1 hour. While the dough rests in the refrigerator, prepare the Chocolate Frangipane & Raspberry Filling.

3   Remove the dough from the refrigerator. Dust your work surface with a little bit of superfine brown rice flour. Place the dough on top and, with a rolling pin, roll it to a ¼-inch thickness. Make sure to keep turning the dough while rolling to ensure that it does not stick to the surface.

4   With a paring knife, cut circles that are approximately 5 inches in diameter. They don't need to be perfect. Dust your fingers with superfine brown rice flour and press the dough into 5 (4½-inch) tart molds. It might break, but do not worry, simply press it into the mold until it is approximately ⅛ inch thick. Cut excess dough from the edges with the help of the paring knife.

5   Refrigerate the tarts for 20 minutes.

prepare the filling and bake the tarts

1   Preheat the oven to 350°F (180°C). Place the finely chopped chocolate in a medium bowl. In a small saucepan, bring the milk to a boil. Pour the boiling milk over the chocolate and stir until it melts together. Set aside.

2   In the bowl of a stand mixer, cream the almond paste and almond flour together with the paddle attachment on medium-high speed. It will be lumpy. Add 1 egg. Continue creaming on high speed until the

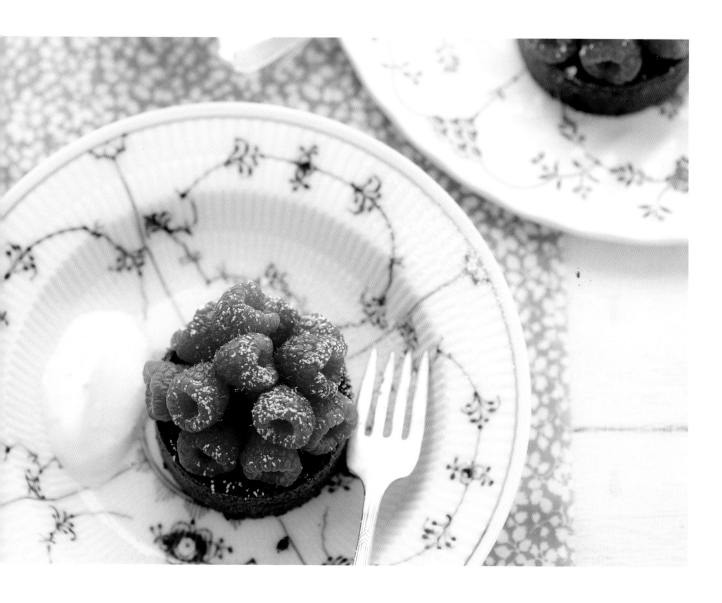

lumps start to break down. Scrape the sides of the bowl. Add the other egg and cream until combined. There might be some small lumps left, which is fine.

3   Add the chocolate-milk mixture and mix until combined. Add the baking powder and salt. Scrape down the sides and bottom of the bowl and mix thoroughly. As the frangipane cools, it will thicken.

4   Fill the tart molds halfway with the frangipane mixture. Insert 1 cup (150 g) of raspberries into the frangipane.

5   Bake the tarts until the center is set and the bottom of the crust is thoroughly baked, 20 to 25 minutes.

6   Let the tarts cool on a rack. Serve topped with the remaining raspberries and a dusting of powdered sugar.

strawberry & pistachio crumble galettes

THESE GALETTES ARE A CROSS BETWEEN a cookie and a tart. They are thin enough that they could be considered a cookie, but with a short crust similar to a tart. It is a great recipe to make with any seasonal fruit.

MAKES eight 3-inch galettes

PASTRY CRUST

½ cup (70 g) superfine brown rice flour, plus more for dusting

½ cup plus 1 tablespoon (70 g) amaranth flour

2 tablespoons potato starch

2 tablespoons tapioca starch

2 teaspoons natural cane sugar

¼ teaspoon salt

1 stick (8 tablespoons or 110 g) cold unsalted butter, cut into ½-inch cubes

6 to 8 tablespoons ice water

STRAWBERRY COMPOTE

4 ounces (110 g) strawberries, hulled and diced

2 tablespoons natural cane sugar

1 teaspoon freshly squeezed lemon juice

PISTACHIO CRUMBLE

⅓ cup (55 g) unsalted natural pistachios

¼ cup (50 g) natural cane sugar

¼ cup (35 g) superfine brown rice flour

2 tablespoons cornstarch

5 tablespoons (70 g) cold unsalted butter, cut into ½-inch cubes

GALETTE ASSEMBLY

2 cups (240 g) thinly sliced strawberries

make the dough

1 Combine the first six ingredients in a food processor. Pulse twice to aerate the ingredients. Add the cold butter and pulse ten times, until the butter is cut into pea-size pieces. Add 6 tablespoons ice water and pulse until the mixture comes together. The dough will not form a ball, so simply press it between your fingers to see if it holds together. Add more water if needed.

2 Turn the dough out onto a work surface and form a disk. Wrap the dough in plastic wrap, flatten it, and refrigerate for 1 hour.

3 Dust your work surface with superfine brown rice flour. Roll the dough to a ¼-inch thickness. Using a 3-inch cookie cutter, cut 8 disks. You might have to re-roll the dough once more to obtain 8 disks. Place them on a baking sheet lined with parchment paper and chill for another 30 minutes.

make the compote

Place all the ingredients in a small saucepan and cook until thick and concentrated, about 7 minutes. Chill until ready to assemble.

make the crumble

1 Place the pistachios in a food processor and pulse until they are finely chopped. Add the sugar, flour, and cornstarch. Pulse to combine.

2 Add the butter and pulse until the mixture forms a crumbly dough. Set aside until ready to use; freeze whatever you don't use in a freezer bag for up to 1 month.

assemble the galettes

1 Preheat the oven to 350°F (180°C). Remove the baking sheet with the pastry disks from the refrigerator. Top each disk with 1 teaspoon Strawberry Compote, ¼ cup thinly sliced strawberries, and some of the Pistachio Crumble.

2 Bake for 25 minutes, until the crust and crumble topping are golden. Let them cool in the pan for 5 minutes before picking them up.

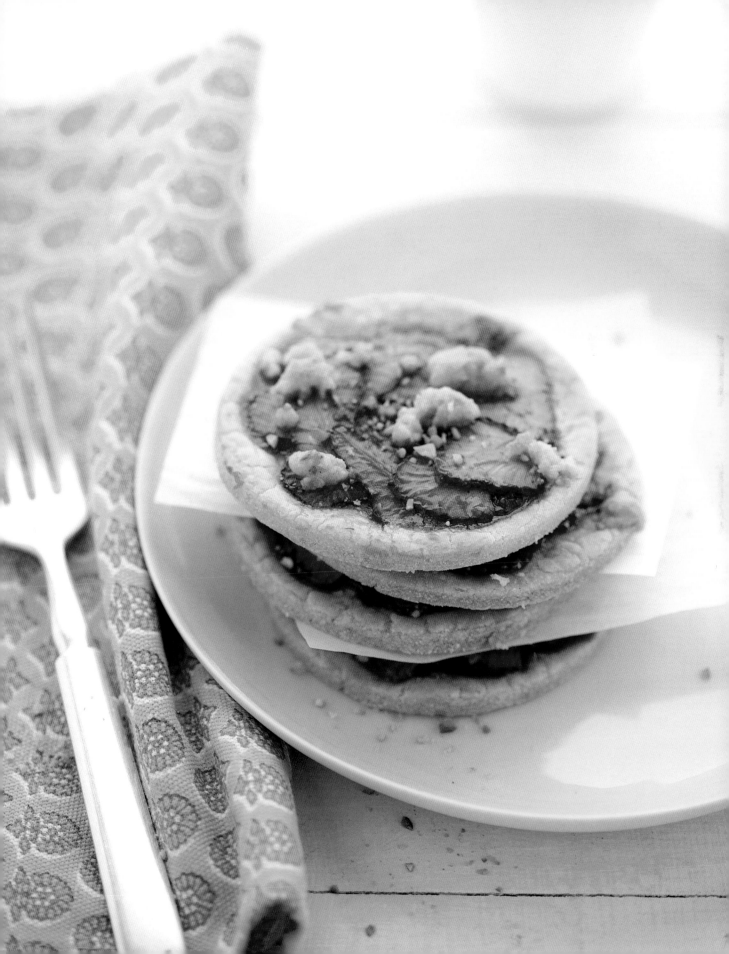

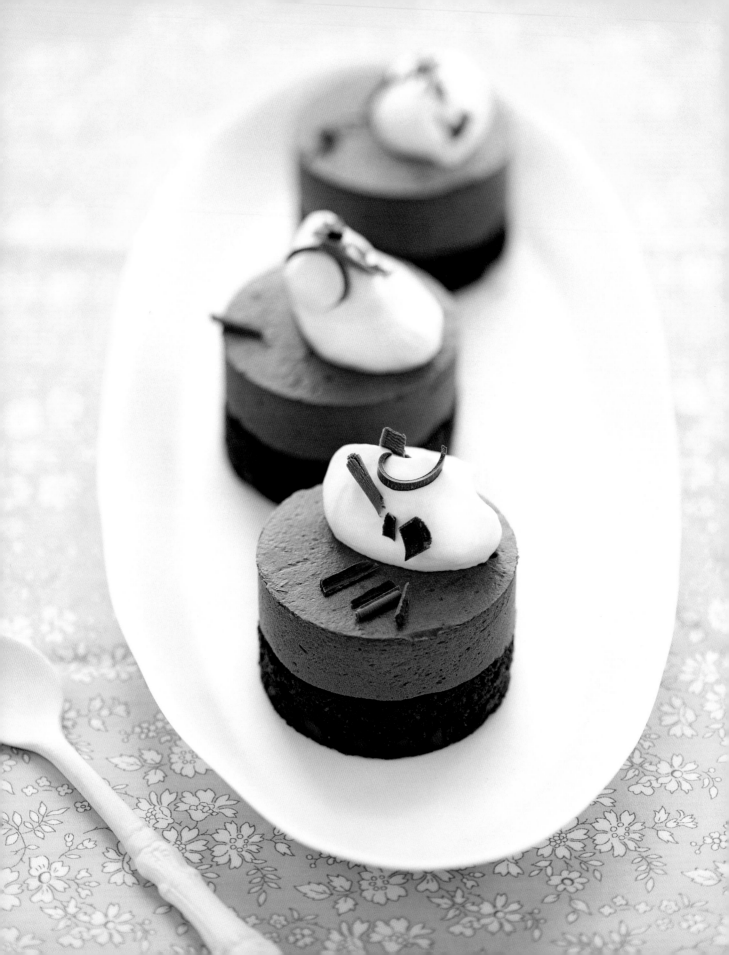

chocolate chunk mousse cakes

THIS WILL SATISFY ANY MIDAFTERNOON chocolate craving. Light chocolate mousse is paired with a dark and intense cake studded with mini chocolate chips.

make the cakes

1 Preheat the oven to 350°F (180°C). Lightly grease a 9-inch springform cake pan and line the bottom with a circle of parchment paper.

2 In a large bowl, whisk together the first five ingredients. In a separate small bowl, whisk together the rest of the ingredients. Add the wet ingredients to the dry and whisk until incorporated.

3 Pour the batter into the greased and lined cake pan. Bake for 18 to 20 minutes, until the center is set. Insert a toothpick to check for doneness. It should come out clean. Remove from the oven and let cool for 15 minutes before inverting onto a cooling rack. Let cool completely.

4 Cut 8 disks of cake using a 2½-inch cookie cutter. Line the inside of 8 (2½-inch) ring molds with a piece of parchment or acetate paper and place them on a baking sheet. Fill each ring mold with a disk of chocolate cake. Proceed with the Chocolate Chunk Mousse.

make the mousse and finish the cakes

1 Place the chopped chocolate in a heatproof bowl. Place the bowl over a pan filled partway with simmering water, but do not let the pan touch the water. Melt the chocolate slowly while stirring. Remove from the heat and let it cool for 10 minutes.

2 Using a stand mixer or a handheld mixer, whip 1½ cups (375 ml) of the heavy cream with the vanilla seeds to soft peaks. Add the melted chocolate and *fleur de sel* to the cream and fold gently until incorporated. Fold in the shaved chocolate.

3 Place the chocolate mousse in a pastry bag fitted with a #5 plain tip. Pipe the mousse all the way to the top of the molds. Using a small offset spatula, flatten the tops.

4 Chill the cakes until the mousse is set. Lift the cakes out of their molds. Remove the parchment or acetate.

5 Using a stand mixer or handheld mixer, whip the remaining ½ cup (125 ml) heavy cream to soft peaks. Top the mousse cakes with a dollop of whipped cream and shaved chocolate.

**CHOCOLATE CHUNK CAKES
(MAKES ONE 9-INCH ROUND CAKE
TO CUT INTO EIGHT 2½-INCH MINI
CAKES)**

1 egg

¼ cup (50 g) natural cane sugar

¼ cup plus 3 tablespoons (105 g)
    unsweetened applesauce

¼ cup (60 ml) olive oil

1 teaspoon vanilla extract

¼ cup (35 g) superfine brown
    rice flour

2 tablespoons quinoa flour

2 tablespoons almond flour

2 teaspoons tapioca starch

2 teaspoons unsweetened cocoa
    powder

¼ teaspoon salt

¼ teaspoon baking soda

2 tablespoons mini chocolate chips

CHOCOLATE CHUNK MOUSSE

12 ounces (340 g) bittersweet
    chocolate, chopped

2 cups (500 ml) heavy cream

½ vanilla bean, split lengthwise
    and seeds scraped

¼ teaspoon *fleur de sel*

1 ounce (30 g) bittersweet
    chocolate, shaved, plus more
    for garnish

coconut & lemon soufflés

MOST PEOPLE THINK THAT MAKING a soufflé is very difficult and time-consuming, when in fact it is not. This soufflé mix can be made 4 hours in advance. Fill the ramekins and leave them at room temperature. Simply bake them when you are ready to serve, and in 10 minutes you will have a tall, hot, and creamy coconut soufflé. Fresh coconut adds a much fresher and nuttier flavor, but you may use dried coconut instead.

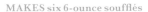

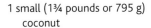

MAKES six 6-ounce soufflés

1 small (1¾ pounds or 795 g) coconut

1 tablespoon (15 grams) unsalted butter, at room temperature, plus more for ramekins

¼ cup (50 g) natural cane sugar, plus more for ramekins

4 egg yolks

2 tablespoons cornstarch

1 tablespoon freshly squeezed lemon juice

2 teaspoons finely grated lemon zest

1 cup (250 ml) unsweetened coconut milk

Pinch of salt

1 teaspoon coconut extract

6 egg whites

¼ teaspoon cream of tartar

Powdered sugar, for dusting

1   Preheat the oven to 325°F (160°C). Crack open and peel the coconut. Grate ½ cup of the flesh and shave the rest with a vegetable peeler. Place the grated coconut on one baking sheet and the shaved coconut on another. Bake for 7 minutes or until golden. This makes more than you need, but the leftovers may be stored in an airtight container for several days.

2   Increase the oven temperature to 400°F (200°C). Using a pastry brush, butter the ramekins in straight vertical motions. Add a generous amount of sugar to one of the ramekins and coat the entire inside of it. Invert and tap out the excess sugar into another ramekin and repeat. Clean the rim of the ramekins with your finger. This coating of butter and sugar will allow the soufflés to rise.

3   In a medium bowl, whisk together the egg yolks and ¼ cup sugar. Add the cornstarch, lemon juice, and lemon zest. Whisk until smooth.

4   Heat the coconut milk and salt in a medium saucepan and bring it to a low simmer over medium-high heat. Pour it into the egg yolk mixture while constantly whisking so that the eggs do not curdle. Return the tempered mixture to the saucepan and cook until it thickens, about 1 minute. Transfer the custard into a clean bowl and add the ½ cup toasted grated coconut and coconut extract.

5   Whip the egg whites with the cream of tartar until they are stiff but not dry. Fold one-third of the whipped whites into the warm custard base. Fold until all the whites have been incorporated and the base is light. Gently fold in the remaining whites without deflating the batter.

6   Spoon the soufflé mixture into the ramekins. Fill them almost to the top. Bake for 8 to 10 minutes, until puffed and golden. Dust with powdered sugar and serve immediately, garnished with toasted coconut shavings.

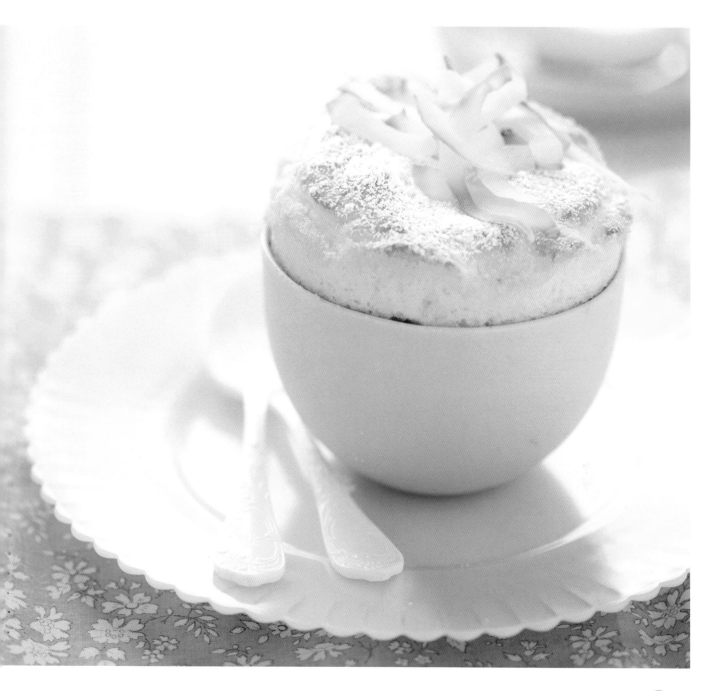

HOW TO OPEN A FRESH COCONUT

To open a fresh coconut, drill two holes on the bottom of the fruit where the dark spots appear. Drain the water. Wrap the coconut in a kitchen towel and place it on a hard surface. Hit it with a hammer until the first crack appears. Hit it again along the crack line. Continue until it opens. Insert a knife in between the shell and the flesh and move it around to release the flesh. Peel the skin with a vegetable peeler. Rinse the coconut. It is ready to eat.

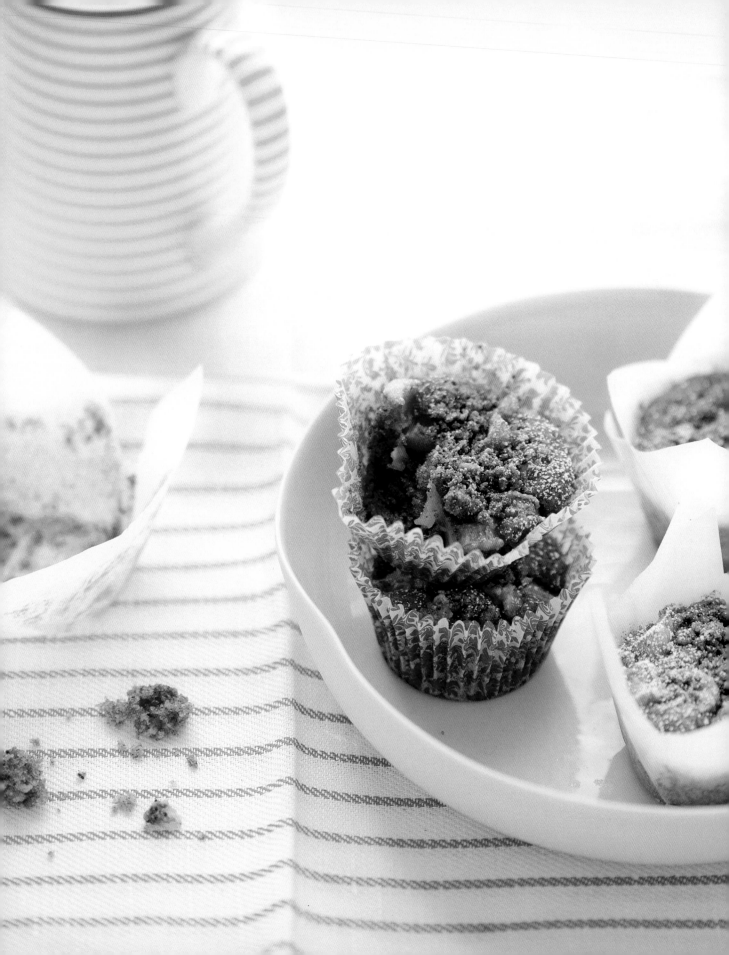

rhubarb & buckwheat crumble cakes

I RECENTLY LEARNED THAT BUCKWHEAT IS not a grain but rather the seed of a plant that is related to rhubarb. I wonder if this is the reason why rhubarb and buckwheat taste perfect together. These cakes are slightly sour and earthy. We like to eat them for breakfast with homemade Strawberry Compote (page 200).

MAKES 12 cakes

make the crumble

In a medium bowl, whisk together the first six ingredients. Add the butter and work it into the flour with your fingers until a crumbly mixture is achieved. Refrigerate the crumble while preparing the dough. You only need ½ cup of the crumble for the cakes; you may freeze the rest of the crumble in a freezer bag for up to 1 month.

make the cakes

1 In a small bowl, combine the rhubarb and cane sugar. Let stand at room temperature for 30 minutes. Add 1 tablespoon of superfine brown rice flour and toss to coat.

2 Preheat the oven to 350°F (180°C). In the bowl of a stand mixer, cream together the butter, powdered sugar, vanilla extract, and lemon zest on medium speed until light. Add the egg and applesauce and mix to combine.

3 In a smaller bowl, whisk together the ½ cup superfine brown rice flour, buckwheat flour, tapioca starch, salt, and baking soda. Add to the butter and sugar mixture and beat until the batter comes together.

4 Line the cups of a muffin pan with baking papers and divide the batter among them. Top with the rhubarb mixture and ½ cup (90 g) of the Buckwheat Crumble. Bake for 22 minutes or until golden. Let the cakes cool in the pan for a few minutes. Transfer them to a rack and let them cool completely.

BUCKWHEAT CRUMBLE

¼ cup (50 g) light brown sugar

2 tablespoons buckwheat flour

2 tablespoons superfine brown rice flour

2 tablespoons potato starch

1 tablespoon almond flour

⅛ teaspoon salt

3 tablespoons (45 g) unsalted butter, at room temperature, cut into pieces

RHUBARB AND BUCKWHEAT CAKES

6 ounces (170 g) rhubarb, cut into ¼-inch pieces

1 tablespoon natural cane sugar

½ cup plus 1 tablespoon (80 g) superfine brown rice flour

1 stick (8 tablespoons or 110 g) unsalted butter, at room temperature

¾ cup (90 g) powdered sugar, sifted

1 teaspoon vanilla extract

1 teaspoon finely grated lemon zest

1 egg, at room temperature

¼ cup (60 g) unsweetened applesauce

2 tablespoons buckwheat flour

2 tablespoons tapioca starch

½ teaspoon salt

½ teaspoon baking soda

roasted apricots with rosemary-lemon ice cream

I LOVE THE COMBINATION OF ROASTED stone fruits and fresh herbs, perfect to serve on top of ice cream or yogurt. Here I've put the herb—rosemary—in the buttermilk ice cream, which is served over roasted apricots.

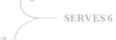

SERVES 6

ROSEMARY-LEMON ICE CREAM

3 tablespoons chopped fresh rosemary

1 tablespoon finely grated lemon zest

⅛ teaspoon salt

¾ cup (150 g) superfine sugar

¼ cup (60 ml) freshly squeezed lemon juice

12 ounces (340 g) crème fraîche or heavy cream

½ cup (125 ml) full-fat buttermilk

ROASTED APRICOTS

3 tablespoons natural cane sugar

1 vanilla bean, split lengthwise and seeds scraped

1 tablespoon freshly grated lemon zest

1 pound (450 g) apricots, halved and pitted

2 tablespoons finely chopped unsalted natural pistachios

make the ice cream

1   Mix the rosemary, lemon zest, salt, and ¼ cup (50 g) of the superfine sugar in a mortar and pestle. You could do it in a food processor, but it will not be the same. Bruise the rosemary until fragrant. Add the lemon juice and let the mixture stand for 30 minutes.

2   Transfer the mixture to a larger bowl and add the crème fraîche, buttermilk, and remaining ½ cup sugar. Whisk to combine. Strain through a fine-mesh sieve into a clean bowl. Churn in an ice cream machine according to the manufacturer's instructions. Transfer to a freezer-safe container and freeze for at least 2 hours before serving.

roast the apricots

1   Preheat the oven to 450°F (230°C). Combine the sugar, vanilla seeds, and lemon zest in a bowl. Rub the mixture between your fingers to combine and to release the oil in the zest.

2   Place the apricots in a baking dish, sprinkle the sugar mixture over the apricots, and bake for 5 to 8 minutes, until the sugar begins to caramelize. Serve warm, topped with the Rosemary-Lemon Ice Cream and chopped pistachios.

TIP: Try this ice cream with fresh tarragon instead of rosemary, and serve it with cooked cherries instead of the roasted apricots.

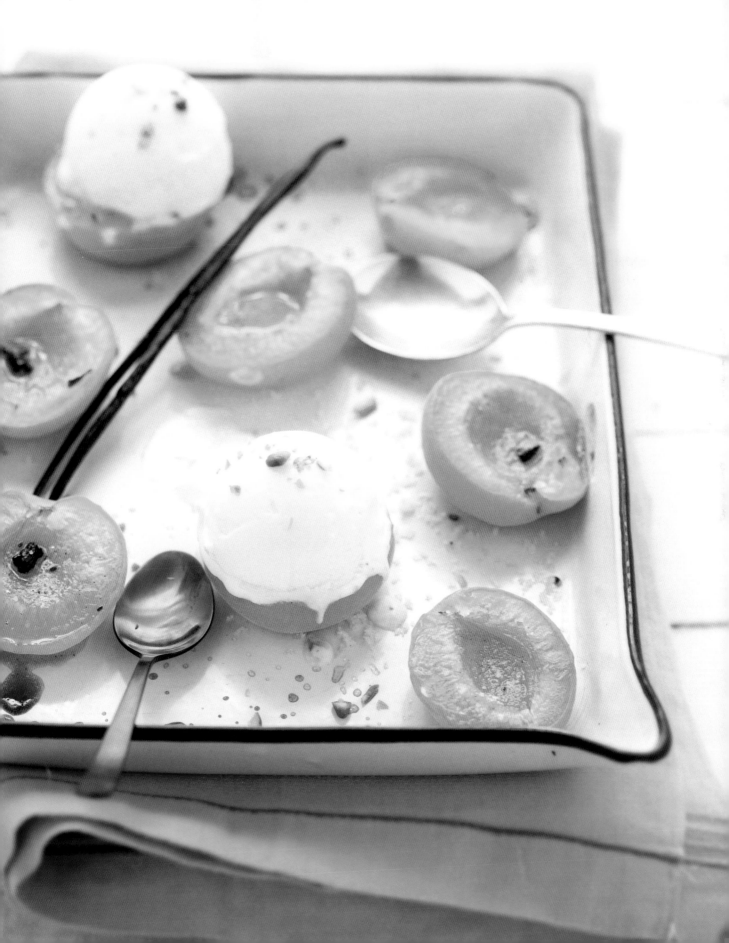

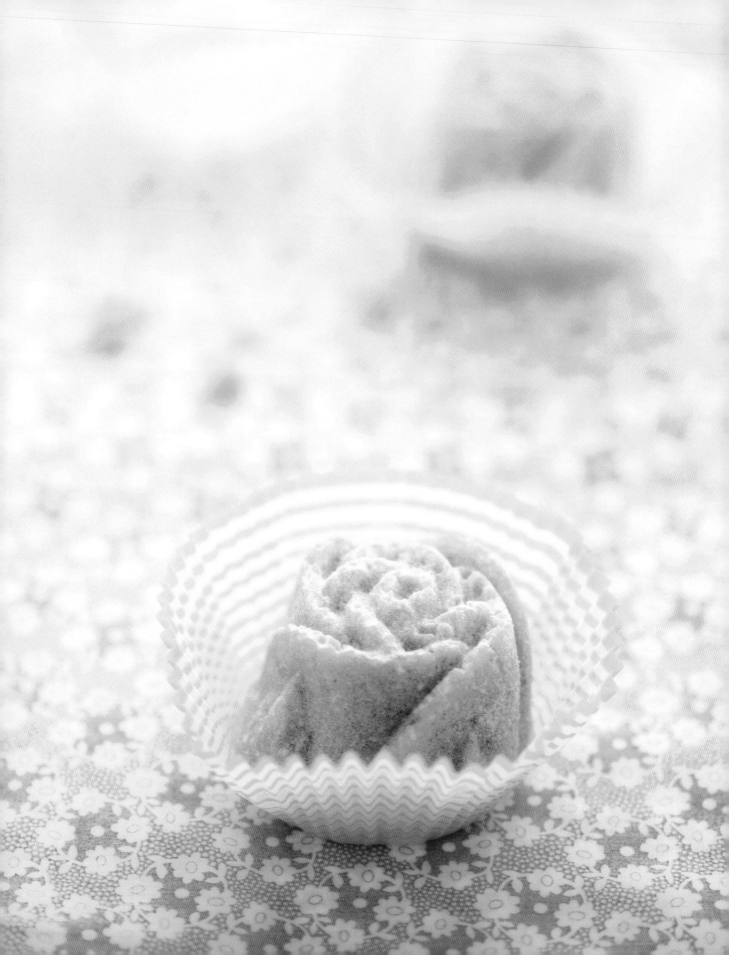

pistachio-rose cakes

THESE ARE THE PERFECT GLUTEN- AND dairy-free little tea cakes. You can bake them in any mold you like, but I love them in rose-shaped Bundt molds, especially during spring. I use really bright green unsalted pistachios that I purchase when I go back home to Europe, which give the cakes' interiors an intense green color.

———— MAKES 12 rose-shaped mini Bundt cakes or muffin-size cakes

1 Preheat the oven to 350°F (180°C). Combine the pistachios, sugar, and lemon zest in a food processor. Pulse until the mixture turns into a fine powder, about 1 minute. Scrape down the sides of the bowl.

2 Add the eggs, coconut milk, and olive oil to the food processor. Pulse to combine. Add the superfine brown rice flour, potato starch, baking powder, and salt and pulse until the batter comes together. Scrape the sides of the bowl to avoid any unmixed chunks. It will be a pourable batter.

3 Transfer the batter to a measuring cup or bowl with a spout. Grease 12 small molds with oil or nonstick spray. Fill the molds halfway. Bake for 18 to 20 minutes, until a toothpick inserted in the center comes out clean. Let the cakes cool in the molds for 10 minutes.

4 Remove the cakes from the molds and dust them with superfine sugar while still warm. The cakes will keep in the refrigerator for up to 3 days. They actually get moister the next day. They may also be stored in the freezer for up to 1 month.

½ cup (80 g) unsalted natural pistachios

¾ cup (150 g) natural cane sugar

1 tablespoon finely grated lemon zest

2 eggs

⅓ cup (80 ml) unsweetened coconut milk

⅓ cup (80 ml) olive oil

½ cup (70 g) superfine brown rice flour

¼ cup (40 g) potato starch

¾ teaspoon baking powder

½ teaspoon salt

Superfine sugar, for dusting

strawberry & amaretti crisps
with mascarpone cream

YOU MIGHT HAVE NOTICED THAT DIFFERENT recipes offer slightly different methods of making crumble toppings. Some call for melted butter, others for diced cold butter, and still others rely on the creaming method. When baking a crumble or a tart crust that contains butter, the butter in the dough should always be cold before going in the oven. This will result in a crisper and lighter topping. So whichever method you begin with, I recommend that the crumble be baked when cold.

Amaretti cookies can be found in specialty shops and Italian markets, especially during the holiday season. If you cannot find them, you can still make this crumble topping by substituting ½ cup (50 g) of almond flour and 2 teaspoons of natural cane sugar for the cookies.

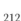

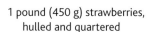 MAKES six 4-ounce ramekins

1 pound (450 g) strawberries, hulled and quartered

¼ cup plus 3 tablespoons (95 g) natural cane sugar

1 vanilla bean, split lengthwise and seeds scraped

4 small (1½ ounces or 45 g) amaretti cookies

⅓ cup (45 g) superfine brown rice flour

⅓ cup (40 g) tapioca starch

¼ cup (30 g) slivered blanched almonds

¼ teaspoon almond extract

¼ teaspoon baking powder

⅛ teaspoon salt

1 stick (8 tablespoons or 110 g) cold unsalted butter, cut into ½-inch cubes

2 teaspoons cornstarch

½ cup (125 ml) heavy cream

4 ounces (110 g) mascarpone cheese

1 Preheat the oven to 350°F (180°C). In a large bowl, toss together the strawberries, 2 tablespoons of the sugar, and vanilla seeds. Allow to macerate for 15 minutes while preparing the topping.

2 Coarsely crumble the amaretti in a food processor. Add ¼ cup of the sugar, superfine brown rice flour, tapioca starch, slivered almonds, almond extract, baking powder, and salt. Pulse to combine. Add the cold butter and pulse three times, until a crumbly dough forms.

3 By now, the strawberries will have released some of their juices. Add the cornstarch to the bowl and toss to combine. Fill the ramekins with the strawberry mixture and top with the crumble.

4 Bake for 25 minutes, until the filling is bubbly and the topping is golden brown. Let the ramekins cool for a few minutes before serving.

5 Using a stand mixer or handheld mixer, whip the heavy cream, mascarpone, and remaining 1 tablespoon sugar together. Top the crisps with a dollop of the cream and serve.

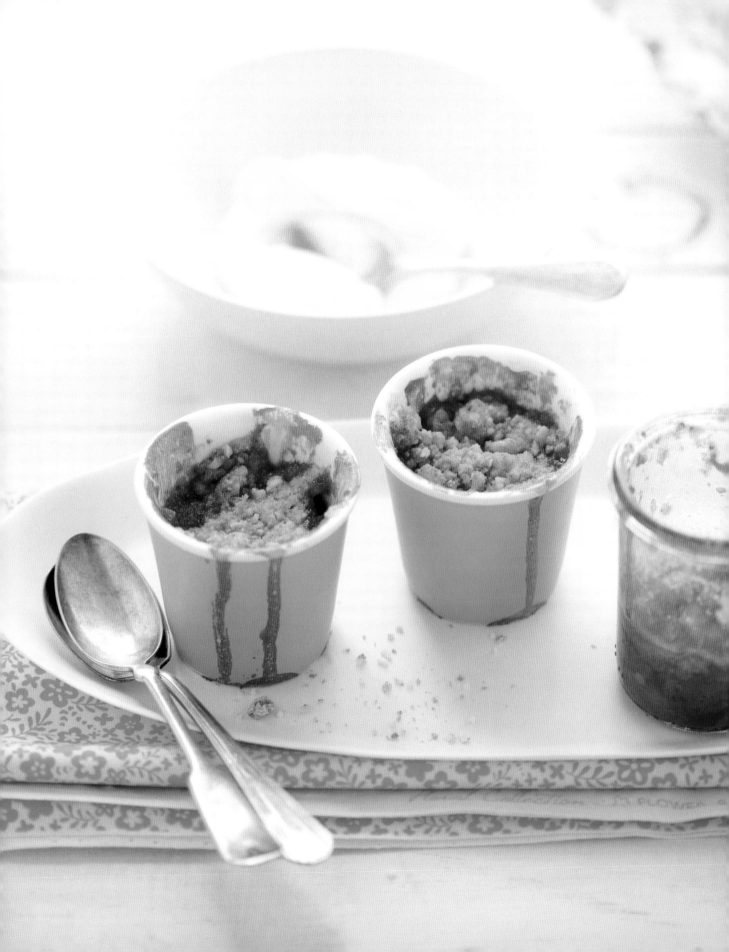

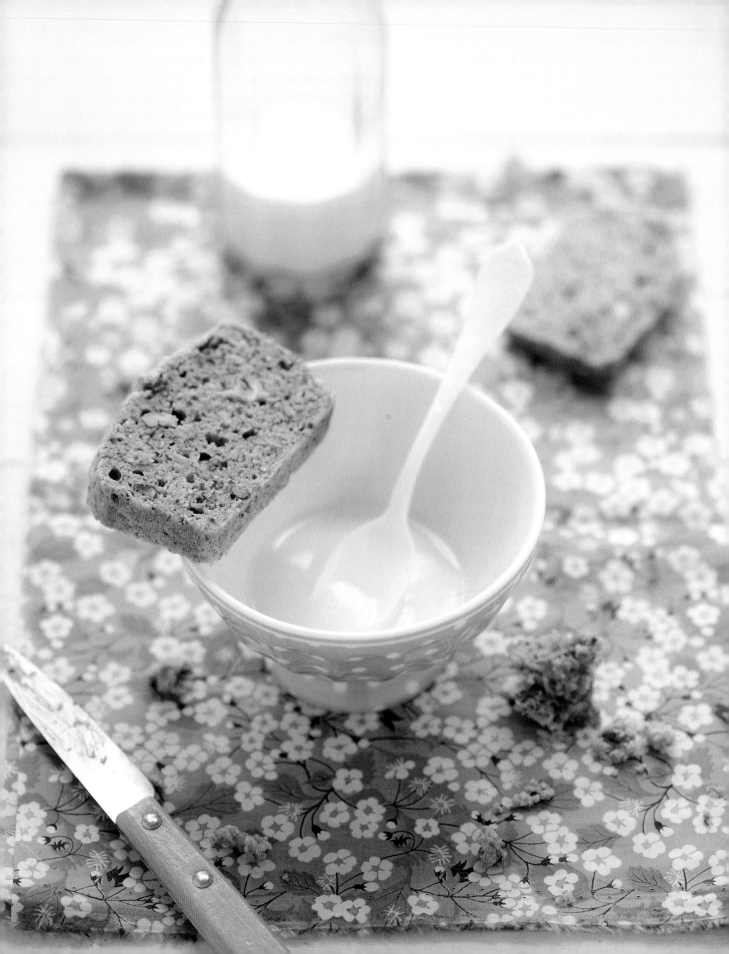

banana, carrot & quinoa bread

THIS QUICK BREAD RECIPE REQUIRES ONLY two bowls and a whisk, which means that my children are right next to me, folding away, whenever I make it. It is another gluten- and dairy-free recipe loaded with nutrients, so a slice usually ends up in their lunch boxes. I love mine with a little bit of coconut oil spread over the top.

———————————————————————— MAKES one 8½ by 4½-inch loaf or 18 muffins

1   Preheat the oven to 350°F (180°C). In a medium bowl, whisk together the banana puree, eggs, sugar, olive oil, and vanilla extract.

2   In a large bowl, whisk together the quinoa flour, superfine brown rice flour, almond flour, tapioca starch, salt, baking soda, and ground cinnamon.

3   Add the wet ingredients to the dry and mix until incorporated. Fold in the pecans and carrots. Pour the batter into a greased loaf pan or muffin cups. Bake for 45 to 55 minutes for the loaf pan or 15 minutes for the muffins. To check doneness, insert a wooden skewer in the middle, and if it comes out clean, they are done. Let cool in the pan for 20 minutes and then invert onto a cooling rack. Cool completely before slicing the loaf.

1½ cups (300 g) mashed banana puree, from about 3 ripe bananas

3 eggs

¾ cup (150 g) natural cane sugar

¾ cup (185 ml) olive oil

2 teaspoons vanilla extract

½ cup (70 g) quinoa flour

½ cup (70 g) superfine brown rice flour

½ cup (50 g) almond flour

3 tablespoons tapioca starch

½ teaspoon salt

½ teaspoon baking soda

¼ teaspoon ground cinnamon

½ cup (50 g) chopped pecans

¾ cup (75 g) grated carrots

buttermilk & honeyed almond crunch ice cream sandwiches

BUTTERMILK, HONEY, AND ALMONDS make these ice cream sandwiches delicate and—why not?—messy. The Honey Lace Cookies are great on their own, too, as after-dinner petits fours.

SERVES 8

HONEY LACE COOKIES
(MAKES 18 COOKIES)

¼ stick (2 tablespoons or 30 g) unsalted butter

2 tablespoons light brown sugar

1½ tablespoons honey

1 tablespoon superfine brown rice flour

1 tablespoon almond flour

⅛ teaspoon salt

HONEY CANDIED ALMONDS

1 cup (120 g) slivered blanched almonds

2 tablespoons honey

2 tablespoons light brown sugar

1 tablespoon (15 g) unsalted butter

BUTTERMILK ICE CREAM

1 cup (250 ml) whole milk

½ cup (100 g) natural cane sugar

4 strips lemon zest

5 egg yolks

1½ cups (375 ml) heavy cream

½ cup (125 ml) full-fat buttermilk

Honey Candied Almonds

make the cookies

1   Combine the first three ingredients in a small saucepan and cook over medium-high heat until melted. When the mixture comes to a boil, continue cooking for 1 minute, stirring once. Remove from the heat.

2   Add the superfine brown rice flour, almond flour, and salt and stir to combine. Pour this mixture into a bowl and cool until it is pliable.

3   Preheat the oven to 350°F (180°C). Roll ½-inch balls and place them 3 inches apart on baking sheets lined with parchment paper or silicone mats.

4   Bake for 6 to 7 minutes. They will spread and turn golden brown. Let the cookies cool completely on the baking sheet, then gently lift them off.

5   Store the cookies at room temperature in an airtight container. Do not refrigerate them or they will become soft and soggy.

make the candied almonds

1   Preheat the oven to 350°F (180°C). Evenly spread the almonds on a baking sheet and bake them for 5 to 8 minutes or until lightly golden but not too dark.

2   Combine the honey, brown sugar, and butter in a small saucepan. Cook it for 2 minutes over medium-high heat. Remove from the heat. Add the toasted almonds and stir to coat them.

3   Spread the mixture on a baking sheet lined with parchment paper or a silicone mat. Bake until the nuts caramelize, 8 to 10 minutes. Let the mixture cool completely and then coarsely chop it. Store in an airtight container.

make the ice cream

1   Combine the milk, ¼ cup of the sugar, and lemon zest in a small saucepan. Heat over medium-high heat until it comes to a low boil.

2   Meanwhile, whisk together the egg yolks, remaining ¼ cup sugar, and heavy cream in a bowl until smooth. Add the warm milk mixture while constantly whisking. Return the mixture to the saucepan and cook,

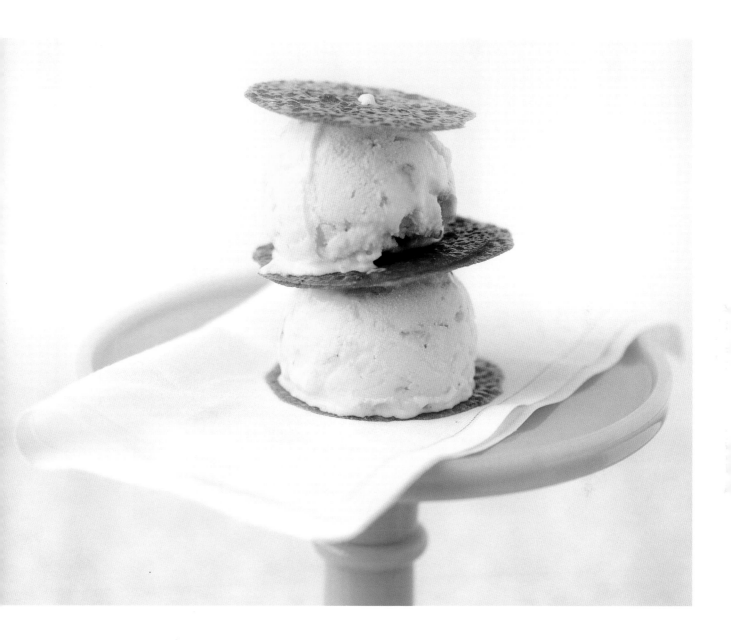

stirring constantly, over medium heat until it starts to thicken, about
3 minutes. Do not let it boil or it will curdle.

   3   Strain the mixture through a fine-mesh sieve into a clean bowl.
Add the buttermilk and stir to combine. Place the bowl over an ice bath
and cool to room temperature, stirring occasionally. Cover the bowl with
plastic wrap and refrigerate for at least 4 hours.

   4   Churn the ice cream base in an ice cream machine according to the
manufacturer's instructions. When it is done, mix in the chopped Honey
Candied Almonds, transfer to a freezer-safe container, and freeze until hard.

   5   Make ice cream sandwiches using the Honey Lace Cookies.

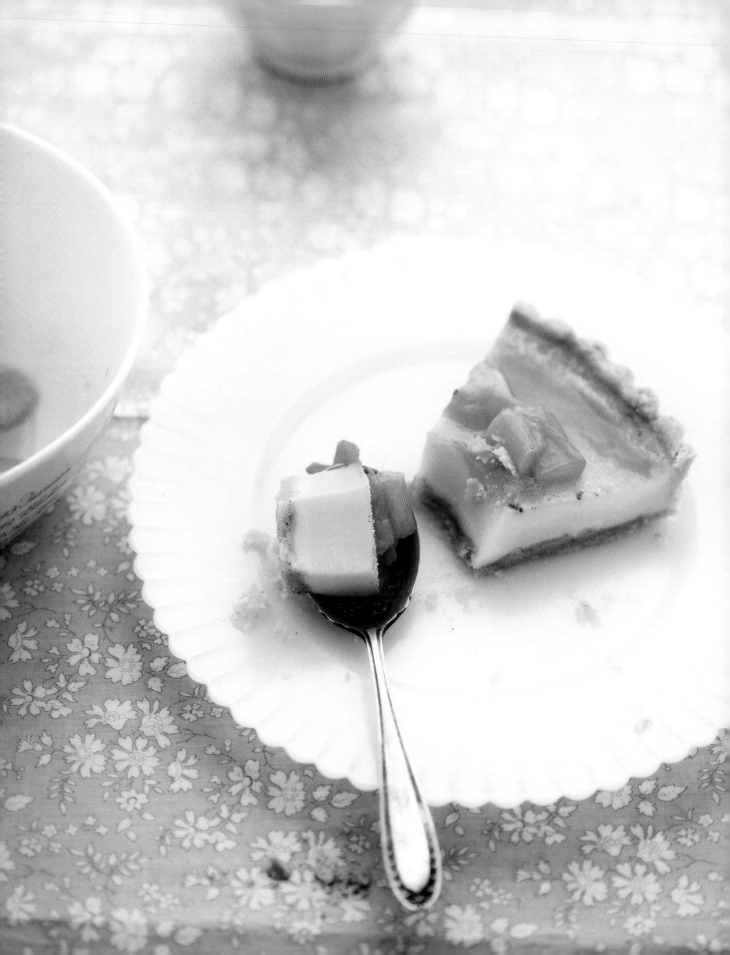

vanilla & orange flower water custard tart

THE BEST-SELLING TART IN MY FAMILY'S pastry shop is *pastel de arroz*. It has always been my favorite. It's a cinnamon-scented custard in a puff pastry shell that crumbles into a thousand buttery flakes. I remember eating them straight out of the oven—so creamy and crisp. This recipe is inspired by the *pastel de arroz* that I knew as a child. It is flavored with vanilla bean seeds and orange flower water, which can be found in many specialty and Middle Eastern markets. You could also flavor it with cardamom, cinnamon, and lemon zest. The possibilities are endless. Serve this with the Rhubarb Compote on page 192, if you like.

MAKES one 9-inch tart

make the crust

1 Combine the first five ingredients in a food processor and pulse to aerate. Add the cold butter and pulse ten times or until the butter is cut into pea-size pieces.

2 In a small bowl, whisk together the egg yolk and 3 tablespoons ice water. Add the mixture to the food processor and mix. It will not form a dough. Simply press the dough between your fingers to see if it holds together. If not, add 1 more tablespoon of ice water at a time.

3 Transfer the dough to a work surface, knead it a couple of times, and form it into a disk. Wrap it in plastic wrap, flatten it, and refrigerate for 1 hour.

4 Dust your (preferably cold) work surface with a little bit of superfine brown rice flour. Roll the dough to a ¼- to ⅛-inch thickness. Fill a 9-inch tart mold with the dough and cut off the excess. The dough tends to crack a bit, but don't worry; simply pinch it back together. Chill for 30 minutes.

prepare the custard and bake the tart

1 Preheat the oven to 425°F (220°C). In a medium bowl, whisk together the eggs, sugar, cornstarch, vanilla seeds, and orange flower water until smooth. Add the heavy cream and milk and whisk.

2 Place the tart mold on a baking sheet. Pour the custard into the mold.

3 Bake for 10 minutes, reduce the oven heat to 350°F (180°C), and bake for another 25 to 25 minutes or until the custard is set and lightly golden.

4 Cool the tart on a cooling rack for 20 minutes before cutting. Serve warm or at room temperature.

PASTRY CRUST

¾ cup (105 g) superfine brown rice flour, plus more for dusting

¼ cup (40 g) potato starch

¼ cup (35 g) sorghum flour

4 teaspoons natural cane sugar

⅛ teaspoon salt

1 stick (8 tablespoons or 110 g) cold unsalted butter, cut into ½-inch cubes

1 egg yolk

3 to 5 tablespoons ice water

VANILLA AND ORANGE FLOWER WATER CUSTARD

4 eggs

½ cup (100 g) natural cane sugar

¼ cup (30 g) cornstarch

1 vanilla bean, split lengthwise and seeds scraped

1 tablespoon orange flower water

1 cup (250 ml) heavy cream

½ cup (125 ml) whole milk

roasted strawberry & coconut milk sherbet

WHEN THE FIRST WARM DAYS OF SPRING roll around, one of our favorite activities is to go strawberry picking. It takes me back to my own childhood, when we picked strawberries from my grandmother's garden. Besides eating them fresh, I like to roast them and serve them with anything from yogurt to my morning porridge. Their flavor becomes deeper and sweeter with roasting.

This makes a small batch, but it can easily be doubled to fit a standard 1-quart ice cream machine.

SERVES 4

1 pound (450 g) strawberries, hulled and halved

¼ cup plus 3 tablespoons (85 g) natural cane sugar

½ vanilla bean, split lengthwise and seeds scraped

¾ cup (185 ml) unsweetened coconut milk

1 tablespoon freshly squeezed lemon juice

1 tablespoon kirsch, optional

¼ teaspoon salt

1   Preheat the oven to 300°F (150°C). Combine the strawberries, 3 tablespoons of the sugar, and the vanilla seeds and pod in an 8-inch square baking pan. Bake for 1 hour. The strawberries will release their juices and create a light syrup. Remove the vanilla bean pod and puree the strawberries with their juices. Let cool and reserve.

2   Meanwhile, combine ¼ cup (60 ml) water and the remaining ¼ cup sugar in a small saucepan. Bring to a boil over medium-high heat and cook until the sugar melts. Remove from the heat and let it cool to room temperature.

3   Whisk the cooled strawberry puree and syrup together. Add the coconut milk, lemon juice, kirsch (if using), and salt. Refrigerate for at least 2 hours.

4   Churn the sherbet base in an ice cream machine according to the manufacturer's instructions. Transfer to a freezer-safe container and freeze until solid. Remove the sherbet from the freezer 10 minutes before serving.

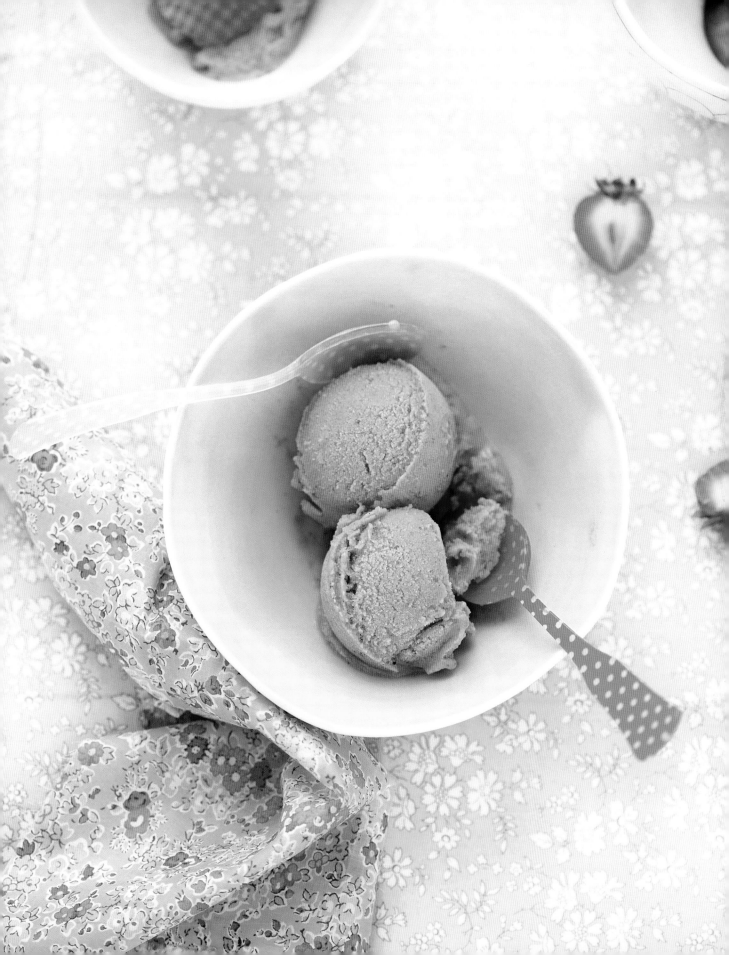

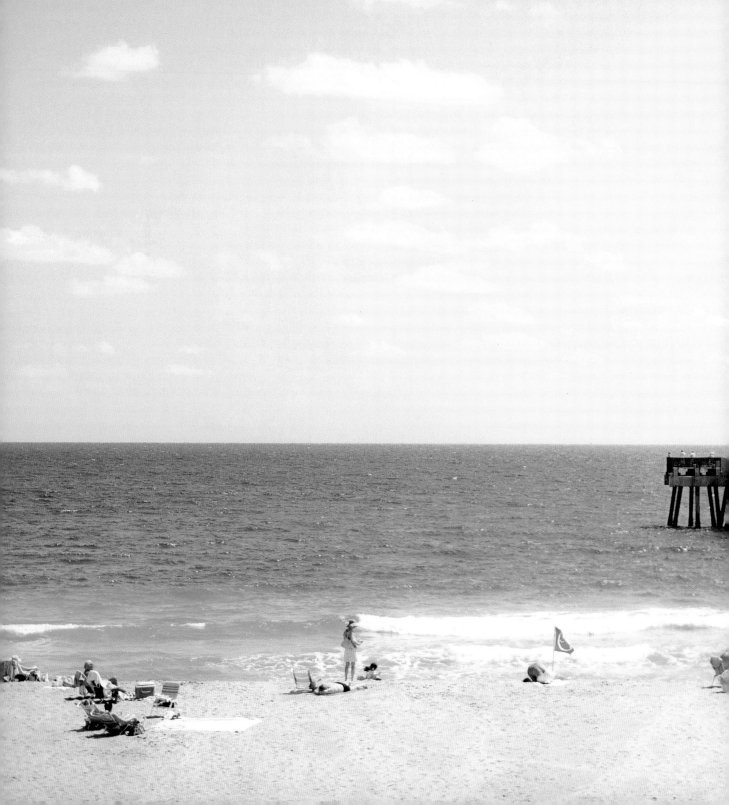

summer

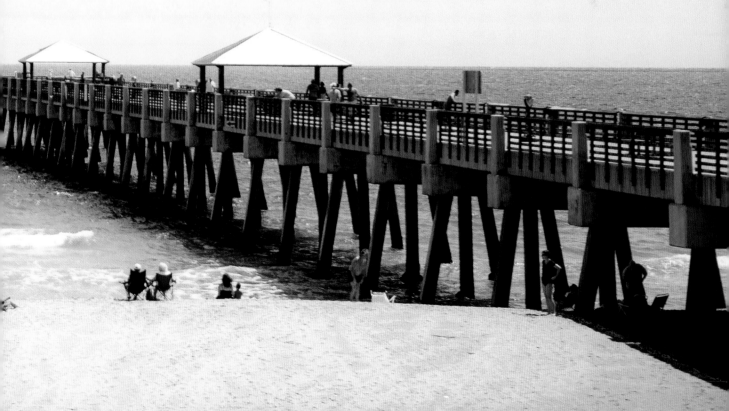

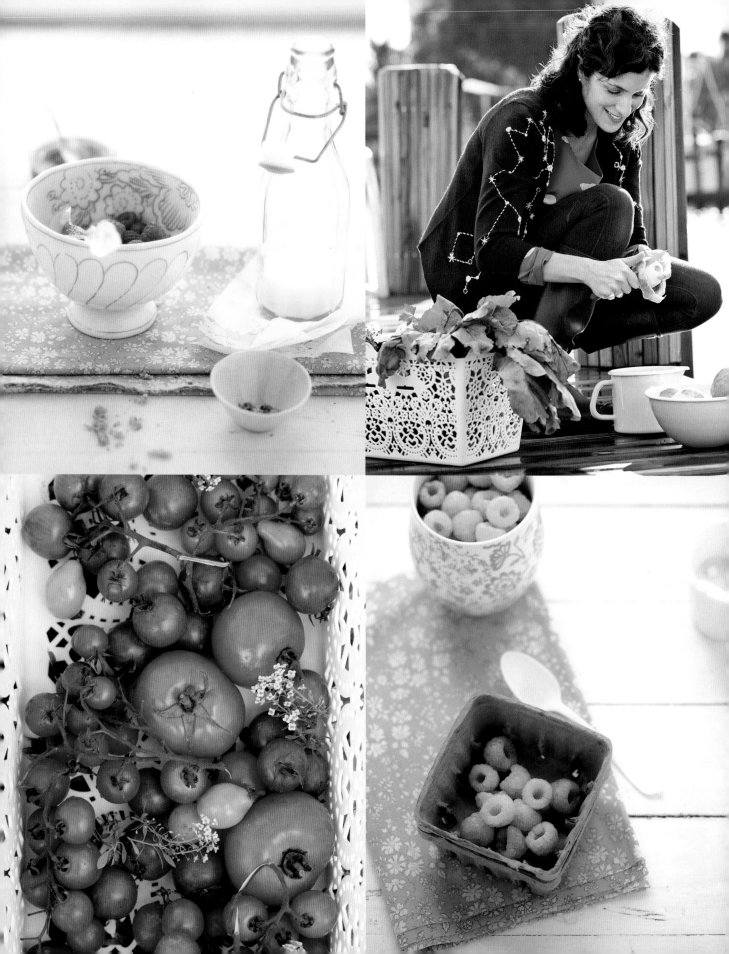

SUMMER
small plates

Heirloom Cherry Tomato Focaccia · *Grilled Corn & Herb Chowder* · *Vegetable* Menestra *with Truffled Polenta* · *Roasted Black Cherry Tomato Soup* · Piperrada, *Ricotta & Tomato Tartlets* · *Potato-and-Egg Salad with Arugula & Chervil Pesto* · *Ivory Lentil, Serrano Ham & Melon Salad* · *Basque Fish Stew (*Marmitako*)* · *Summer Lobster & Apple Salad* · *Chicken, Zucchini & Gruyère Clafoutis* · *Roasted Red Snapper with Potatoes, Shaved Fennel & Shiso* · *Chilled Watermelon, Tomato & Almond Soup* · *Eggplants Stuffed with Millet & Serrano Ham* · *Quinoa Spaghetti with Garlicky Squid & Niçoise Olives* · *Potato, Zucchini & Watercress Tortilla*

IN MY FAMILY, SUMMER IS ALL ABOUT long days at the beach, sun-kissed cheeks, afternoon ice cream sandwiches, and outdoor dinners with grilled fish. Fire and outdoor cooking are a central part of our summer. "Can we go fishing again, Dad?" Jon asks. We hear this all the time, ever since he caught his first pompano last summer. We pack our tiffin box with wedges of Potato, Zucchini & Watercress Tortilla (page 255), Ivory Lentil, Serrano Ham & Melon Salad (page 238), and some watermelon wedges, and we head to Juno Beach for an afternoon of fishing. The children chase after birds, we collect shells, and we hope we will be lucky enough to catch some more pompano to take home.

When I was growing up, our summers officially started on June 23, on the evening of San Juan (St. John's Day). Neighbors and friends spent days gathering old wood, old clothes, and things that needed to be forgotten. We would create bonfires that symbolized new beginnings and the cleansing of bad spirits. It was the celebration of summer solstice. As with all celebrations, there was lots of food—a potluck of sorts with *pintxos* and nibbles.

My approach to entertaining in the summer comes out of this tradition. Gathering friends around an outdoor table in the cool shade, I serve simple, no-fuss meals that focus mainly on summer produce and local-caught fish.

heirloom cherry tomato focaccia

THIS FOCACCIA IS SOFT AND THICK. Top it with small heirloom tomatoes on the vine for a beautiful presentation. Make sure your tomatoes are juicy and plump. If you cannot find heirloom cherry tomatoes, use colorful tomatoes. Slice them and drain them on a paper towel to remove some of their water (too much moisture will make the focaccia soggy and it will not cook thoroughly). Serve this focaccia as a savory snack or as a side for a bowl of soup or salad.

MAKES one 11 by 8½-inch pan

1 tablespoon active dry yeast

¾ to 1 cup (185 to 250 ml) water, heated to 110°F (43°C)

1 teaspoon sugar

2 tablespoons ground chia seeds

3 tablespoons boiling water

1 cup (160 g) potato starch

1 cup (140 g) sorghum flour

½ cup (70 g) millet flour

1½ teaspoons salt

1½ teaspoons freshly ground black pepper

¼ cup (60 ml) olive oil

1 tablespoon honey

1 egg, lightly beaten

12 ounces (340 g) cherry tomatoes

1 teaspoon *fleur de sel*

Fresh basil, for garnish

Fresh oregano, for garnish

1   In a small bowl, whisk together the yeast, ¾ cup (185 ml) warm water, and sugar. Let the yeast activate for 10 minutes. It will be very foamy.

2   In a small bowl, whisk together the ground chia seeds and the boiling water to form a thick paste. Reserve.

3   In the bowl of a stand mixer, using the paddle attachment on medium speed, combine the potato starch, sorghum flour, millet flour, salt, 1 teaspoon of the pepper, 2 tablespoons of the olive oil, honey, egg, yeast mixture, and chia seed paste. Mix for 1 minute. The dough should have the consistency of thick cake batter. Add the reserved warm water if needed.

4   Transfer the dough into a greased 11 by 8½-inch baking pan. Wet your fingers and evenly spread the dough. Cover the pan with a sheet of greased plastic wrap and let the dough ferment for 40 to 50 minutes, until it has doubled in volume. The time will vary depending on the temperature in your kitchen.

5   Preheat the oven to 375°F (190°C). Gently brush the top of the dough with most of the remaining 2 tablespoons olive oil. Place the cherry tomatoes on top. Gently press them into the dough and brush a bit more olive oil on top of them. Sprinkle with the *fleur de sel* and remaining ½ teaspoon black pepper. Bake for 35 to 40 minutes, until light golden and the tomatoes are slightly bursting. Garnish with the fresh herbs.

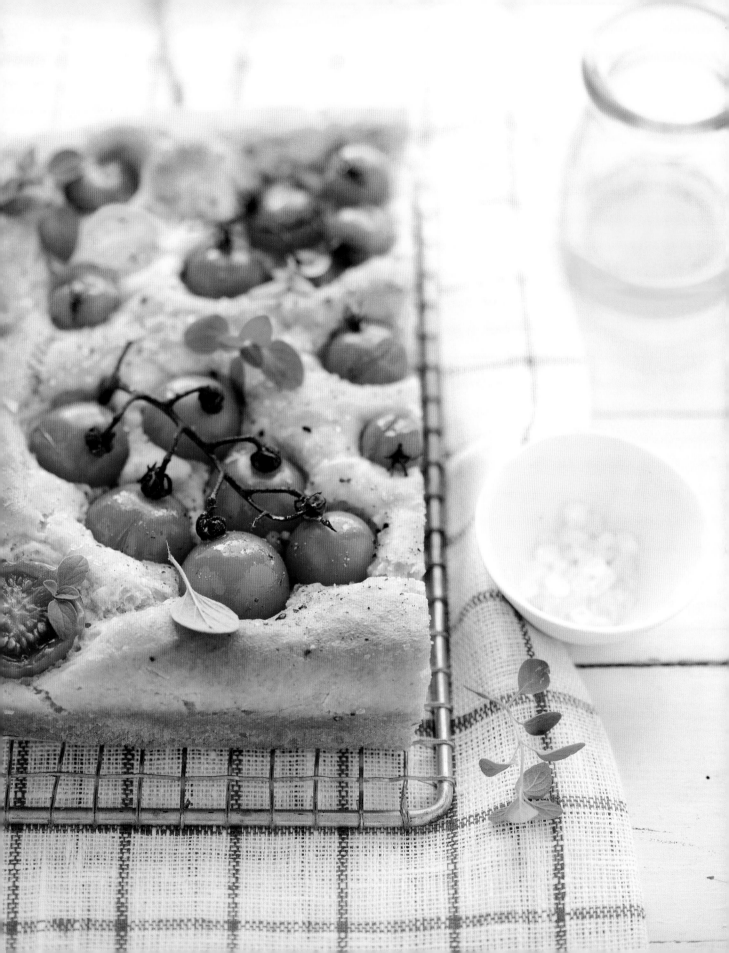

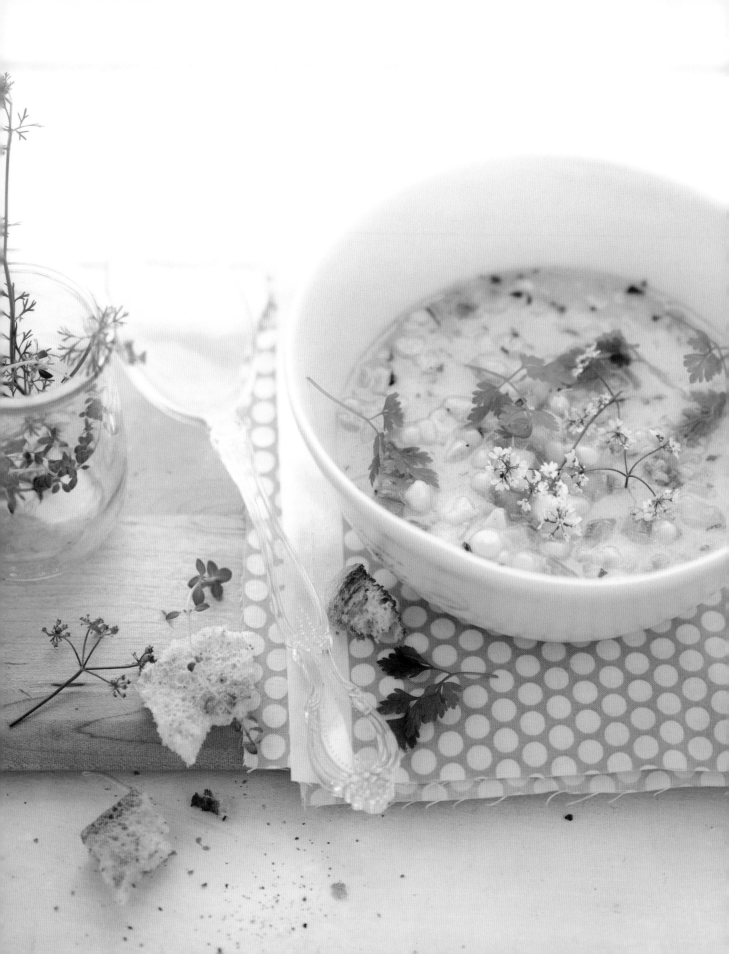

grilled corn & herb chowder

"I CAN'T WAIT TO GO BACK TO THE CORN festival!" Jon says. "That was so much fun." A day spent under the sun with Ferris wheel rides, cotton candy, and grilled corn on the cob. I didn't grow up eating corn. Honestly, it was always considered animal food—grown and harvested mainly to feed the livestock. It was when I came to the United States for the first time that I started to appreciate its sweetness and texture. I love this creamy chowder, with the smoky flavor of grilled corn and cumin combined with the freshness of the cilantro and chervil.

SERVES 4

1   Preheat the grill or a grill pan. Peel and rinse the corn. Grill the corn over medium-high heat, lightly charring the outside. It should take 8 to 10 minutes. Let the corn cool slightly and then cut off the kernels. You should have about 3 cups of grilled kernels.

2   In a medium saucepan, combine the coconut milk, vegetable broth, thyme, and corn kernels. Bring to a simmer over medium-high heat. Turn the heat off and let it steep for 15 minutes.

3   In a large pot, heat the olive oil. Add the garlic, onion, celery, ½ teaspoon of the salt, ½ teaspoon of the black pepper, ground cumin, and ground coriander. Cook the vegetables over medium heat for 5 minutes or until soft but not brown. Add the coconut milk–corn mixture. Bring the soup to a low simmer and cook for 10 minutes. Season with the remaining ½ teaspoon salt and ½ teaspoon black pepper.

4   Add the cilantro and chervil and stir. Serve warm.

4 ears corn

2 cups (500 ml) unsweetened coconut milk

1½ cups (375 ml) vegetable broth

3 sprigs thyme

3 tablespoons olive oil

2 cloves garlic, minced

1 medium yellow onion, diced

2 celery stalks, diced

1 teaspoon salt

1 teaspoon freshly ground black pepper

½ teaspoon ground cumin

½ teaspoon ground coriander

1 tablespoon chopped fresh cilantro

1 tablespoon chopped fresh chervil

FOOD STYLING

I am often asked for food styling tips. The truth is that my approach to food styling is very natural, and everything that I photograph is ready to be eaten. I use very few tricks.

I find that one of the most beautiful ways to dress up a dish is through the addition of garnishes. Herbs, microgreens, different salts, and coarsely ground pepper add texture and color to a dish. However, those garnishes must make sense with the flavors of the dish. I find that herb flowers are delicate, carry the flavor of the leaves, and are easy to grow. So instead of buying packaged herbs, try planting your own in tiny pots that can be kept by a windowsill.

I also pay close attention to the dishes in which I choose to photograph each recipe. Think of how colors complement each other or the texture of the bowl against the food. When food is colorful, I rely on white dishes. Vintage pieces also add a lot of texture and character to a shot.

vegetable *menestra* with truffled polenta

MENESTRA, A MEDLEY OF SEASONAL VEGETABLES that are blanched and then finished in a light broth, is a traditional dish of the region of Navarre, in the Basque Country, where some of the best vegetables of the Iberian Peninsula grow. My aunt Marijo is a master of this dish. She blanches each vegetable separately, coats them in an egg batter, and then quickly sautés them in olive oil. She finishes the vegetables in a light sauce with thin slices of Serrano ham. It's immensely time-consuming to make but amazingly good.

My version is a little bit different. It is inspired by a vegetarian *bollito misto* dish I had a few years ago at the restaurant Rendezvous, in Boston. I serve it with truffled polenta and some shaved Idiazabal cheese.

SERVES 4

4 sprigs thyme

1 small bunch parsley

1 bay leaf

2¼ teaspoons salt

6 small new potatoes

8 ounces (225 g) white asparagus, trimmed, peeled, and cut into 2-inch pieces

8 baby carrots

8 ounces (225 g) green beans, ends trimmed and cut into 2-inch pieces

1 cup (150 g) fava beans (from about 1 pound or 450 g of pods), peeled

1 cup (160 g) quick-cooking polenta

1 tablespoon white truffle oil

1 ounce (30 g) Idiazabal or Parmesan cheese, finely grated, plus more, shaved, for garnish

3 tablespoons olive oil

1 purple spring onion or medium leek, thinly sliced

½ teaspoon freshly ground black pepper

Olive oil, for serving

1 Tie the thyme, parsley, and bay leaf together with some butcher's twine. In a medium saucepan, bring 2 quarts (2 L) water, 1 teaspoon of the salt, and the herbs to a boil over medium-high heat.

2 Place the potatoes in the boiling water, reduce the heat to medium, and cook for 8 to 10 minutes or until the tip of a paring knife goes easily into the center of a potato. Remove the potatoes from the water with a slotted spoon and let them cool. Slice them into ¹/₂-inch-thick rounds.

3 Add the white asparagus to the simmering water. Cook the tips for 7 minutes and the stalks for 8 to 9 minutes. Remove with a slotted spoon and shock in an ice water bath to stop the cooking. When the vegetables are cool, drain on paper towels.

4 Add the carrots to the water and cook for 5 to 7 minutes. Remove with a slotted spoon and shock in an ice water bath. When cool, drain on paper towels.

5 Add the green beans to the water and cook for 5 minutes. Shock in ice water and drain.

6 Finish with the fava beans. Cook them for 1 minute, shock them in ice water, and drain them. Do not discard the cooking water, which by this point has turned into a vegetable broth, as you will use this to cook the polenta.

7 Measure 3¹/₂ cups (875 ml) of the broth used to cook the vegetables. Discard the herbs. If there isn't enough broth, add water to make up the difference.

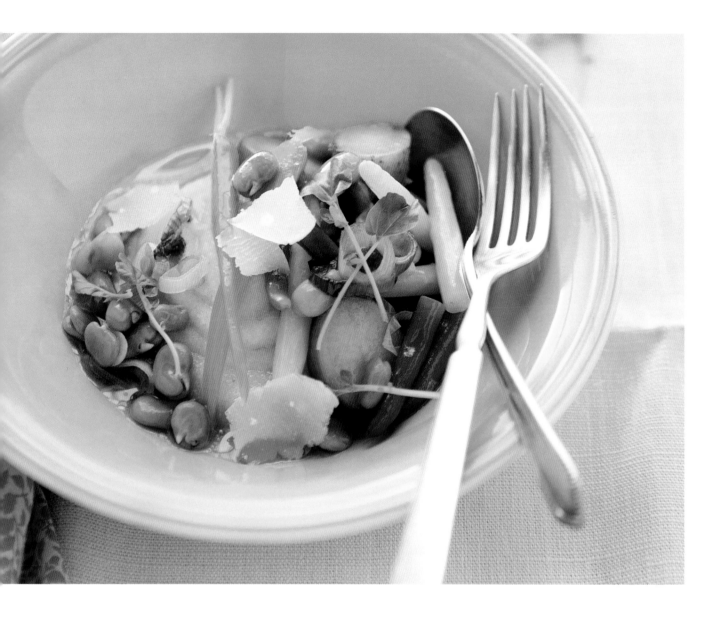

8   Add 3 cups (750 ml) of this liquid to a medium saucepan and bring
it to a boil over medium-high heat. In a steady stream, add the polenta
while whisking. The polenta will thicken in 1 minute. Remove from the
heat and add the truffle oil, grated cheese, and ¾ teaspoon of the salt.
Spoon the cooked polenta into a serving bowl.

9   Heat a large sauté pan over medium-high heat. Add the olive oil,
the sliced spring onion, and all the blanched vegetables. Season with the
remaining ½ teaspoon salt and the black pepper. Toss the vegetables in
the oil for 1 minute, add the remaining ½ cup (125 ml) cooking liquid, and
spoon the mixture over the polenta. Serve with a drizzle of olive oil and
topped with shaved cheese.

roasted black cherry tomato soup

ROASTING TOMATOES WITH SHALLOTS and garlic really brings out their sweetness. Make sure to use ripe tomatoes. If heirloom black cherries are not available, use whatever cherry tomato variety you have—or even larger tomatoes sliced. Larger tomatoes tend to be juicier and will release more juices while roasting. They will take a bit longer to roast and will possibly yield a soup that is not as thick. Adjust the amount of coconut milk to achieve the desired consistency.

SERVES 4

3 pounds (1.5 kg) black cherry tomatoes, halved

2 medium shallots, diced

4 cloves garlic, crushed but left whole

6 sprigs thyme

¼ cup (60 ml) olive oil

1 teaspoon salt

1 teaspoon freshly ground black pepper

1 to 1½ cups (250 to 375 ml) unsweetened coconut milk

¼ cup (60 ml) whole-milk plain yogurt

Fresh herbs of your choice, for garnish

1 Preheat the oven to 400°F (200°C). Divide the tomatoes, shallots, garlic, and thyme between two large rimmed baking sheets. Drizzle with the olive oil and sprinkle the salt and pepper on top. Toss the vegetables to coat them with the oil.

2 Roast for 25 minutes, until the vegetables have softened, released their juices, and begun to caramelize. Remove the baking sheets from the oven and discard the thyme leaves. Reserve a few cherry tomatoes to use as garnish.

3 Transfer the vegetables and their juices to a food processor and puree in two batches. Strain the puree into a large pot through a medium-mesh sieve that will catch the skin and seeds. Add the coconut milk and heat until it is warm all the way through. Adjust seasoning if necessary.

4 Serve warm or at room temperature with a dollop of yogurt and fresh herbs. The soup will keep in the refrigerator for up to 3 days.

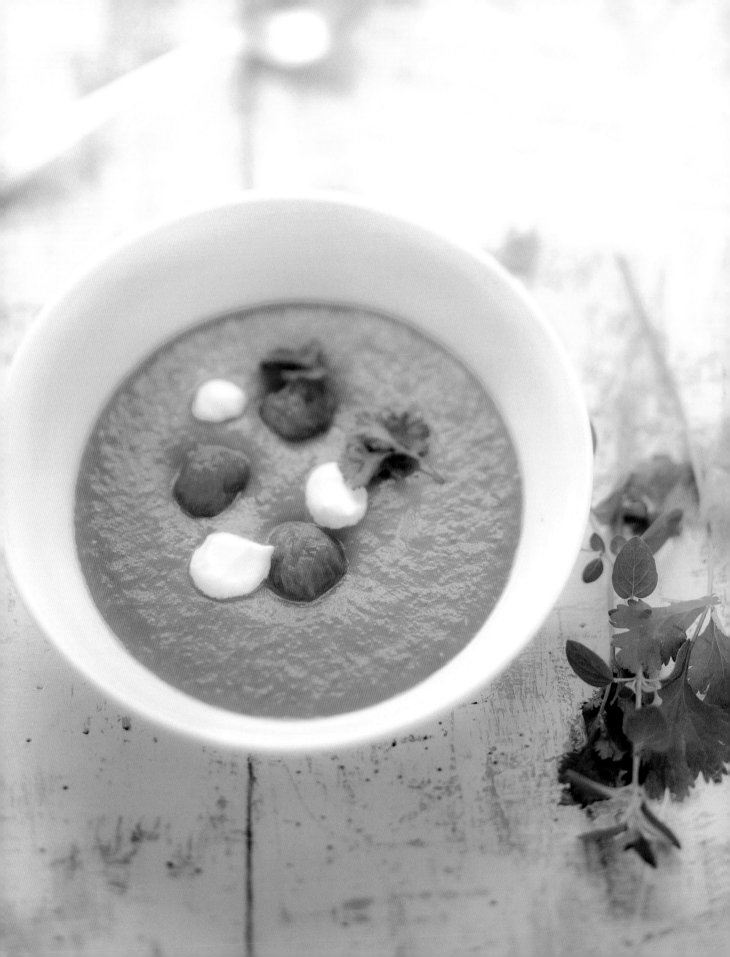

piperrada, ricotta & tomato tartlets

"I DON'T FEEL LIKE COOKING TONIGHT," my mom said one evening after we came back from the beach. It was Saturday afternoon, and we had just spent two hours stuck in traffic. Our cheeks were rosy from the sun and sand still stuck to our knees. "How about peppers with fried eggs?" *Piperrada* is one of my favorite summertime Basque dishes. It literally means "bunch of peppers" and consists of onions, garlic, and lots of sweet bell peppers slowly cooked and lightly caramelized. It is often served with eggs that are poached right in the pan with the peppers.

These are flaky tartlets filled with caramelized peppers and ricotta and bursting cherry tomatoes.

MAKES one 9-inch tart or six 4-inch tartlets

PASTRY CRUST

½ cup (70 g) superfine brown rice flour, plus more for dusting

¼ cup (40 g) potato starch

¼ cup (30 g) amaranth flour

⅓ cup (35 g) almond flour

½ teaspoon salt

½ teaspoon freshly ground black pepper

1 stick (8 tablespoons or 110 g) cold unsalted butter, cut into ½-inch cubes

1 egg, lightly beaten

1 to 2 tablespoons ice water

PIPERRADA, RICOTTA, AND TOMATO FILLING

3 tablespoons olive oil, plus more for drizzling

1 medium yellow onion, thinly sliced

2 cloves garlic, minced

3 medium sweet bell peppers (assorted colors), cut into 2-inch thin strips

2 sprigs thyme

1 teaspoon salt, plus more for garnish

make the crust

1   Combine the first six ingredients in a food processor. Pulse twice to aerate them. Add the cold butter and pulse ten times, until the butter is cut into pea-size pieces.

2   Whisk together the egg and 1 tablespoon ice water. Add to the food processor and pulse until the dough comes together. The dough will not form a ball; simply press it between your fingers to see if it comes together. Add 1 more tablespoon ice water if needed.

3   Turn the dough out onto a work surface, knead it a couple of times, and form a disk. Wrap the disk in plastic wrap, flatten it with your hands, and refrigerate for 1 hour.

4   Dust your work surface with a little bit of superfine brown rice flour. Place the dough on top and roll it to a ⅛-inch thickness. If using a large tart pan, gently roll the dough around the rolling pin and lift it over the mold. Press it in lightly and cut off the excess. If using tartlet pans, cut 5½-inch circles and fill the tartlet molds. You should get 4 circles. Re-roll the leftover dough and repeat. Cut off excess dough. Place the tart pan(s) on a baking sheet and refrigerate for 20 minutes.

5   Preheat the oven to 375°F (190°C). Cover the tart crust(s) with parchment paper and fill the tart pan(s) with dried beans or pie weights. Blind-bake the tart(s) for 20 minutes. Remove the crust(s) from the oven, but leave the oven on. Remove the pie weights and the parchment and proceed with the filling.

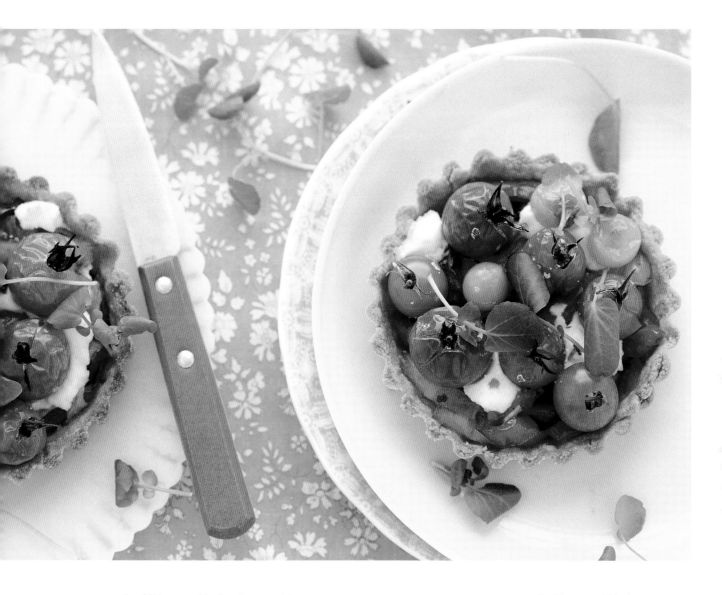

prepare the filling and bake the tart(s)

1   Increase the oven temperature to 400°F (200°C). In a large sauté pan, heat the olive oil over medium heat. Add the onion, garlic, bell peppers, thyme, salt, black pepper, and red pepper flakes. Cook the vegetables until tender, stirring occasionally, about 15 minutes. You want them soft and slightly caramelized but not too dark.

2   Divide the pepper mixture over the partly baked tart crust(s). Top with the ricotta and cherry tomatoes. Drizzle the top(s) with a little bit of olive oil and salt.

3   Bake the tart(s) for 15 minutes or until the tomatoes start to soften and burst. Season the watercress with olive oil and salt. Serve warm, topped with the watercress salad.

½ teaspoon freshly ground black pepper

⅛ to ¼ teaspoon red pepper flakes, depending on how spicy you like it

3 ounces (90 g) whole-milk ricotta, drained

12 ounces (340 g) cherry tomatoes, cut in half if they are large

Watercress, for garnish

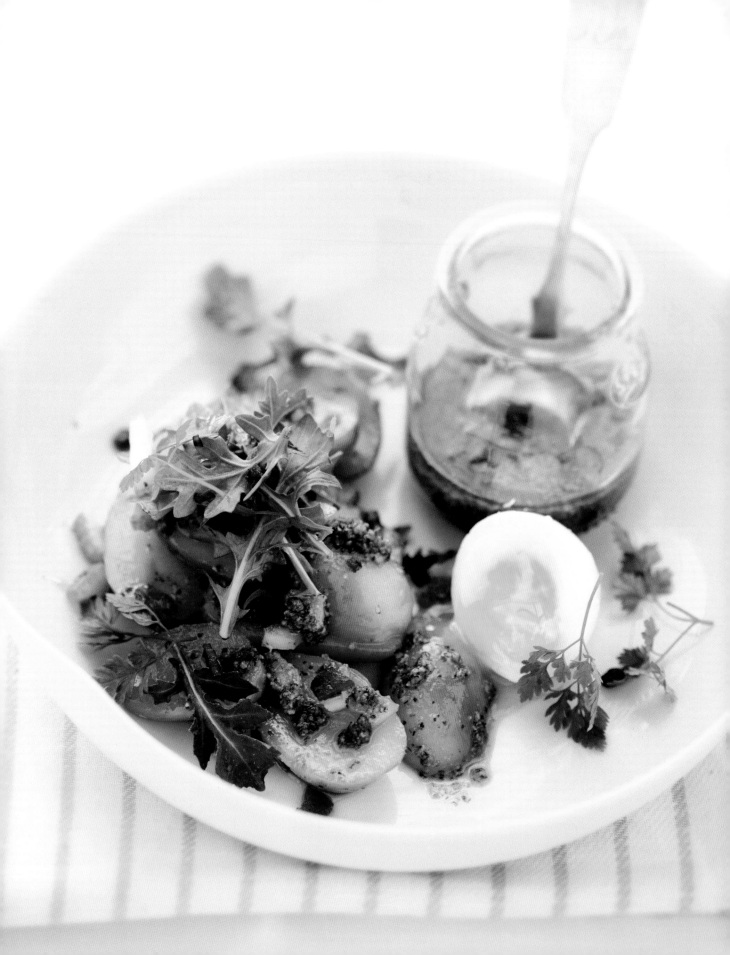

potato-and-egg salad with arugula & chervil pesto

THIS SALAD MUST BE THE quintessential summer potluck and cookout dish. My version combines arugula and chervil pesto with warm potatoes and soft-boiled eggs.

SERVES 4 to 6

make the pesto

1   In a food processor, chop the garlic and pine nuts to a fine powder. Add the arugula and chervil and process until finely chopped. Add the celery salt, black pepper, and Parmesan cheese and blend. While the machine is running, add in the olive oil in a steady stream until the pesto comes together.

2   Store the pesto in the refrigerator for up to 3 days or freeze in an airtight container for up to 1 month.

make the salad

1   Preheat the oven to 350°F (180°C). Brush the slices of bacon with the maple syrup. Place the bacon on a baking sheet and cook for 15 to 20 minutes, until golden. Reserve.

2   Add the potatoes to a large pot and cover them with cold water. Bring the water to a boil over high heat. Once the water comes to a boil, reduce the heat to medium, cover the pot, and cook the potatoes for 7 to 10 minutes, or until the tip of a paring knife pierces through easily. Drain the potatoes and let them cool for 5 minutes. When they are cool enough to handle, peel them and slice them in half.

3   In a bowl, toss together the potatoes, celery, crumbled bacon, and Arugula & Chervil Pesto.

4   Cook the eggs according to the instructions for soft-boiled eggs (see sidebar). Cut the eggs in half and serve them next to the salad.

ARUGULA AND CHERVIL PESTO (MAKES ¾ CUP)

1 clove garlic, minced

3 tablespoons pine nuts

1 cup (30 g) arugula

¼ cup (10 g) fresh chervil or parsley leaves

1 teaspoon celery salt

½ teaspoon freshly ground black pepper

1 ounce (30 g) Parmesan cheese, finely grated

½ cup (125 ml) olive oil

POTATO-AND-EGG SALAD

4 slices (3 ounces or 90 g) bacon

1 tablespoon maple syrup

1½ pounds (680 g) red new potatoes

1 celery stalk, diced

4 eggs, at room temperature

COOKING SOFT-BOILED EGGS

Bring a large pot of water to a boil. With a large spoon, swirl the boiling water around for a few seconds. Carefully add rooom-temperature eggs to the water and continue to swirl them around for a few more seconds. Cook the eggs for 5 minutes, then immediately transfer them to a bowl filled with ice water. When they are cool, peel the eggs, and they will be ready to eat, with a perfect runny yolk in the center.

ivory lentil, serrano ham & melon salad

"WE ARE GOING ON A ROAD TRIP," my dad said on a sunny day in August. The kids and I were visiting for the summer and looked forward to day trips with my dad, who knows the Basque Country like the palm of his hand. "Let's make sure we have some *jamón*, bread, and that melon we got at the market yesterday." We drove to the small town of Zugarramurdi to visit the prehistoric caves and learn about the Basque folklore surrounding them. I love listening to my dad tell us stories of witches and mythological characters. The kids listen intently, with a measure of fear in their eyes, a feeling I remember very well myself. After exploring, we sit on a park bench with a loaf of bread and some Serrano ham wrapped around slices of green melon—all fears gone. Summer delight.

SERVES 4 to 6

2 teaspoons grainy Dijon mustard

2 teaspoons honey

2 tablespoons champagne vinegar or apple cider vinegar

1 tablespoon pistachio oil, optional

¼ cup (60 ml) olive oil

2 teaspoons salt

1 cup (200 g) ivory lentils, rinsed

½ cup (50 g) thinly sliced radishes

1 cup (30 g) arugula

1 cup (40 g) watercress

6 slices (3 ounces or 90 g) thinly sliced Serrano ham or prosciutto

½ small cantaloupe, peeled and sliced into 6 wedges

1   To make the vinaigrette, whisk together the mustard, honey, vinegar, pistachio oil (if using), olive oil, and 1 teaspoon of the salt. Set aside.

2   In a medium saucepan, combine the lentils, 3 cups (750 ml) water, and the remaining 1 teaspoon salt. Bring to a boil over medium-high heat, reduce the heat to medium-low, and cook, covered, for 15 minutes or until the lentils are tender. Drain and rinse in cold water.

3   Toss together the cooked lentils, radishes, arugula, and watercress with half of the vinaigrette on a platter. Wrap the prosciutto slices around the cantaloupe wedges. Place the melon wedges around the salad and drizzle the rest of the vinaigrette over the salad and cantaloupe slices. Serve immediately.

TIP: Ivory lentils are great for salads. They cook quickly and have a nice bite. If ivory lentils are not available, you could use red lentils, quinoa, millet, or any legume you prefer.

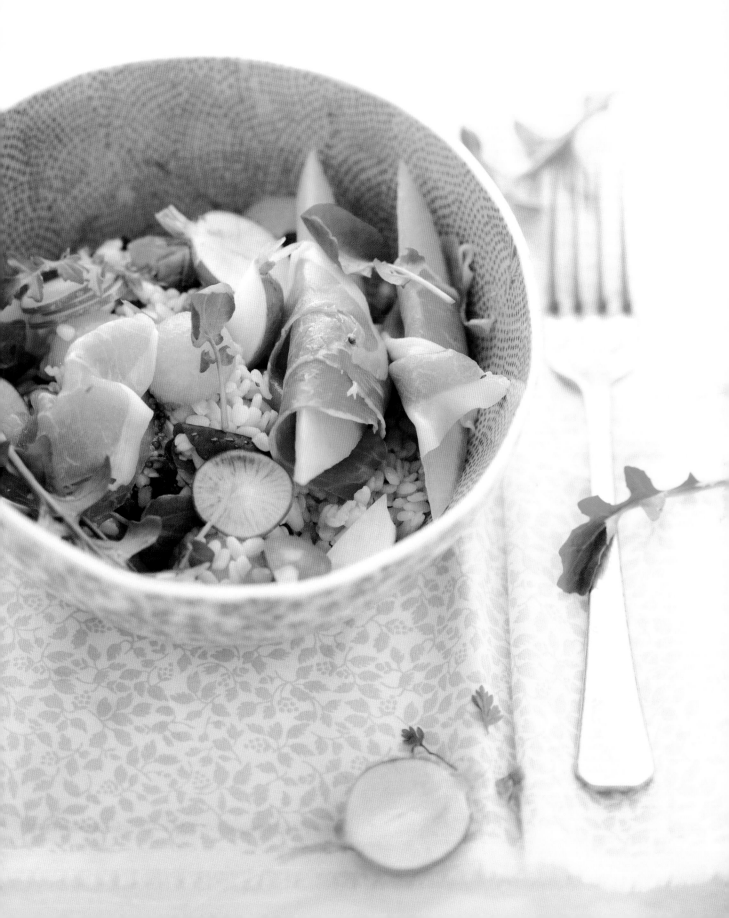

basque fish stew (*marmitako*)

THIS CLASSIC SUMMER FISH STEW is called *marmitako* in Basque. Fresh tuna and potatoes are cooked in a light fish stock and flavored with lots of paprika. The trick to a great *marmitako* is the fish broth. Ask your fishmonger for fish bones and skin, preferably tuna. If tuna bones are not available, opt for fish such as snapper or grouper. Fattier fish such as sea bass will also work, but they will result in a fattier-tasting broth. For the stew itself, tuna steaks will work, but traditionally the more flavorful meat closer to the head or belly is used.

SERVES 4

FISH BROTH (MAKES ABOUT 3 CUPS)

1 pound (450 g) fish bones and skin

½ medium leek, root end trimmed and diced

½ medium yellow onion, peeled but left whole

1 carrot, peeled and halved

¼ cup (10 g) fresh parsley leaves

¼ cup (10 g) fresh chervil leaves

1 teaspoon salt

½ teaspoon freshly ground black pepper

FISH STEW

1 medium tomato

2 tablespoons olive oil

½ medium yellow onion, diced

2 cloves garlic, minced

1 cubanelle pepper or ½ green bell pepper, diced

½ red bell pepper, diced

½ teaspoon salt

1½ pounds (680 g) Yukon gold potatoes, peeled and cut into chunks (see sidebar)

1 teaspoon Spanish *pimentón* or smoked paprika

⅛ teaspoon red pepper flakes

3 cups Fish Broth

1 pound tuna, skinned, boned, and cut into 1½-inch cubes

Chopped fresh parsley, for garnish

Chopped fresh chervil, for garnish

make the broth

1   Combine all the ingredients in a large pot along with 4 cups (1 L) water. Bring to a boil over medium-high heat. Reduce the heat to medium-low, cover, and simmer for 30 minutes.

2   Strain the liquid into a clean bowl, discard the fish bones and vegetables, and reserve the broth.

make the stew

1   Score the tip of the tomato with a paring knife. Bring a small pot of water to a boil. Add the tomato, cook for 30 seconds, and immediately transfer it to an ice bath to stop the cooking process. This will help you peel the skin easily. Skin the tomato and remove the stem. Chop it into medium pieces. Reserve.

2   In a large pot, heat the olive oil, onion, garlic, green pepper, and red pepper. Add the salt and cook the vegetables for 5 minutes over medium heat. Stir occasionally. When the vegetables are soft, add the diced tomato. Cook for 2 minutes.

3   Add the potatoes, *pimentón*, and red pepper flakes. Stir and cook for 1 minute. Add the fish broth. Bring the liquid to a boil, reduce the heat to medium, cover the pot, and cook for 15 minutes or until the potatoes are tender.

4   Add the tuna, stir, and turn off the heat. Let the tuna gently cook in the broth for about 2 minutes or until the outside is no longer pink. Adjust the seasoning if necessary. Sprinkle with the fresh herbs and serve immediately.

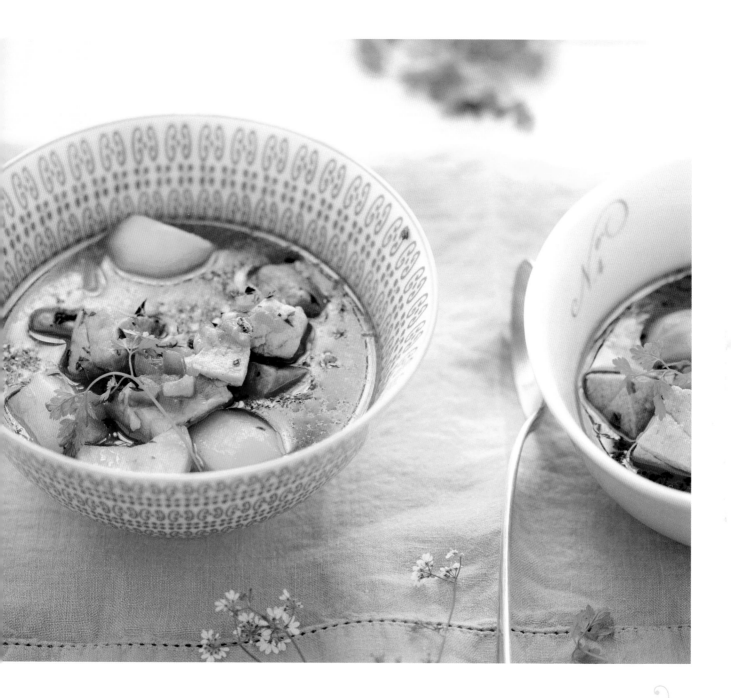

HOW TO CUT POTATOES FOR A STEW THE BASQUE WAY

One of the first cooking tips I learned from my grandmother was how to cut potatoes for stews and soups. "Never cut potatoes on a chopping board. They will release all their good starch and it will be left behind on the cutting board," she said. Instead, she suggested holding the peeled potatoes over the pot in one hand and a paring knife in the other. Cut into the potato ever so slightly and then break off a chunk. It will make a "click" sound. Then let the potatoes fall into the soup. This releases much more starch and ends up thickening the soup beautifully.

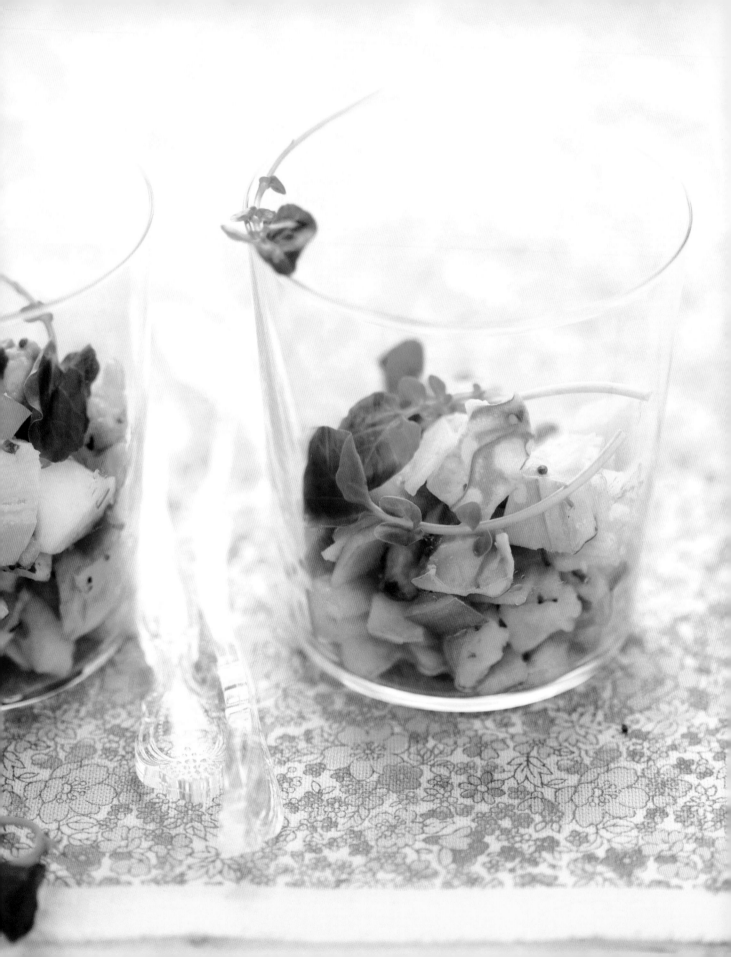

summer lobster & apple salad

THIS IS A VERY COLORFUL SALAD composed of some of my favorite summer ingredients. It can be served completely chilled, but I tend to like warm salads, especially this one. The slightly warm lobster and tomatoes paired with the crunchy apples and creamy avocado make a wonderful salad that's full of texture.

SERVES 4 to 6

1 In a small saucepan, combine the potatoes with enough cold water to cover. Bring them to a boil over medium-high heat. Reduce the heat to medium, cover the pot, and cook for 20 minutes or until the tip of a paring knife pierces through easily. Drain the potatoes. When they are cool enough to handle, peel and cut them into bite-size pieces.

2 Fill a medium saucepan with water. Season the water with a handful of salt so it tastes like seawater. Bring the salted water to a boil, add the lobster tail, and cover with a lid. Cook over medium heat for 10 minutes. Remove the lobster from the pot, set on a clean plate, and let it cool slightly. Cut the shell with scissors and remove the meat. Cut into bite-size pieces and reserve.

3 In a large bowl, gently toss together the potatoes, lobster, apples, avocado, yellow tomato, red bell pepper, red onion, and lemon juice.

4 To make the vinaigrette, whisk together the mustard, apple cider vinegar, parsley, olive oil, and salt. Pour the vinaigrette over the lobster mixture and gently toss it together. Spoon into chilled glasses or cups and serve immediately.

2 medium Yukon gold potatoes

1 (12-ounce or 340 g) lobster tail

2 medium Pink Lady apples or any other tart variety, cored and diced

1 avocado, pitted, peeled, and diced

1 medium yellow tomato, diced

½ medium red bell pepper, diced

¼ small red onion, diced

2 tablespoons freshly squeezed lemon juice

1 teaspoon grainy Dijon mustard

1 tablespoon apple cider vinegar

2 tablespoons finely chopped fresh parsley

3 tablespoons olive oil

½ teaspoon salt, plus more to cook the lobster

SUMMER ENTERTAINING

I like to keep summer menus uncomplicated and easy to serve. Because I live in Florida, where summers are very warm, I try to stay away from the oven as much as possible. This also allows me to keep the house cool for guests. I recommend preparing dishes that you can make ahead and saving larger items, like whole roasted fish, for the grill outside.

This lobster-and-apple salad is one of my favorites. Prepare it in advance and chill until 15 minutes before serving time. Add the vinaigrette then and let it come to room temperature. I tend not to like salads that are too cold.

I would serve it with Chilled Watermelon, Tomato & Almond Soup (page 248), which can also be made ahead of time; a great cheese platter; and some refreshing drinks.

chicken, zucchini & gruyère clafoutis

IN OUR FAMILY, WE MAKE CLAFOUTIS and frittatas out of everything, especially leftovers. This is a great dish to make if you have leftover roasted chicken and vegetables, for example. It is also very portable and great for potluck gatherings. If you want to make a vegetarian version of this dish, replace the chicken with the same amount of cooked garbanzo beans.

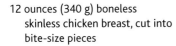

MAKES one 13 by 9-inch pan or 8 individual ramekins

12 ounces (340 g) boneless skinless chicken breast, cut into bite-size pieces

1½ teaspoons salt

1 teaspoon freshly ground black pepper

2 tablespoons olive oil, plus more if needed

1 small yellow onion, diced

2 cloves garlic, minced

½ medium fennel bulb, diced

1 medium zucchini, thinly sliced

6 eggs

2 egg yolks

1 tablespoon cornstarch

1 cup (250 ml) unsweetened coconut milk

2 ounces (60 g) Gruyère cheese, grated

⅓ cup (20 g) finely chopped fresh herbs (any combination of parsley, chervil, thyme, sorrel, tarragon, and/or oregano)

1 Preheat the oven to 350°F (180°C). Season the chicken with ½ teaspoon of the salt and ¼ teaspoon of the black pepper.

2 Heat the olive oil in a medium sauté pan over medium-high heat. Add the diced chicken. Cook the chicken on both sides until the pieces start to brown, about 5 minutes. Transfer the chicken to a bowl.

3 Add another tablespoon of olive oil to the sauté pan, if needed. Add the onion, garlic, and fennel. Stir the vegetables and scrape up the brown bits left on the bottom of the pan from sautéing the chicken. Reduce the heat to medium-low. Cook the vegetables for 5 minutes, until soft but not mushy.

4 Add the zucchini, and season with ½ teaspoon of the salt and ¼ teaspoon of the black pepper. Cook for 2 minutes. Add the chicken back to the pan. Stir and remove from the heat.

5 In a large bowl, whisk together the eggs, egg yolks, cornstarch, coconut milk, grated Gruyère, herbs, remaining ½ teaspoon salt, and remaining ½ teaspoon black pepper. Spread the sautéed vegetable-and-chicken mixture in a 13 by 9-inch baking pan or spoon into 8 individual ramekins. Pour the custard on top.

6 Bake the clafoutis for 30 to 35 minutes (20 minutes for the individual ramekins) or until the center is set and the top is lightly golden. Serve immediately.

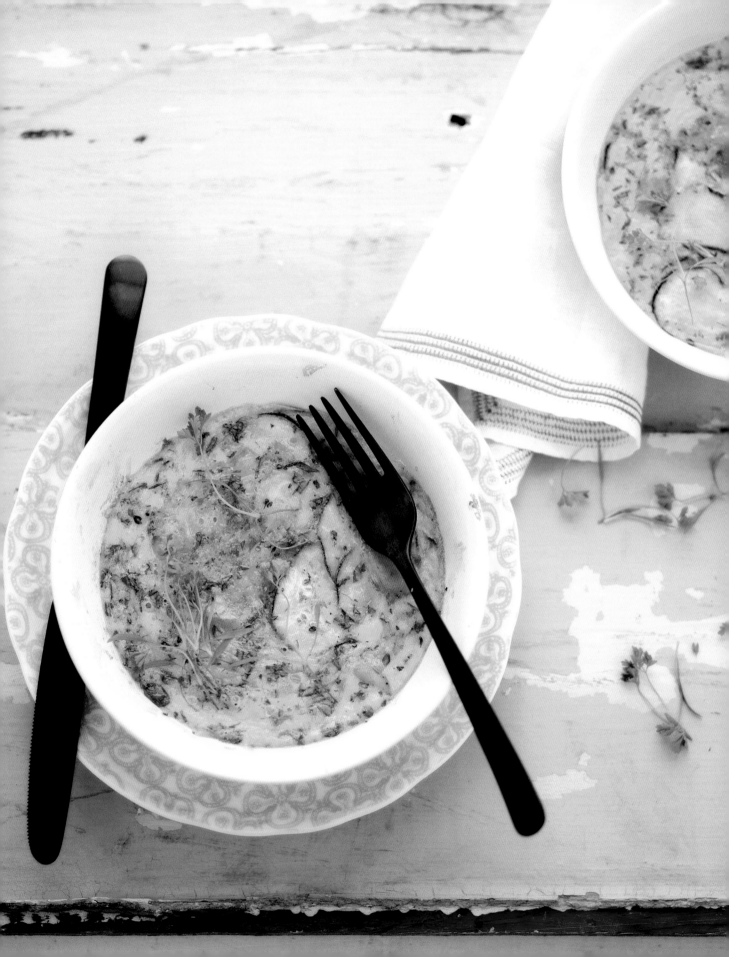

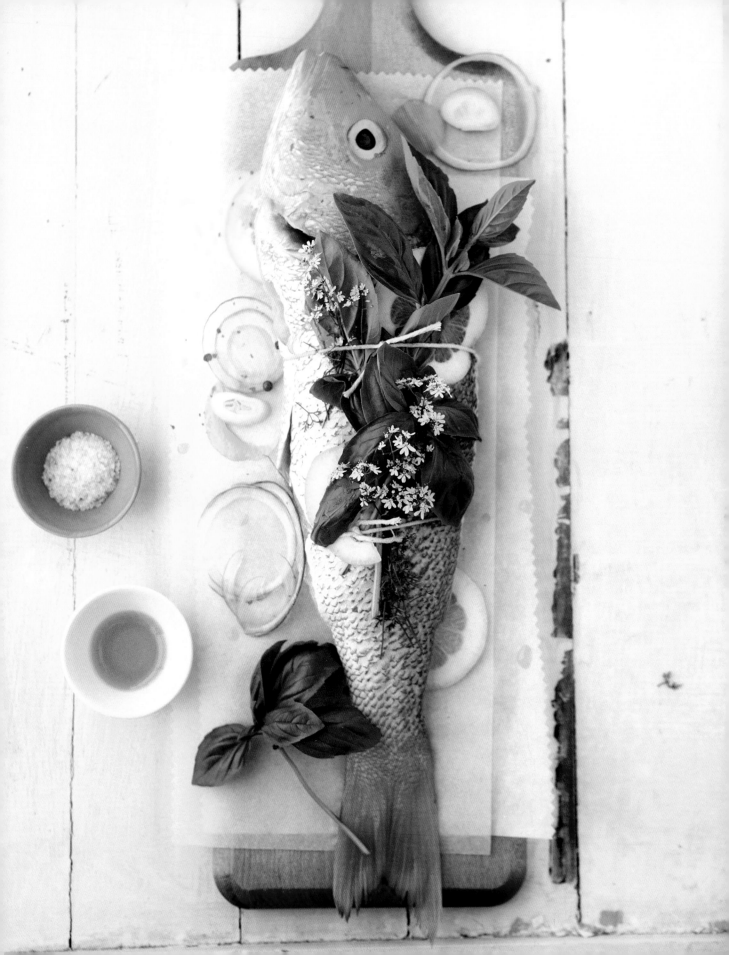

roasted red snapper with potatoes, shaved fennel & shiso

I LOVE THE SMELL OF SALTY AIR in the small fishing towns all along the Basque coastline. Watching the fishing boats arrive early in the morning is one of our favorite summertime activities. We drive to Getaria to get the freshest catch of the day.

This roasting method works for any medium fish such as snapper, John Dory, or Mediterranean sea bass. Ask your fishmonger to clean it for you, but keep the head on if you can. There is lots of flavor there.

SERVES 4 to 6

prepare the fennel

Toss all the ingredients together and refrigerate while you prepare the fish. If you cannot find shiso, you may use a combination of fresh mint, basil, and tarragon.

roast the fish

1   Preheat the oven to 400°F (200°C). Arrange the sliced potatoes in a single layer in a baking pan large enough to hold the fish. Drizzle the potatoes with 1 tablespoon of the olive oil and ¼ teaspoon of the salt. Bake the potatoes for 20 to 25 minutes, or until they are just starting to turn golden.

2   Meanwhile, season the inside and outside of the red snapper with the remaining 1 teaspoon salt. Stuff the belly area with the lemon slices.

3   Remove the baking pan from the oven. Place the red snapper on top of the potatoes. Pour the wine in the baking pan. Drizzle the top of the fish with 1 tablespoon of the olive oil. Return the pan to the oven and roast for 20 to 25 minutes, depending on the thickness of the fish. To check for doneness, insert the tip of a knife in the belly of the fish, close to the spine, and lift it to see if the flesh separates from the bones. If it doesn't, it needs a few more minutes.

4   Let the fish rest for 5 minutes while you prepare the vinaigrette. Heat the remaining 1 tablespoon olive oil in a sauté pan. Add the sliced garlic and cook it for 1 minute while swirling it around in the oil. Do not let it burn. Stand back and add the vinegar. It will splatter, so be careful!

5   Insert the tip of a chef's knife into the top of the spine of the fish. Cut along the entire spine, keeping the knife very close to the bone. Open the fish in half with the help of a spatula and pour the vinaigrette over it. Serve it immediately with the potatoes and Shaved Fennel with Shiso.

SHAVED FENNEL WITH SHISO

- 1 medium fennel bulb, thinly sliced
- ½ medium red onion, thinly sliced
- ¼ cup purple shiso, torn into pieces
- 2 tablespoons fresh chervil or parsley leaves, torn into pieces
- ½ teaspoon salt
- 2 tablespoons freshly squeezed lemon juice
- 3 tablespoons olive oil

ROASTED RED SNAPPER WITH POTATOES

- 2 medium russet potatoes, peeled and sliced into ¼-inch-thick pieces
- 3 tablespoons olive oil
- 1¼ teaspoons salt
- 1 (2-pound or 1 kg) whole red snapper, gutted, scales and fins removed
- 1 lemon, thinly sliced
- ¼ cup (60 ml) Txakoli or other dry white wine
- 2 cloves garlic, thinly sliced
- 2 tablespoons apple cider vinegar

chilled watermelon, tomato & almond soup

THIS RECIPE IS A VARIATION ON THE classic tomato gazpacho, using watermelon and almonds. It is what I call a "blender soup." Place all the ingredients in the blender and it is ready in seconds. Serve it in chilled shot glasses as an amuse-bouche or in bowls as a first course.

If you are not a fan of raw garlic, you could omit it, but I find that it adds a bit of spice to the soup, which I like.

SERVES 4 to 6

2 cups (300 g) diced seedless watermelon

2 medium very ripe tomatoes, peeled (optional) and diced

¼ small red onion, diced

2 tablespoons almond flour

1 tablespoon red wine vinegar

1 tablespoon olive oil

¾ teaspoon salt

¼ teaspoon finely grated garlic (optional)

1 ounce (30 g) feta cheese, crumbled, for garnish

2 tablespoons olive oil, for garnish

Fresh herbs of your choice, for garnish

1 Puree the first eight ingredients in a food processor or blender. Pour into a pitcher and refrigerate the soup for 1 hour. The soup may be stored in the refrigerator for up to 2 days. Stir before serving, as it tends to separate.

2 Serve the chilled soup with crumbled feta cheese, a drizzle of olive oil, and fresh herbs.

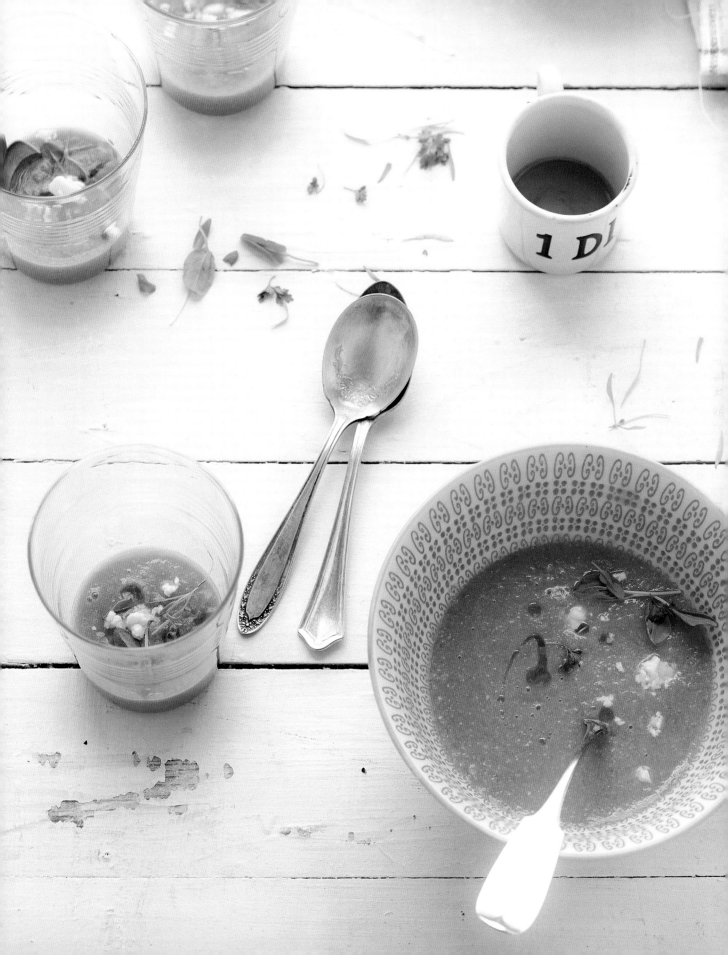

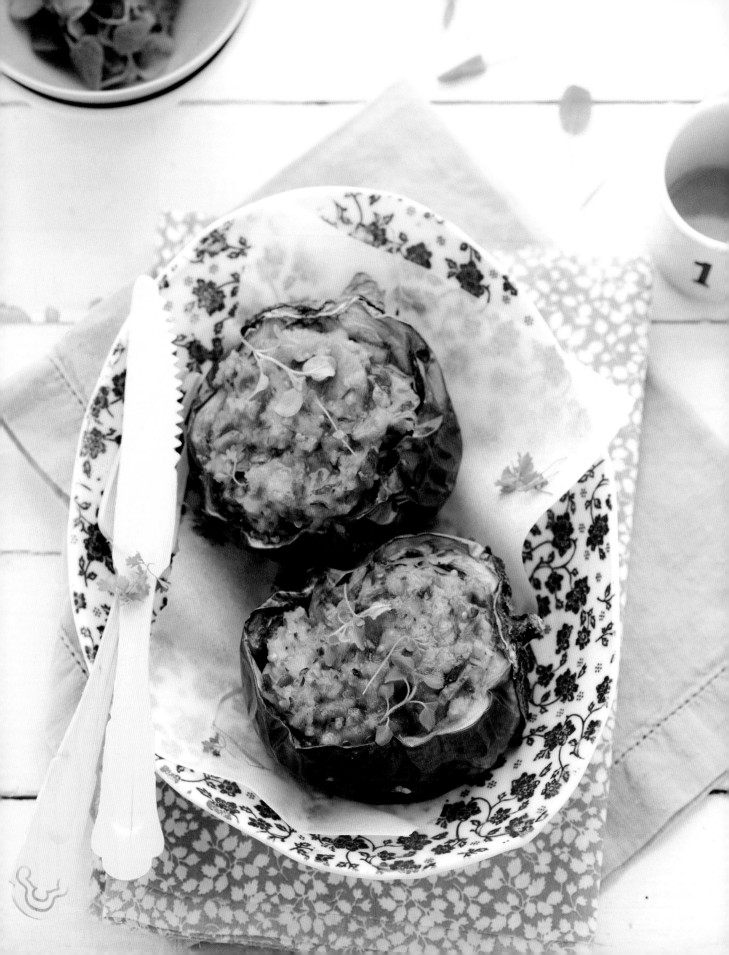

eggplants stuffed with millet & serrano ham

I HAVE TO ADMIT THAT IT TOOK ME MANY years to start appreciating eggplant. My mom never cooked it much; zucchini seemed to be far more abundant in our area. Eggplant tasted bitter to me, with a strange aftertaste. I wondered if it was something we were doing wrong. Then, the first time I visited New York City as a teenager, I had the most delicious eggplant stuffed with lamb and tomato at a Middle Eastern restaurant. I couldn't believe what I had been missing all those years.

Millet makes this filling hearty and rich in nutrients. Omit the Serrano ham and use vegetable broth to make it vegetarian.

SERVES 4 to 6

1 Preheat the oven to 400°F (200°C). Place the eggplants on a baking sheet, cut side up. Brush them with 1 tablespoon of the olive oil and sprinkle with ½ teaspoon of the salt. Bake the eggplants for 20 to 30 minutes, until the flesh has softened. Let the eggplants cool for 15 minutes and then scoop out the flesh, leaving a ¼-inch rim around the outer shell. Dice the eggplant flesh and reserve.

2 In a small saucepan, combine the millet, chicken stock, and ¼ teaspoon of the salt. Bring to a boil, reduce the heat to low, and simmer, covered, for 25 minutes or until the millet is soft but still has a bite. Reserve.

3 In a large sauté pan, heat 3 tablespoons of the olive oil over medium heat. Add the shallot, leek, garlic, green pepper, and remaining ½ teaspoon salt. Cook the vegetables for 5 minutes or until soft, stirring occasionally.

4 Add the reserved eggplant, diced tomato, Serrano ham or prosciutto, red pepper flakes, and herbs. Cook the mixture for 3 minutes, stirring occasionally.

5 Remove the mixture from the heat and add the cooked millet, mascarpone, Parmesan, and beaten egg. Stir to combine. Adjust the seasoning if needed.

6 Reduce the oven heat to 375°F (190°C). Spoon the filling into the hollowed eggplants and place them in a baking pan. Drizzle the tops with the remaining 1 tablespoon olive oil. Pour ¼ cup (60 ml) hot water into the baking pan. Bake the eggplants for 30 minutes. Serve immediately.

3 medium (1 pound or 450 g each) eggplants, halved

¼ cup plus 1 tablespoon (75 ml) olive oil

1¼ teaspoons salt

¼ cup (45 g) millet

½ cup (125 ml) chicken stock

1 medium shallot, minced

1 medium leek, white and tender green parts only, diced

1 clove garlic, minced

½ medium green bell pepper, seeded and diced

1 ripe tomato, peeled, seeded, and diced

4 thin slices (2 ounces or 60 g) Serrano ham or prosciutto

⅛ to ¼ teaspoon red pepper flakes, depending on how spicy you like it

1 tablespoon finely chopped fresh parsley

1 tablespoon fresh thyme leaves

1 tablespoon finely chopped fresh oregano

3 tablespoons mascarpone cheese

1 ounce (30 g) Parmesan cheese, finely grated

1 egg, lightly beaten

quinoa spaghetti with garlicky squid & niçoise olives

SQUID IS ONE OF THE STAPLES on the Basque summer menu. Grilled with caramelized onions, stuffed, or cooked in a black sauce made with their own ink, squid remains one of my favorite summer ingredients. This dish takes 15 minutes to cook from start to finish. It's very simple and flavorful, but be careful not to overcook the squid or it will turn rubbery.

Serve it with the same chilled Txakoli that is used in the dish. Txakoli is a young, slightly sparkling, and very dry white wine that is produced in different provinces of the Basque Country. Each region or city has specific regulations and strict labeling policies. If you have trouble finding Txakoli, use any dry white wine of your choice.

SERVES 4

8 ounces (225 g) quinoa spaghetti (or any other spaghetti you prefer)

¼ cup plus 1 tablespoon (75 ml) olive oil, plus more for garnish

2 slices stale gluten-free bread, crust removed and crumbled (about ⅔ cup or 35 g crumbled)

½ teaspoon salt, plus more for the spaghetti

8 ounces (225 g) cleaned squid tubes and tentacles, tubes cut into ½-inch rings

½ teaspoon freshly ground black pepper

4 cloves garlic, thinly sliced

¼ cup (15 g) chopped fresh parsley, plus more for garnish

1 tablespoon chopped fresh cilantro

¼ to ½ teaspoon red pepper flakes, depending on how spicy you like it

½ cup (80 g) Niçoise olives (I leave the pits in, as I find it enhances flavor, but you can remove them if you're concerned about someone biting into a hard pit)

½ cup (125 ml) Txakoli or other dry white wine

1 Fill a large pot with water and bring it to a boil. Generously season the water with salt. Add the spaghetti and cook according to the package instructions. Drain and set aside.

2 Meanwhile, in a small sauté pan, heat 2 tablespoons of the olive oil, bread crumbs, and ¼ teaspoon of the salt over medium heat. Cook until the bread is toasted, about 5 minutes, stirring often. Set aside.

3 In a large sauté pan, heat 3 tablespoons of the olive oil over medium-high heat. Season the squid with the remaining ¼ teaspoon salt and the pepper. Add the sliced garlic and squid to the hot oil and stir for 1 minute, until cooked. Do not overcook the squid or it will become very rubbery. Add the chopped parsley, cilantro, red pepper flakes, and olives. Stir for a few seconds.

4 Deglaze the pan with the wine. Cook for 30 seconds so some of the alcohol cooks off.

5 Add the drained spaghetti to the pan and cook in the sauce for a few seconds. Serve immediately with the toasted bread crumbs, fresh parsley, and a drizzle of olive oil.

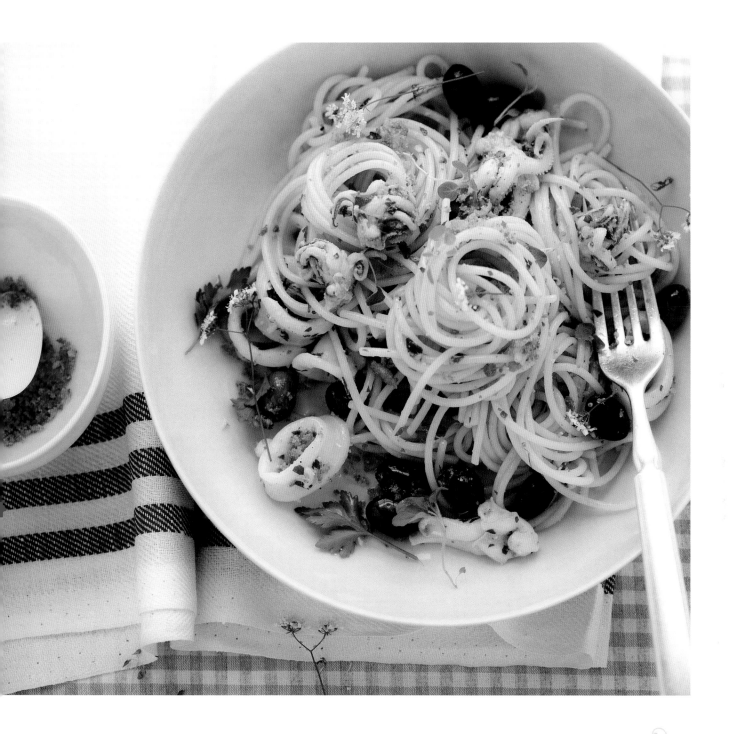

GARLIC TIP

A trick my grandmother taught me when I first began cooking was to always remove the core of the garlic before cooking it. She claimed that by removing the core, garlic was easier to digest and I would never, ever get garlic breath. True or false? I'm not sure, but it has stuck with me all these years. To do this, cut the garlic clove lengthwise and remove the core or stem from both halves.

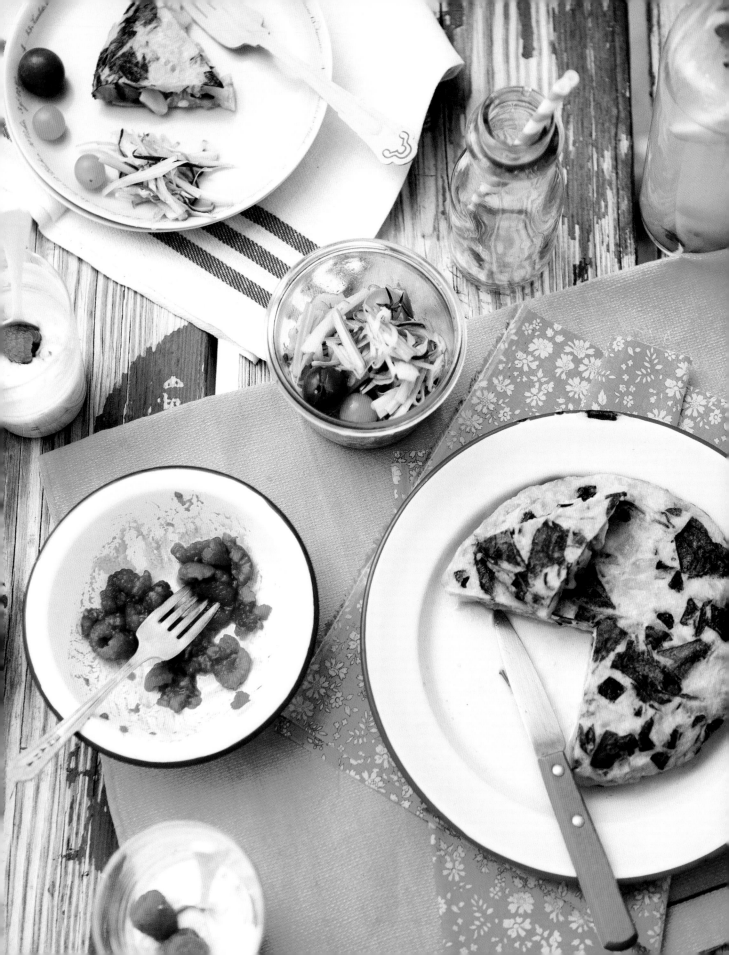

potato, zucchini & watercress tortilla

MY FRIEND CASTOR SAID THIS TO ME recently: "When someone you love comes over for dinner, you make them *tortilla de patata* because it takes time and love to make it. When someone who means nothing to you comes over for dinner, you buy the most expensive fish and just stick it in the oven." I couldn't agree more.

The traditional tortilla consists simply of eggs, onions, potatoes, and excellent olive oil. Here I have added some diced zucchini and peppery watercress for an extra kick.

SERVES 4

1   Locate a plate or pan lid that measures about 8 inches, or the same circumference as the nonstick skillet you will be using. This will help you flip the tortilla.

2   Heat the olive oil in a deep 7- to 8-inch nonstick skillet over medium heat. Add the onion and cook it for 2 minutes or until softened but not brown. Add the potatoes and ½ teaspoon of the salt. Cook the potatoes for 5 minutes, stirring occasionally. Add the zucchini and cook for an additional 5 minutes or until soft, stirring occasionally. Initially, the pan might look overcrowded with vegetables, which is fine. They will cook down.

3   With a slotted spoon, transfer the cooked potatoes and zucchini to a plate lined with paper towels. Pour the leftover hot olive oil from the pan into a heatproof bowl and reserve.

4   In a medium bowl, whisk together the eggs and remaining ¼ teaspoon salt. Add the drained potatoes, zucchini, and watercress. Stir them with the eggs.

5   Pour 1 tablespoon of the reserved olive oil back into the nonstick skillet. Heat the oil over medium heat. Pour the egg mixture into the pan. Stir the center of the egg mixture with a wooden spoon in a circular motion for a few seconds to set it. Gently round the edges of the tortilla with the help of the wooden spoon. Cook for 1 to 2 minutes.

6   Place the plate or lid over the pan. Hold it tight with one hand and flip the tortilla over onto the plate. The cooked side of the tortilla will be facing up. Gently slide it back into the pan to finish cooking the other side. Again, round the edges to get a nice circle. Cook for another 1 to 2 minutes, depending on how runny you like the inside.

7   Gently slide the tortilla onto a clean plate. Let it cool for 10 minutes before cutting into it. Serve warm or at room temperature.

½ cup (125 ml) olive oil

½ cup (60 g) small-diced yellow onion (about ¼ medium onion)

2 cups (300 g) peeled and medium-diced russet potato (about 2 medium potatoes)

¾ teaspoon salt

1½ cups (225 g) medium-diced zucchini (1 medium zucchini)

4 eggs

½ cup (30 g) coarsely chopped watercress

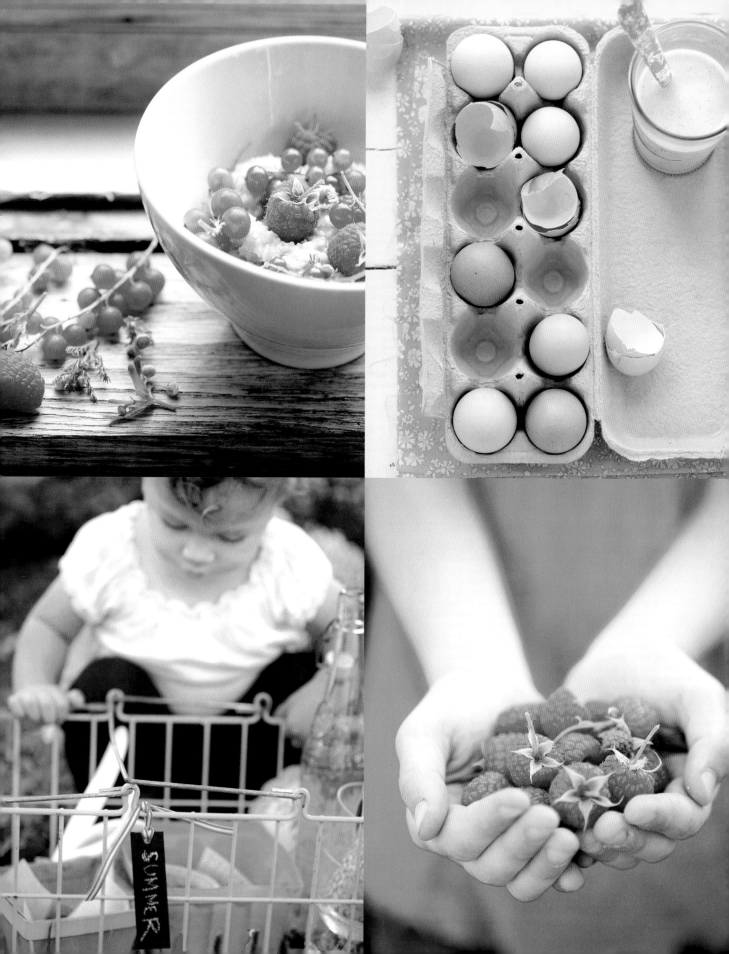

SUMMER
sweet treats

WHEN I THINK OF SUMMER, I think of ice cream pops, crushed berries in vintage enamel bowls, and midafternoon nectarine cakes. I think of late summer mornings spent in the kitchen, canning crate after crate of peaches, and tall metal pots with blackberries and burning sugar splattering.

On warm days we take the children berry picking. We wend our way among prickly blackberry bushes surrounded by fields of wild chamomile. Jon likes to lead the way, walking briskly with wooden stick in hand. "I spot some over there," he says, running ahead. Miren is not far behind. Once back home, we eat the berries by the handful. Most do not even make it into the refrigerator. For those that do, quick compotes and galettes will make the best summer treats. We try to save some for canning to preserve the taste of summer.

One of my earliest summer memories revolves around my grandfather Angel whisking a batch of vanilla ice cream by hand over a bath of ice and coarse salt. I watched him in awe as he stirred the deep yellow custard back and forth for what seemed like an eternity. "Now come have a taste," he whispered. The cold, thickened ice cream was lightly sweet, with a million specs of vanilla. "We will serve it with some of the blackberries we picked behind the school," he added. Perhaps this is why I love making ice cream with my children these days. It is all about building memories.

The dessert recipes in this chapter are simple and mostly inspired by the fruits of summer. There's not much one can do to improve upon a perfectly ripe peach. Except, perhaps, to add a bit of vanilla ice cream.

red velvet apricot &
hazelnut shortbread tartlets

APRICOTS ARE AMONG THE FIRST FRUITS of summer. If you're lucky, they start to appear at the end of spring. They tend to be a bit tart when they're not fully ripe, so you might want to add a bit more sugar if that is the case, but overall this is not intended to be a very sweet dessert.

I recently discovered red velvet apricots. They have a deep burgundy skin with bright orange flesh and are slightly sweeter than the traditional variety. I love their pop of color, especially for a tart this simple.

The hazelnut shortbread crust is very flaky and tender. Use the best artisanal salted butter you can find; it's the butter that makes it so wonderful. This is a press-in dough, so no need to worry about rolling it out. I don't recommend baking it in a large tart pan, because it is so delicate that it might fall apart. This recipe makes perfect individual tartlets that will melt in your mouth.

MAKES six 4½-inch tartlets

1 cup (140 g) superfine brown rice flour

⅓ cup (55 g) potato starch

⅓ cup (40 g) tapioca starch

⅓ cup (35 g) hazelnut flour

1 vanilla bean, split lengthwise and seeds scraped

2 sticks (16 tablespoons or 225 g) good-quality salted butter, at room temperature

2 tablespoons whole milk

7 or 8 red velvet apricots

1 tablespoon almond flour

½ cup (60 g) white or red currants

1 tablespoon natural cane sugar, or more depending on how tart the apricots are

Finely chopped natural pistachios, for garnish

1   In a large bowl, whisk together the superfine brown rice flour, potato starch, tapioca starch, hazelnut flour, and vanilla seeds. Dice the soft butter into the flour and work it between your fingers until the butter and the flour form a sandy mixture. Add the milk and mix with your hands until it forms a soft dough.

2   Divide the dough into 6 pieces and press each piece of dough into the tart molds, starting from the bottom and working your way up the sides, until the dough is evenly distributed and about ¼ inch thick. Dust your fingers with a little bit of superfine brown rice flour if the dough becomes too sticky. Remove excess dough with your fingers by pressing against the edges of the mold. Refrigerate the tart bases for 30 minutes.

3   Preheat the oven to 400°F (200°C). Cut the apricots in half. Remove the pit and slice each half into thin wedges.

4   Sprinkle the almond flour over the crust. Arrange the apricot slices tightly around the edges of the tart mold, forming a flower pattern. Top with the currants. Sprinkle the tops with the sugar.

5   Bake the tartlets for 30 minutes, until the crust is golden and the fruit starts to lightly bubble. Let the tartlets cool in the pan for 20 minutes and then lift them out of the mold. Serve warm or at room temperature, garnished with pistachios.

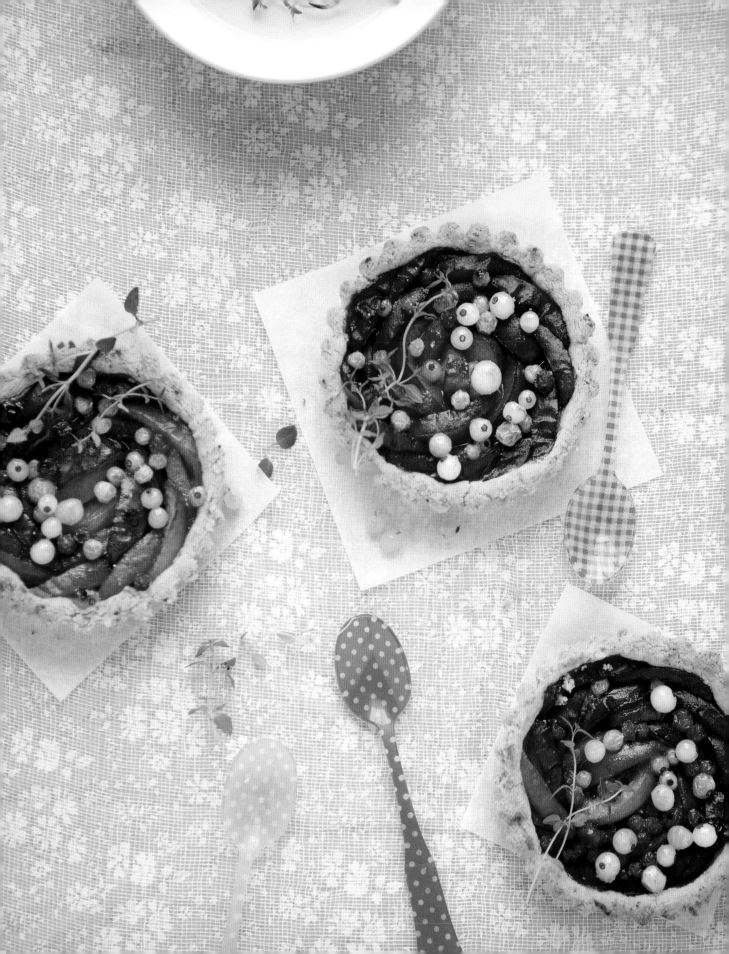

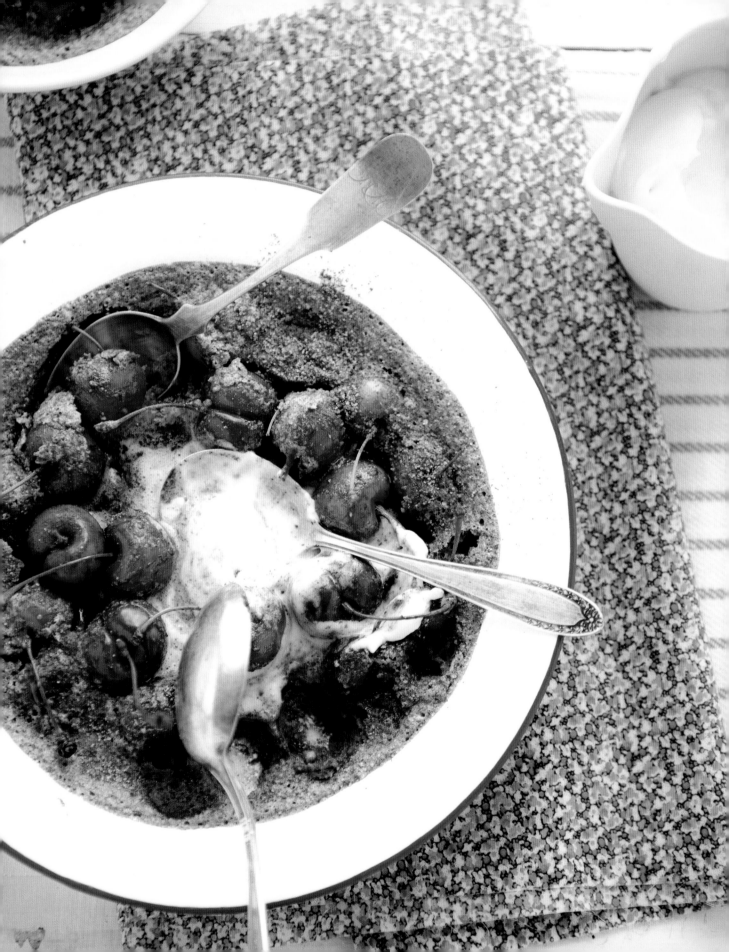

chocolate-cherry gratin

CHERRIES HAVE ALWAYS BEEN one of my favorite summer fruits. We grew up surrounded by cherry trees and always had the boys in the neighborhood jump fences to fetch some for us. Many times we had to run for our lives after being caught stealing cherries from those trees.

As wonderful as they are fresh, I believe roasted is my favorite way of eating cherries. In this recipe, they are baked in a rich yet light custard of chocolate, almonds, and mascarpone. The topping is crunchy and the interior creamy. Normally, I leave the cherries whole both for visual effect and because the pits add an almond extract–like flavor, but they may be pitted to make the gratin easier for guests to eat.

SERVES 6

1 Preheat the oven to 425°F (220°C). Place the chopped chocolate in a heatproof bowl and set it over a pot filled partway with simmering water. Do not let the water boil. Stir the chocolate and melt it over the water bath. Set aside to cool.

2 In the bowl of a stand mixer, using the whip attachment, combine the eggs, egg yolk, ¼ cup (50 g) of the sugar, and almond extract. Whip on high speed for 5 minutes, until the mixture is thick and light.

3 Gently fold in the mascarpone, melted chocolate, almond flour, and salt until it is a homogeneous batter.

4 Pour the batter into a 10-inch soufflé or pie dish. Stud the batter with the cherries.

5 In a small bowl, combine the remaining 2 teaspoons sugar and the cocoa powder. Sprinkle this mixture over the cherries.

6 Bake for 20 minutes, until the top is crunchy but the interior remains creamy. Serve lukewarm or at room temperature. If you like, whip the cream to soft peaks and serve with the gratin.

2 ounces (60 g) bittersweet chocolate, finely chopped

2 eggs, at room temperature

1 egg yolk, at room temperature

¼ cup plus 2 teaspoons (60 g) natural cane sugar

½ teaspoon almond extract

4 ounces (110 g) mascarpone cheese, at room temperature

⅓ cup (35 g) almond flour

¼ teaspoon salt

1 pound (450 g) Bing cherries (stemmed and pitted, if desired)

1 teaspoon unsweetened cocoa powder

½ cup (125 ml) heavy cream, optional

crushed blueberry
eton mess

"**I KNOW WHAT WE WILL BE EATING FOR** dessert tomorrow!" says my husband, Chad, as he watches me separate eggs to make ice cream. There are usually three things I make when I have leftover egg whites: *financiers*, macarons, and baked meringues. I love the texture and the messiness of this dessert, which includes meringues—it's crunchy and creamy in one bite.

SERVES 6

1 cup (150 g) blueberries

1 tablespoon natural cane sugar

1 tablespoon freshly squeezed
    orange juice

4 egg whites, at room temperature

½ teaspoon cream of tartar

⅛ teaspoon salt

1 cup (200 g) superfine sugar

4 teaspoons cornstarch, sifted

1 cup (250 ml) heavy cream

1   Combine the blueberries, natural cane sugar, and orange juice in a small saucepan. Cook on medium heat for 2 minutes, until the blueberries release some juices. Do not cook them to mush. Remove and reserve 2 tablespoons of the blueberry juice.

2   Preheat the oven to 225°F (110°C). Line a baking sheet with parchment paper. Place the egg whites in the bowl of a stand mixer. Whip on medium speed with the whisk attachment. Add the cream of tartar and salt. Turn the speed to high and whip the whites until light and peaks start to form.

3   In a small bowl, mix the superfine sugar and cornstarch. Gradually, while whipping, add 1 tablespoon at a time of this mixture to the whites; adding it too fast will deflate the meringue. Finish adding all of the sugar mixture and whip until stiff peaks form.

4   Add the 2 tablespoons reserved blueberry juice to the bowl and fold it into the meringue with three strokes. Make six mounds of meringue on the baking sheet. Bake for 1 hour, until dry on the outside but still soft. Let them cool for 15 minutes.

5   Place the heavy cream in the bowl of a stand mixer and whip to soft peaks.

6   Serve the cooled meringues with the blueberry sauce and whipped cream.

TIP: If you cannot find superfine sugar, pulse granulated sugar in a food processor until it turns into a fine powder.

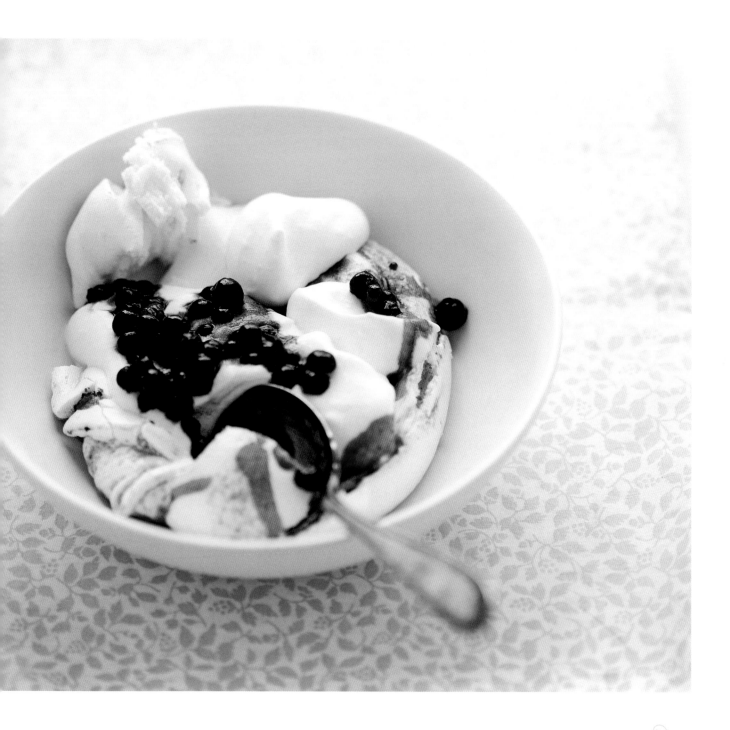

LEFTOVER EGG WHITES

Egg whites keep in the refrigerator for up to 1 week. When making meringue, I find that the older the egg whites, the better they whip. As they age, they lose moisture and become more acidic, which aids with meringue stability. So never throw away egg whites. They can also be frozen, but I find they do not whip well after they have been thawed out. Use them for another purpose, such as *financiers*.

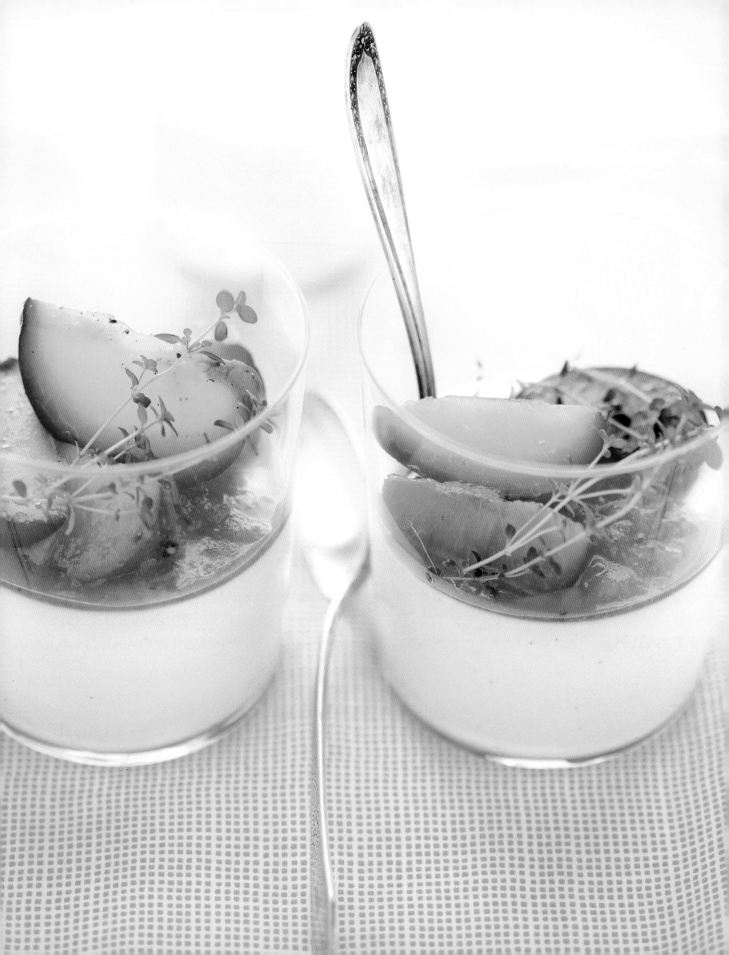

coconut & yogurt panna cotta
with roasted plums

ROASTED FRUIT, stone fruit in particular, is a favorite in our family. Simply prepared with a little bit of sugar, vanilla, and lemon thyme, it is the perfect topping for yogurt or vanilla ice cream. It is also a great last-minute dessert for an impromptu dinner party.

SERVES 8

make the panna cotta

1   In a medium saucepan, heat the coconut milk, sugar, and vanilla bean and seeds over medium heat until it reaches a low boil. Remove from the heat and remove the vanilla bean.

2   Meanwhile, in a small bowl, sprinkle the gelatin over the whole milk and whisk until there are no lumps. Let the gelatin bloom for 5 minutes. Add the gelatin to the hot coconut milk mixture and stir. Add the yogurt and gently whisk to break up any lumps.

3   Pour the panna cotta into 8 (4-ounce) jars or bowls and chill in the refrigerator for at least 2 hours. Store the panna cotta in the refrigerator for up to 3 days or freeze in tightly wrapped jars for up to 1 month. While it is chilling, prepare the roasted fruit.

roast the plums

1   Preheat the oven to 400°F (200°C). Arrange the plums on a baking sheet, cut side up. In a bowl, mix the sugar with the vanilla seeds. Sprinkle the sugar over the plums. Top with the leaves from the lemon thyme sprigs and the butter.

2   Bake for 10 to 15 minutes, until the plums are soft but still keep their shape. Let cool, and serve over the chilled panna cotta.

COCONUT AND YOGURT PANNA COTTA

1½ cups (375 ml) unsweetened coconut milk

½ cup (100 g) natural cane sugar

1 vanilla bean, split lengthwise and seeds scraped

2 teaspoons unflavored powdered gelatin

½ cup (125 ml) whole milk

1½ cups (375 ml) whole-milk plain yogurt

ROASTED PLUMS

1½ pounds (680 g) red plums or any kind you prefer, halved and pitted

¼ cup (50 g) natural cane sugar

1 vanilla bean, split lengthwise and seeds scraped

5 sprigs lemon thyme

1 tablespoon (15 g) unsalted butter, cut into pieces

HOW TO MAKE YOGURT AT HOME

Heat 4 cups (1 L) fresh, organic whole milk to 170°F (76°C). Transfer the milk to a clean bowl and let it cool to 110°F (43°C), or a little bit over body temperature. Add ½ cup (125 ml) of this milk to ½ cup (125 ml) store-bought unsweetened organic whole-milk plain yogurt (as a starter). Whisk to combine. Add the yogurt mixture back into the milk and stir. Pour into yogurt jars. Transfer the jars to a large baking dish and place this in the oven with the pilot light on overnight; if you have an electric oven, leave the oven light on. After 8 hours, cover the jars and store them in the refrigerator. The yogurt will thicken a bit more once cooled, and it will keep in the refrigerator for 10 days.

nectarine, yogurt & poppy seed cake

THERE ARE THREE THINGS THAT I LOOK for in pound cake: I like for it to be moist, not overly sweet, and to have texture. This cake has all three elements. The sliced nectarines and yogurt add moistness to the cake, the addition of quinoa flour balances the sweetness, and the poppy seeds add texture. It is perfect to take on a picnic, to the beach, or to have with tea as a midafternoon snack.

MAKES one 8-inch pound cake

1½ sticks (12 tablespoons or 170 g) unsalted butter, at room temperature

¾ cup (150 g) muscovado or dark brown sugar

½ cup (100 g) natural cane sugar, plus more for topping

2 teaspoons vanilla extract

1 teaspoon finely grated lemon zest

2 eggs, at room temperature

¾ cup (185 ml) whole-milk plain yogurt

¾ cup (105 g) superfine brown rice flour

⅓ cup (45 g) quinoa flour

¼ cup (25 g) almond flour

2 tablespoons tapioca starch

1 tablespoon poppy seeds

2 teaspoons baking powder

1 teaspoon ground ginger

½ teaspoon salt

4 nectarines, halved, pitted, and sliced

1 tablespoon slivered almonds

1 Preheat the oven to 350°F (180°C). Grease an 8-inch tube pan and line the bottom with parchment paper. Set aside.

2 Using a stand mixer, cream the butter, muscovado sugar, cane sugar, vanilla extract, and lemon zest on medium speed until light, about 3 minutes. Add the eggs, one at a time. Mix until combined. Stop the mixer and scrape the bowl. Add the yogurt and mix until combined.

3 In a medium bowl, whisk together the superfine brown rice flour, quinoa flour, almond flour, tapioca starch, poppy seeds, baking powder, ground ginger, and salt. Add the dry ingredients to the bowl of the mixer and mix on medium speed until it comes together into a creamy batter.

4 Scoop the batter into the greased pan and spread it evenly. Smooth out the top with a spatula as much as possible. Top with the sliced nectarines and sprinkle with the slivered almonds and more cane sugar.

5 Bake for 1 hour to 1 hour and 15 minutes, until a toothpick inserted in the center comes out clean. Let the cake cool in the pan completely before inverting it onto a cooling rack. Store at room temperature for up to 1 day, or refrigerate for up to 3 days. The cake may also be frozen for up to 1 month.

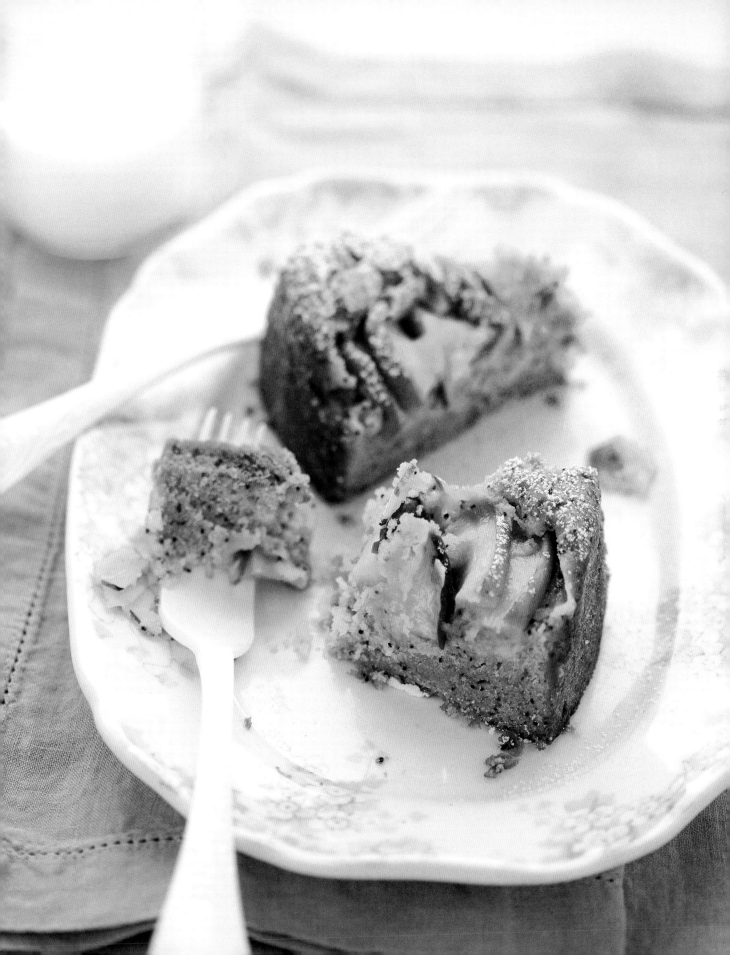

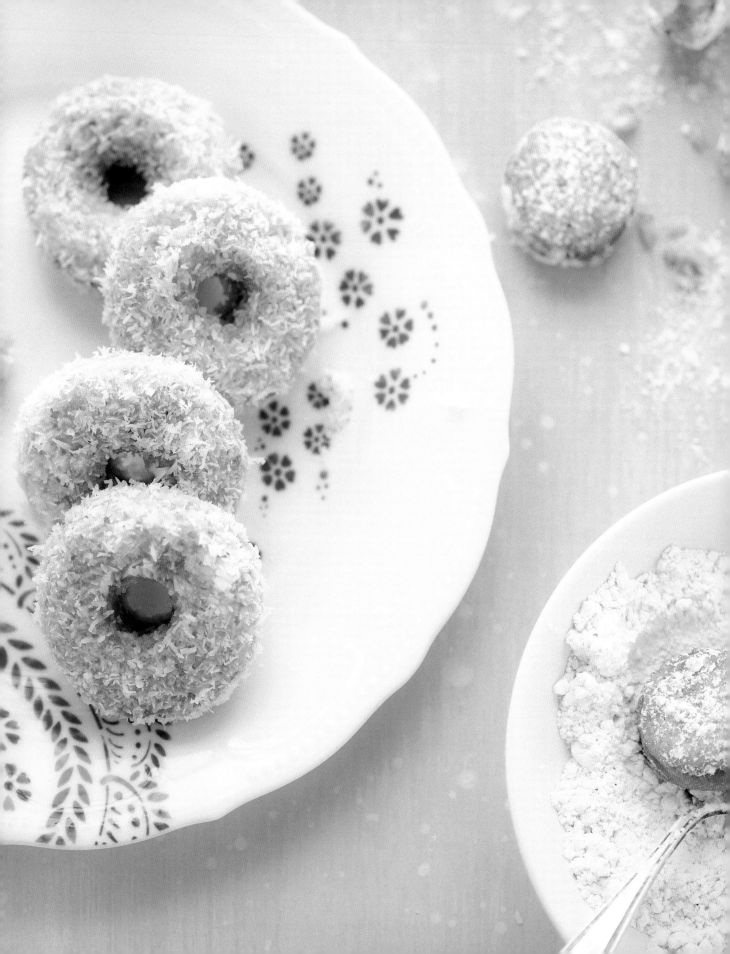

coconut doughnuts

THESE DOUGHNUTS ARE INSANELY MOIST. I promise you, they melt in your mouth. My friends can never get enough of them. This cake doughnut recipe is very simple to make. I store the doughnuts glazed in the freezer for sugar-craving moments.

Once the doughnuts are fried, they can be glazed with Coconut Glaze or any other glaze you like, or dusted with superfine sugar.

MAKES twenty 2-inch doughnuts and 20 doughnut holes

make the doughnuts

1   In a medium bowl, whisk together the first six ingredients. In a large bowl, whisk together the superfine brown rice flour, almond flour, potato starch, coconut flour, tapioca starch, baking powder, baking soda, and salt. Add the wet ingredients to the dry and whisk until the dough comes together. Knead it with your hands a couple of times. It will be soft.

2   Dust a work surface with a generous amount of superfine brown rice flour. Turn the dough out onto your work surface and dust another bit of flour on top of the dough. Pat the dough down a bit. As the dough sits, it will start to get a bit more compact and will be easier to work with. If it feels too soft, you can refrigerate the dough for 15 minutes. Roll the dough to a ¾-inch thickness.

3   Dust a 2-inch cookie cutter or doughnut cutter with additional flour. Cut out circles and place them on a baking sheet lined with parchment paper. If you are using a cookie cutter, cut out ½-inch holes from the center of the disks. You can re-roll the scraps once to make more doughnuts.

4   Chill the doughnuts in the refrigerator for 15 minutes. Meanwhile, fill a shallow cast-iron pan with 2 inches of vegetable oil. Heat the oil until it reads 340°F (170°C) on a candy thermometer or instant-read thermometer.

5   Carefully add the doughnuts to the oil in batches; do not overcrowd the pan. The doughnuts will sink and then rise when they are almost done. Cook to golden brown, turning the doughnuts once. Transfer to a baking sheet lined with paper towels. Repeat the frying process with the doughnut holes. Let them cool slightly.

make the glaze and finish the doughnuts

In a medium bowl, whisk together all the glaze ingredients. Dip the doughnuts in the glaze and cover with the shredded coconut.

COCONUT DOUGHNUTS

2 eggs, at room temperature

½ cup (100 g) natural cane sugar

1¼ cups (310 ml) unsweetened coconut milk

2 tablespoons freshly squeezed lemon juice

2 teaspoons coconut extract

¼ cup (60 ml) coconut oil, melted

1¼ cups (175 g) superfine brown rice flour, plus more for dusting

1 cup plus 1 tablespoon (110 g) almond flour

½ cup (80 g) potato starch

½ cup (60 g) coconut flour

¼ cup (30 g) tapioca starch

2 teaspoons baking powder

1 teaspoon baking soda

1 teaspoon salt

Vegetable oil, for frying

COCONUT GLAZE

2 cups (240 g) powdered sugar, sifted

¼ cup plus 1 tablespoon (75 ml) unsweetened coconut milk

Pinch of salt

2 cups (165 g) unsweetened shredded coconut

cardamom & vanilla bean yogurt pops with red berry consommé

THIS IS THE PERFECT DESSERT TO MAKE with help from your children. Have them help stir the yogurt into the simple syrup and pour it into the molds. Inserting the sticks seems to be my kids' favorite part of the entire process. Serve the pops as is or on top of the refreshing berry consommé and garnished with fresh berries.

SERVES 6

CARDAMOM AND VANILLA BEAN YOGURT POPS

¾ cup (100 g) ripe strawberries, hulled and diced

½ cup plus 2 tablespoons (130 g) natural cane sugar

2 teaspoons freshly squeezed lemon juice

1 vanilla bean, split lengthwise and seeds scraped

4 cardamom pods, crushed

1 cup (250 ml) whole-milk Greek-style yogurt

RED BERRY CONSOMMÉ

1 pound (450 g) ripe red berries (strawberries work well; raspberries and/or currants may be mixed in)

¼ cup (50 g) natural cane sugar

1 tablespoon freshly squeezed lemon juice

make the pops

1   Place six shot glasses in the freezer to chill. In a small saucepan, toss together the strawberries, 2 tablespoons of the sugar, and the lemon juice. Let the mixture sit at room temperature for 15 minutes, until the strawberries start to release their juices. Bring the saucepan to the stove and cook over medium heat for 3 minutes. Puree the mixture in a food processor or blender and strain it into a clean bowl. Refrigerate for 15 minutes.

2   Pour small amounts of the chilled strawberry puree along the insides of the frozen shot glasses. Return to the freezer.

3   In a small saucepan, combine ½ cup (125 ml) water, the remaining ½ cup (100 g) sugar, vanilla bean and seeds, and cardamom pods. Cook over medium-high heat until the sugar dissolves. Remove the pan from the heat and let the syrup steep for 15 minutes. Strain the syrup and discard the cardamom and vanilla bean.

4   Whisk the yogurt into the syrup and refrigerate the mixture for 15 minutes. When chilled, carefully pour the yogurt mixture into the frozen shot glasses. Return the shot glasses to the freezer for 15 minutes. Then insert Popsicle sticks and freeze until solid.

make the consommé

1   Combine all the ingredients in a medium heatproof bowl. Tightly cover the bowl with plastic wrap. Place the bowl over a pot filled partway with simmering water and let the mixture cook for 1 hour. The plastic wrap will poof up, which is fine, but make sure the bowl continues to be tightly wrapped. The berries will start to release their juices.

2   Remove the plastic wrap and strain the liquid into a clean bowl. The juice will be bright red and clear. Do not press the fruit against the strainer or the consommé will become cloudy with the fruit pulp. You want to keep it clear. Chill the consommé for 30 minutes.

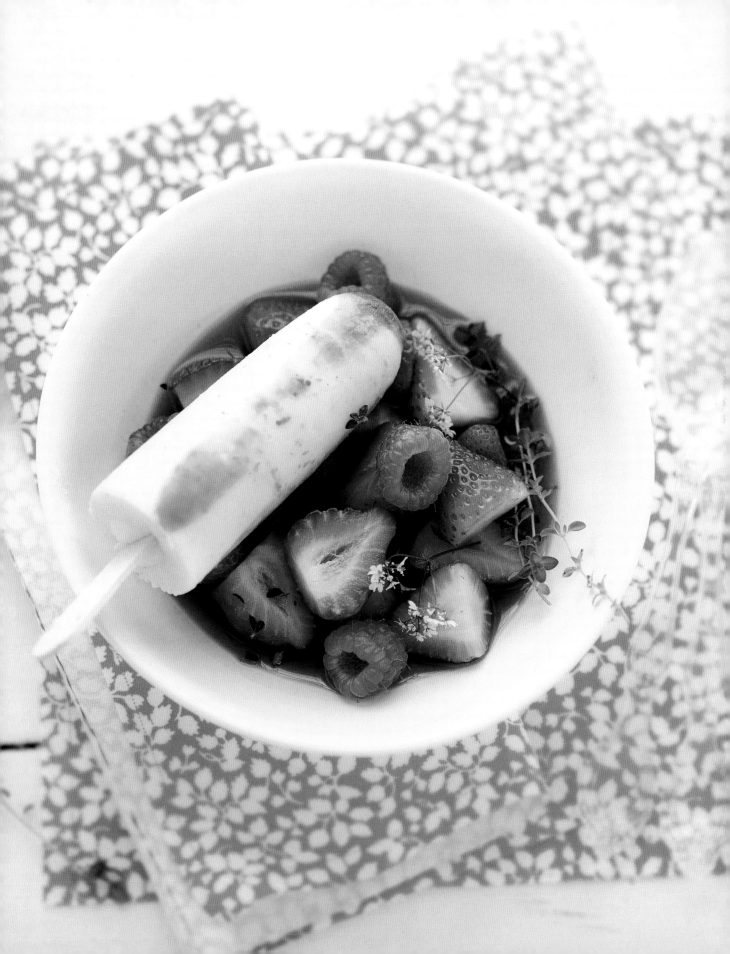

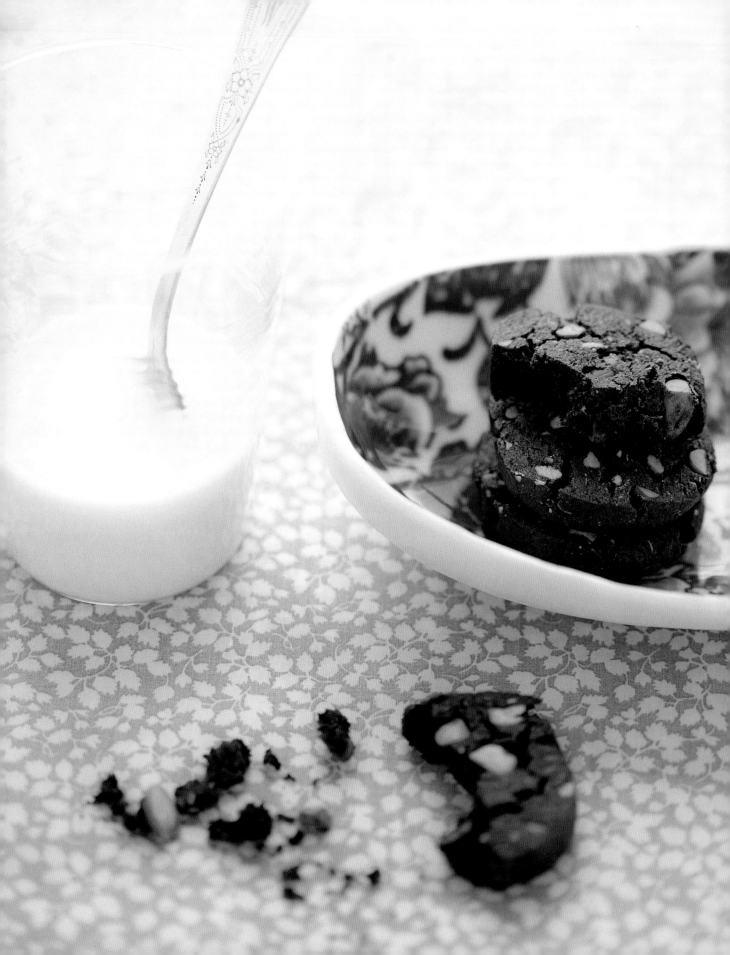

chocolate, quinoa & pistachio chunk cookies

DURING THE SUMMER, MOST OF MY BAKING involves all the wonderful stone fruits and berries that are available, but every so often I get intense chocolate cravings. This recipe satisfies those cravings: rich, deep chocolate cookies flavored with buckwheat and studded with pistachios and quinoa flakes.

I use a combination of Dutch-process and black cocoa powders. The black cocoa powder adds a darker color, as well as extra moistness and a fudgy texture. It can be found at specialty shops. I order mine online from King Arthur Flour. If you cannot find black cocoa powder, use Dutch-process for the entire amount of cocoa powder needed.

This recipe may easily be halved, although it is always great to have extra dough in the freezer for sudden cookie cravings.

MAKES about 33 cookies

1   In the bowl of a stand mixer, using the paddle attachment, cream together the butter, cane sugar, and brown sugar for about 2 minutes on medium speed. Add the eggs one at a time and continue mixing. Add the vanilla extract. Stop the mixer and scrape the sides and bottom of the bowl.

2   In a medium bowl, whisk together the superfine brown rice flour, buckwheat flour, quinoa flour, cocoa powders, tapioca starch, baking soda, and salt. Add to the wet ingredients and mix until it forms a dough.

3   Add the pistachios and quinoa flakes. Mix until incorporated.

4   Turn the dough out onto a work surface. Divide the dough in two and place each half over a sheet of parchment paper. Roll into logs that are approximately 11 inches long and 1½ inches in diameter. Roll the logs in the parchment and chill them for 30 minutes to 1 hour or until firm. The raw cookie logs may also be frozen for up to 3 months, tightly wrapped with plastic wrap.

5   Preheat the oven to 350°F (180°C). Cut each log into disks that are about ⅓ inch thick. Place the cookies on baking sheets lined with parchment paper or silicone mats. Bake for 8 to 10 minutes. They might not look like they are done, but as they cool, they will harden. It is best to slightly underbake them. They will be moist and fudgy. Let them cool on the baking sheet. Store in an airtight container at room temperature for up to 3 days.

1 stick (8 tablespoons or 110 g) unsalted butter, at room temperature

¾ cup (150 g) natural cane sugar

½ cup (100 g) light brown sugar

2 eggs

1 teaspoon vanilla extract

1 cup (140 g) superfine brown rice flour

½ cup (70 g) buckwheat flour

½ cup (70 g) quinoa flour

¼ cup (25 g) Dutch-process cocoa powder

¼ cup (25 g) black cocoa powder

¼ cup (30 g) tapioca starch

1½ teaspoons baking soda

½ teaspoon salt

1 cup (160 g) unsalted natural pistachios, coarsely chopped

½ cup (50 g) quinoa flakes

summer berry & buckwheat galette

THIS IS ONE OF THE SIMPLEST WAYS to make a delicious fruit tart. No need for a mold. I personally love the look of a messy galette. For this version I use golden, red, and black raspberries, as well as wild strawberries that I grow in my garden.

SERVES 6 to 8

BUCKWHEAT CRUST

¾ cup (105 g) superfine brown rice flour, plus more for dusting

¼ cup (40 g) potato starch

¼ cup (35 g) buckwheat flour

4 teaspoons natural cane sugar

⅛ teaspoon salt

1 stick (8 tablespoons or 110 g) cold unsalted butter, cut into ½-inch cubes

1 egg yolk

3 to 5 tablespoons ice water

SUMMER BERRY FILLING

3½ cups (450 g) assorted berries

¼ cup (50 g) natural cane sugar

1 vanilla bean, split lengthwise and seeds scraped

1 teaspoon finely grated lemon zest

GALETTE ASSEMBLY

¼ cup (25 g) almond flour

make the crust

1   Combine the first five ingredients in a food processor. Pulse once or twice to combine. Add the cold butter and pulse ten times. You will end up with small pieces of butter that are visible throughout.

2   In a small bowl, whisk together the egg yolk and 3 tablespoons ice water. Add it to the dough and pulse until it comes together. Add up to 2 more tablespoons ice water, if needed.

3   Turn the dough out onto a work surface, knead it a couple of times, and form a disk. Wrap in plastic wrap, flatten it, and refrigerate for 1 hour. Meanwhile, prepare the filling.

prepare the filling

Toss together the berries, sugar, vanilla bean seeds, and lemon zest in a medium bowl. Let macerate while the dough chills.

assemble the galette

1   Remove the chilled dough from the refrigerator, unwrap it, and place it on a work surface that has been dusted with superfine brown rice flour. Roll the dough to a circle that is ¼ inch thick. Keep rotating the dough while rolling to prevent it from sticking to the surface. Transfer to a baking sheet lined with parchment paper.

2   Cut a circle of dough that is approximately 10 inches in diameter.

3   Sprinkle the almond flour in the center of the dough. Pile the filling on top of the almond flour, leaving 2 to 3 inches of space around the border. Fold the edges over the filling. If the dough cracks, simply pinch it back together. Chill the galette in the refrigerator for 15 minutes.

4   Preheat the oven to 425°F (220°C). Bake the galette for 30 to 40 minutes, until the filling is bubbling and the crust fully baked. Let it cool on the baking sheet for 10 minutes before cutting. Serve warm or at room temperature.

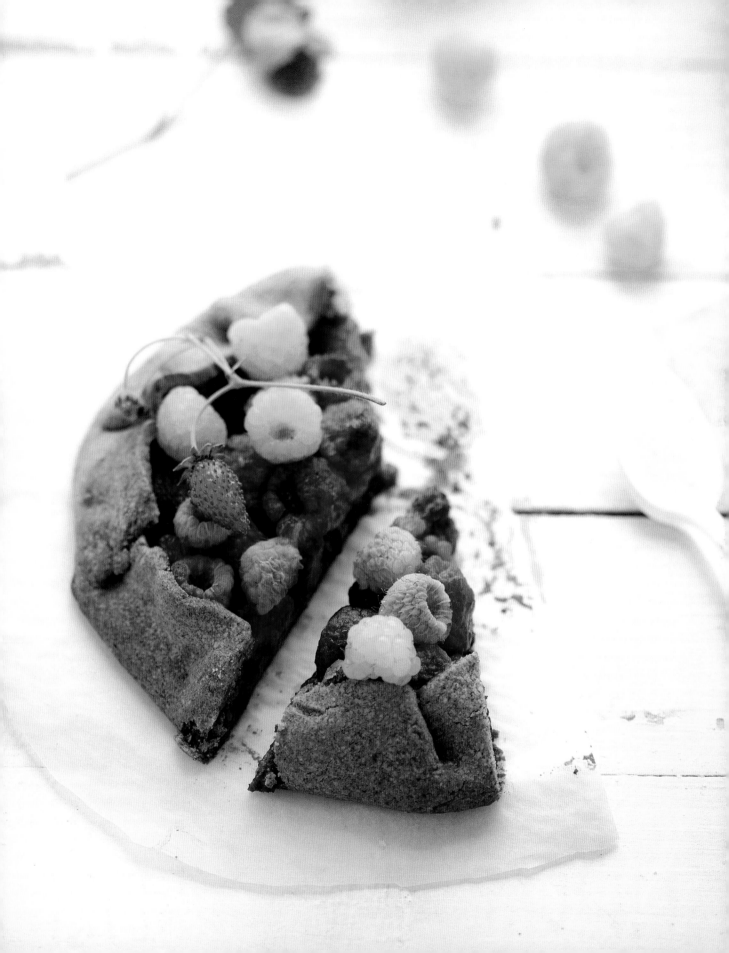

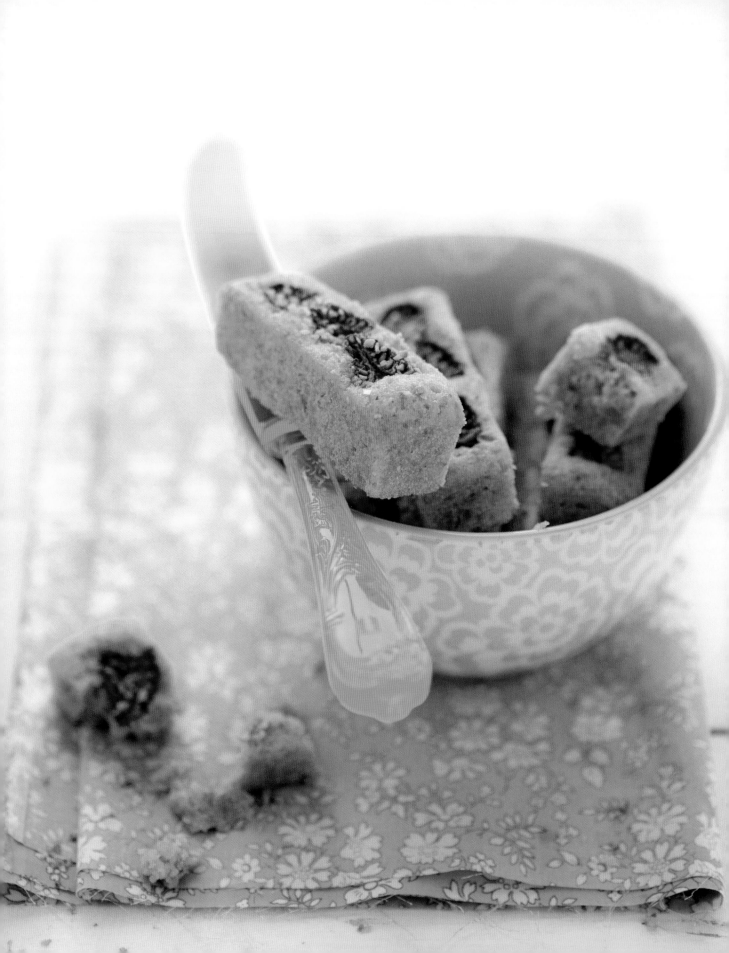

raspberry, pistachio & oat *financiers*

FINANCIERS **ARE THE EASIEST CAKES** to make gluten-free, as their main ingredients are ground-up nuts. Traditionally, ground almonds are used, but in this recipe I use pistachios and oats. The mini rectangular cakes are baked in a silicone mold, but you may also use a muffin pan lined with baking papers.

MAKES 12 rectangular or 10 muffin-size *financiers*

1 Preheat the oven to 350°F (180°C).

2 In a small saucepan, heat the butter over medium-high heat until the milk solids start to brown on the bottom and the butter smells nutty. Strain the brown butter through a fine-mesh sieve and let it cool to room temperature.

3 Combine the sugar, pistachios, oat flour, lemon zest, and salt in a food processor. Pulse until the pistachios are chopped to a fine powder. Transfer to a clean bowl, add the egg whites, and whisk to combine. Add the cooled brown butter and whisk until a uniform mixture forms.

4 Spoon the batter into the molds, filling them halfway full. Gently press in the raspberries.

5 Bake for 20 to 25 minutes, until the tops are lightly golden. Let the *financiers* cool at room temperature before unmolding. They may be stored at room temperature for 1 day and will keep in the refrigerator for up to 3 days. They may also be frozen, tightly wrapped, for up to 1 month.

1¼ sticks (10 tablespoons or 140 g) unsalted butter

½ cup (100 g) natural cane sugar

½ cup (80 g) unsalted natural pistachios

½ cup (50 g) gluten-free oat flour

1 teaspoon finely grated lemon zest

¼ teaspoon salt

4 egg whites

¾ cup (110 g) raspberries

peach & buttermilk sherbet

I HAVE MANY DIFFERENT SHERBET RECIPES in my repertoire and had a difficult time selecting which ones would make the cut here. However, there was never any doubt about this recipe. I absolutely love the tang and creaminess that buttermilk adds to this sherbet. I make multiple variations on this recipe using other stone fruits and even raspberries.

SERVES 6 to 8

1 cup (200 g) natural cane sugar

4 large (1¾ pounds or 795 g) peaches, peeled, pitted, and quartered

3 tablespoons freshly squeezed lemon juice

1½ cups (375 ml) low-fat buttermilk

½ teaspoon salt

1   In a small saucepan, cook the sugar and ½ cup (125 ml) water until the sugar is dissolved. Pour into a bowl and let it cool to room temperature.

2   In a food processor or blender, puree the peaches with the lemon juice. Transfer to a large bowl. Add the sugar syrup, buttermilk, and salt. Whisk to combine. Cover with plastic wrap and chill in the refrigerator for 2 hours.

3   Churn in your ice cream machine according to the manufacturer's instructions. Transfer to a freezer-safe container and freeze for at least 4 hours, until solid. Before serving, place the sherbet in the refrigerator for 15 minutes to soften.

PEELING PEACHES

My family has always been big into canning and preserving. We always had glass jars of preserved food at home, whether it was jam made from fresh-picked blackberries or fresh tomatoes poached in olive oil. I have vivid memories of spending summer mornings making peach jam with my mom, peeling and cutting cases of ripe peaches, the old wooden cutting board covered in golden, peachy juice.

This is a trick my mother taught me for peeling large amounts of stone fruits and tomatoes:

Find a large pot that will hold all your fruit. If you do not have one, you will have to do it in batches, which is fine. Fill the pot with water and bring it to a boil over high heat. In the meantime, cut a small cross on the bottom of the fruit with a paring knife. Fill a large bowl with ice water.

Carefully place the fruit into the boiling water, making sure it is fully submerged. Blanch the fruit for anywhere from 30 seconds to 1 minute, depending on how ripe and soft the fruit is (the softer the fruit, the shorter the blanching time). Immediately drain the fruit in a large colander and transfer to the ice bath to stop the cooking process. Once the fruit is cooled, remove it from the ice bath. The skin should then come right off.

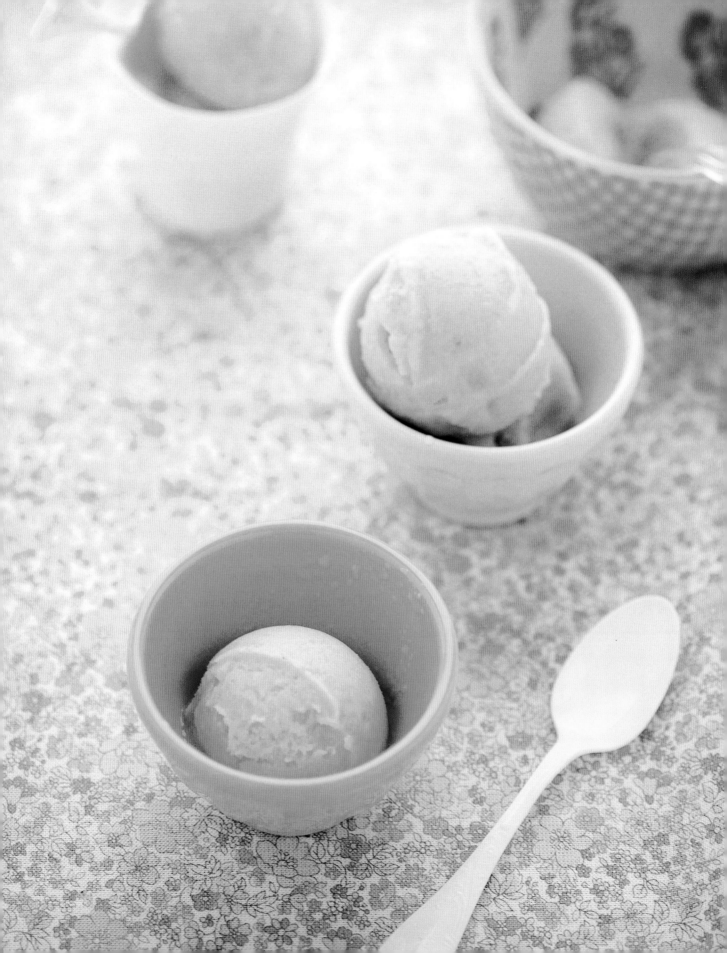

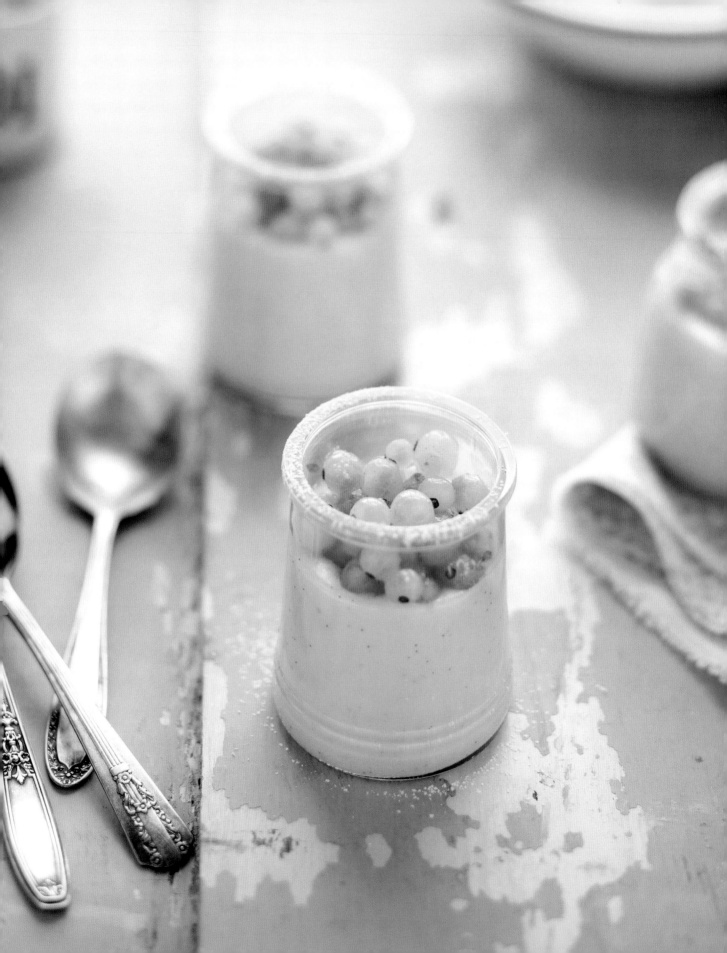

basque vanilla pudding

THIS BASQUE VERSION of the traditional vanilla pudding is called *natillas*. We craved it as kids. My grandmother used to make it with raw milk and fresh eggs from the farm. The milk is infused with a million tiny vanilla specks, lemon zest, and a slight hint of cardamom.

SERVES 8

1 In a medium saucepan, combine the whole milk, ¼ cup (50 g) of the sugar, vanilla bean and seeds, cardamom pods, and lemon zest. Bring this mixture to a simmer over medium heat.

2 Meanwhile, whisk together the egg yolks, the remaining ½ cup sugar, and cornstarch in a medium bowl. Add the heavy cream and whisk until combined.

3 Pour the hot milk mixture a little at a time into the egg yolk mixture while whisking. Strain this custard back into the saucepan. Discard the vanilla bean, zest, and cardamom. Heat the custard over medium heat while stirring with a wooden spoon until it reaches a boil. Continue cooking until it thickens, about 2 minutes. It will be thinner than standard vanilla pudding. Pour the hot custard immediately into 8 (4-ounce) ramekins or jars.

4 Let the custard cool at room temperature for 30 minutes, cover the jars with plastic wrap, and chill in the refrigerator for 2 hours. The custard might develop a thin skin, which is fine.

5 The puddings will keep in the refrigerator for up to 3 days. Serve topped with berries and chopped pistachios.

2 cups (500 ml) whole milk

½ cup (100 g) natural cane sugar

1 vanilla bean, split lengthwise and seeds scraped

2 cardamom pods, cracked

Zest of ½ lemon

6 egg yolks

4 teaspoons cornstarch

1 cup (250 ml) heavy cream

1 cup (150 g) assorted berries (currants, raspberries, strawberries, and so on), for garnish

Unsalted natural pistachios, chopped, for garnish

SUBSTITUTING DAIRY

When I was first diagnosed with an autoimmune disorder, I was advised to remove all gluten and casein proteins from my diet to reduce inflammation in my body. I quickly found alternatives to both.

When it comes to substituting dairy in desserts, I find that unsweetened coconut milk is the best option. I use it often for its high fat content, creaminess, and natural sweetness.

For custard and ice cream recipes, I like to use a combination of unsweetened coconut and almond milks. Coconut and olive oils can easily be substituted for butter in cake recipes and non-hydrogenated shortening in tart crusts.

I often make a dairy-free version of this *natillas* recipe. I use 2 cups (500 ml) unsweetened coconut milk and 1 cup (250 ml) almond milk in place of the milk and heavy cream.

cherry cheesecake ice cream & ice cream sandwiches

WHEN I WAS SIXTEEN, I CAME TO THE United States to spend a summer with the Bryant family in Colorado Springs. After my first week there, I knew that "summer" would turn into a year. I fell in love with the family, and even though my parents were a bit sad to be apart from me for so long, they allowed me to stay. In many ways, I wouldn't be here today if it weren't for the Bryants. They taught me not to take myself so seriously, and most important, they introduced me to my husband, Chad.

Aside from love, Robyn also introduced me to her blueberry cheesecake. Hers was nothing like the baked, rich, dark cheesecake I grew up with. It was a light, no-bake version, filled with cream cheese and heavy cream. I could not get enough. When that year ended and I returned home to my family, I took her blueberry cheesecake recipe with me. Friends still ask me about it twenty years later.

Later I found an ice cream version of the same cheesecake. My recipe uses a combination of mascarpone cheese and crème fraîche. I love that little bit of tanginess and richness that the crème fraîche adds and the texture of the crumbled cookies inside. Serve it scooped into a cup or as an ice cream sandwich with the shortbread cookies, which is how my kids like it.

SERVES 6 to 8

ALMOND SHORTBREAD
(MAKES 48 COOKIES)

1 stick (8 tablespoons or 110 g) unsalted butter, at room temperature

1 cup (200 g) natural cane sugar

2 teaspoons vanilla extract

1 egg, at room temperature

1¼ cups (175 g) superfine brown rice flour, plus more for dusting

1 cup plus 2 tablespoons (115 g) almond flour

¼ cup plus 2 tablespoons (60 g) potato starch

¼ cup (30 g) tapioca starch

½ teaspoon salt

make the shortbread

1   In a stand mixer, using the paddle attachment, cream the butter and sugar on medium speed until light and fluffy, about 2 minutes.

2   Add the vanilla extract and the egg. Mix until combined. Scrape the bottom and sides of the bowl.

3   In a separate bowl, whisk together the dry ingredients. Add them to the butter mixture on low speed. Mix until the dough comes together.

4   Divide the dough into two disks. Wrap each disk in plastic wrap and flatten it with your palms. You will need only one of the disks for this recipe, so the other one may be frozen at this point. Chill the other disk in the refrigerator for 30 minutes.

TIP: This recipe makes more shortbread than you will need for the ice cream. Freeze half of it for another time, or crumble it and use it as a pastry crust for a tart.

recipe continues

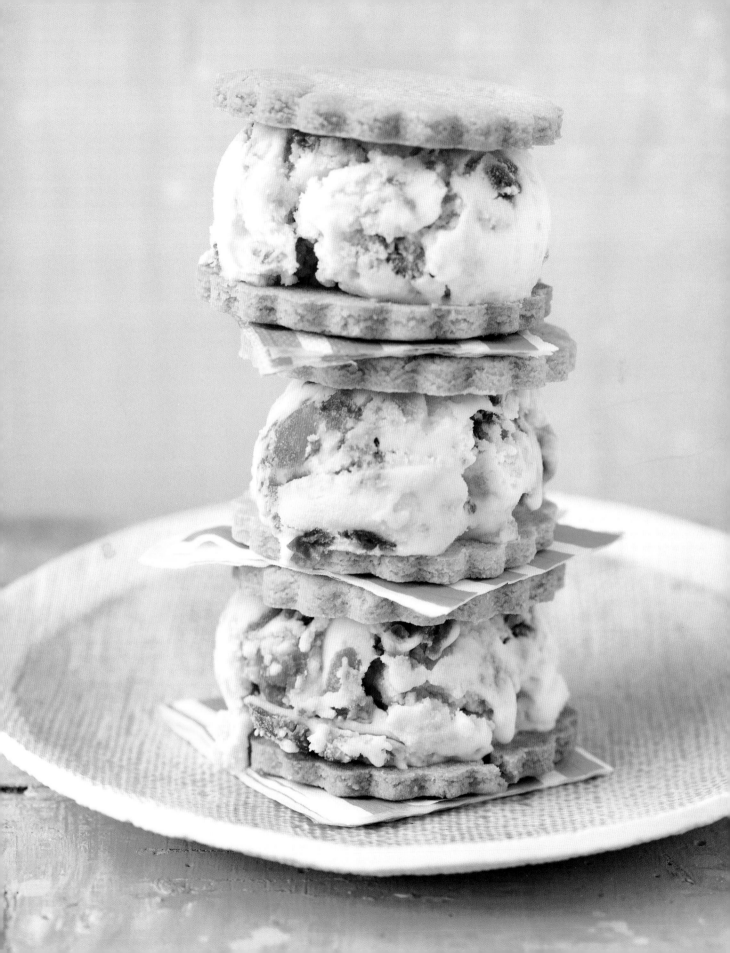

12 ounces (340 g) Bing cherries, stemmed and pitted

¼ cup (50 g) natural cane sugar

Juice of ½ lemon

CHERRY CHEESECAKE ICE CREAM (MAKES 1 QUART)

8 ounces (225 g) mascarpone cheese

8 ounces (225 g) crème fraîche

½ cup (125 ml) whole milk

½ cup plus 2 tablespoons (120 g) superfine sugar

Finely grated zest of ½ lemon

1 teaspoon vanilla extract

¼ teaspoon salt

6 Almond Shortbread cookies, crumbled

Cherry Sauce, drained and chopped

5 Preheat the oven to 350°F (180°C) with racks set on the upper and lower thirds. Remove the dough from the refrigerator and place it on a cold surface dusted with a bit of superfine brown rice flour. Using a rolling pin, roll the dough to a ¼- to ⅛-inch thickness. Move the dough around while rolling so that it doesn't stick to the work surface.

6 Cut circles using a 2-inch fluted cookie cutter and place them on two baking sheets lined with parchment paper. Re-roll the dough if necessary and cut more circles. You should end up with approximately 24 cookies.

7 Bake the cookies for 10 to 12 minutes, until lightly golden, rotating the pans halfway through. Let them cool completely.

8 Crush 6 cookies. You will fold these crumbs into the Cherry Cheesecake Ice Cream. Reserve the rest to make ice cream sandwiches.

make the cherry sauce

1 Combine all the ingredients in a medium saucepan. Cook over medium heat for about 7 minutes, until the cherries soften and the juices form a light syrup.

2 Transfer the cherry sauce to a clean bowl and refrigerate for 2 hours.

make the ice cream

1 Combine the mascarpone, crème fraîche, milk, sugar, lemon zest, vanilla, and salt in a blender and mix until smooth. Transfer to a bowl and refrigerate for 2 hours.

2 Churn the ice cream base in an ice cream maker according to the manufacturer's instructions. When it is done freezing, swirl in the cookie crumbs and the cherries. Do not over-fold or you will lose the swirl patterns.

3 Transfer to a freezer-safe container and freeze for at least 2 hours. Serve as is, or sandwich between Almond Shortbread cookies to make ice cream sandwiches.

peach & pistachio tart

THE FILLING IN THIS TART is a cross between frangipane and flan. It's soft and tender, and I love the bright, summery colors of green and peach.

MAKES one 9-inch tart

make the crust

1   In the bowl of a stand mixer, combine the butter and powdered sugar. Cream the mixture at medium speed for 2 minutes, until light and well combined. Add the vanilla seeds and lemon zest. Mix well.

2   Scrape the sides of the bowl. Add the egg and mix until well incorporated.

3   In a bowl, quickly whisk together the dry ingredients. Add them to the butter-egg mixture. Mix on medium speed until a soft dough forms (it will be similar to a soft cookie dough). Scrape the sides of the bowl well and mix until all the ingredients are well combined.

4   Divide the dough in two. Scrape each piece of dough onto a piece of plastic wrap and form it into a disk. Wrap the dough tightly and press down to flatten it slightly. Chill one of the disks in the refrigerator for at least 1½ hours. The other dough disk may be frozen at this time for later use. This is a versatile tart dough recipe and it is great to have on hand. To thaw out, simply leave it in the refrigerator overnight.

5   Dust a cold work surface, such as marble, with a bit of superfine brown rice flour. Place the dough disk on the surface and lightly dust the top with some more flour. Roll the dough to a ⅛-inch thickness. Make sure to rotate and move the dough around so it does not stick to the work surface. Fill a 9-inch tart mold with the dough. Gently press down the edges and cut off excess dough.

6   Refrigerate the dough for 30 minutes. Meanwhile, prepare the filling.

recipe continues

VANILLA SHORT DOUGH

- 2 sticks (16 tablespoons or 225 g) unsalted butter, at room temperature
- ¾ cup plus 1 tablespoon (100 g) powdered sugar, sifted
- 1 vanilla bean, split lengthwise and seeds scraped
- ½ teaspoon finely grated lemon zest
- 1 egg, at room temperature
- 1 cup (140 g) superfine brown rice flour, plus more for dusting
- ¾ cup (105 g) sorghum flour
- ½ cup (80 g) potato starch
- ½ cup (60 g) tapioca starch
- ½ teaspoon baking powder
- ¼ teaspoon salt

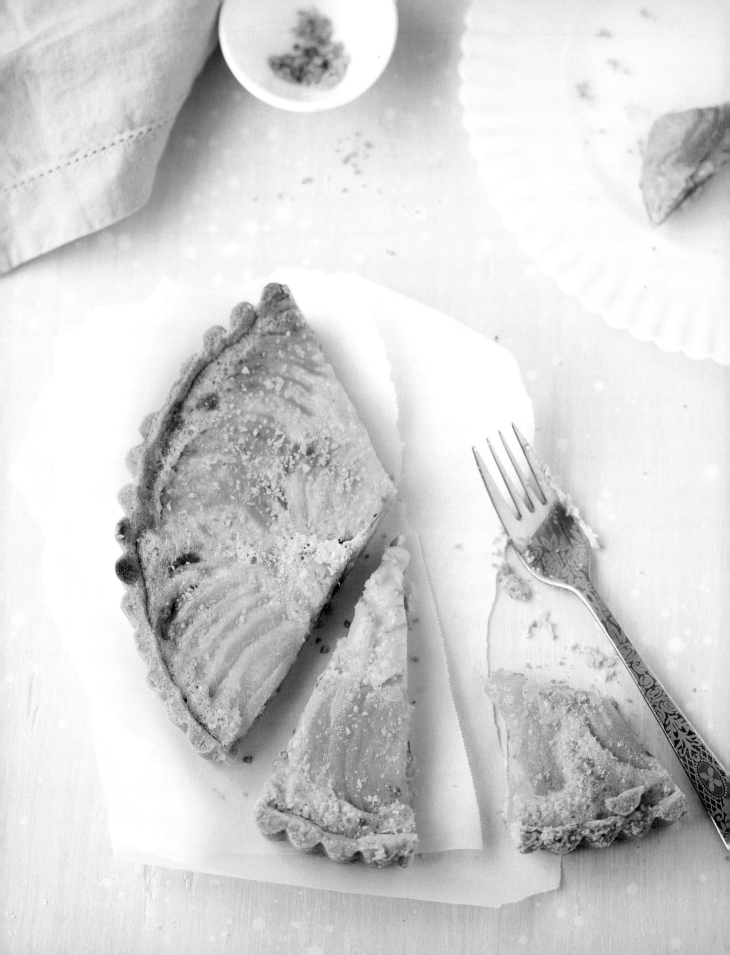

prepare the filling and bake the tart

1   Preheat the oven to 400°F (200°C).

2   Melt the butter in a small saucepan over medium heat and let it cool to room temperature.

3   Combine the pistachios, tapioca starch, and salt in the bowl of a food processor. Grind the mixture to a fine powder.

4   In a medium bowl, whisk together the eggs, sugar, ground-up pistachio mixture, and melted butter. Pour the pistachio filling into the prepared tart crust. Top with the sliced peaches.

5   Bake for 10 minutes. Reduce the oven heat to 350°F (180°C) and bake for an additional 30 minutes or so, until the filling is set and light golden brown.

6   Cool the tart on a cooling rack for 30 minutes before slicing. It may be refrigerated for up to 3 days or frozen for up to 1 month.

PEACH AND PISTACHIO FILLING AND TART ASSEMBLY

7 tablespoons (95 g) unsalted butter

¼ cup plus 1 tablespoon (50 g) unsalted natural pistachios

2 tablespoons tapioca starch

¼ teaspoon salt

2 eggs

¼ cup (50 g) natural cane sugar

5 small (1 pound or 450 g) ripe yet firm peaches, peeled, halved, pitted, and thinly sliced

red currant &
white chocolate slice

THIS IS THE SHEET CAKE RECIPE that I use when I want to have some basic cake for trifles, birthday cakes, or simple strawberry shortcake. I always have some of this in the freezer so I can throw together a last-minute dessert. I have added red currants and shaved white chocolate pieces to this cake, making it slightly sweet-and-sour. It is moist and perfectly crumbly.

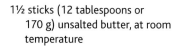

MAKES one 13 by 9-inch pan

1½ sticks (12 tablespoons or 170 g) unsalted butter, at room temperature

1 cup (200 g) natural cane sugar

⅓ cup (70 g) light brown sugar

3 eggs, at room temperature

1 teaspoon vanilla extract

1 cup (140 g) superfine brown rice flour

½ cup (80 g) potato starch

⅓ cup (45 g) sorghum flour

¼ cup (30 g) tapioca starch

¼ cup (25 g) almond flour

1¼ teaspoons baking powder

1 teaspoon salt

3 ounces (90 g) white chocolate, chopped

1½ cups (225 g) red currants

1 Preheat the oven to 350°F (180°C). In the bowl of a stand mixer, cream the butter, cane sugar, and light brown sugar together on medium-high speed until light, about 3 minutes. Add the eggs, one at a time, and mix until combined. Add the vanilla extract and mix well. Scrape the sides of the bowl and mix well.

2 In a separate bowl, whisk together the superfine brown rice flour, potato starch, sorghum flour, tapioca starch, almond flour, baking powder, and salt. Add the dry ingredients to the butter mixture and mix until it comes together. Add the chopped white chocolate and 1 cup (150 g) of the red currants. Gently fold them into the batter.

3 Transfer the batter to a greased 13 by 9-inch cake pan. Spread the batter evenly and smooth out the top with an offset spatula. Stud the cake with the remaining ½ cup (75 g) red currants.

4 Bake the cake for 35 to 40 minutes, until golden brown and a toothpick inserted in the center comes out clean. Let the cake cool in the pan completely before cutting. The cake will keep in the refrigerator for 3 days, or it may be tightly wrapped and frozen for up to 3 months.

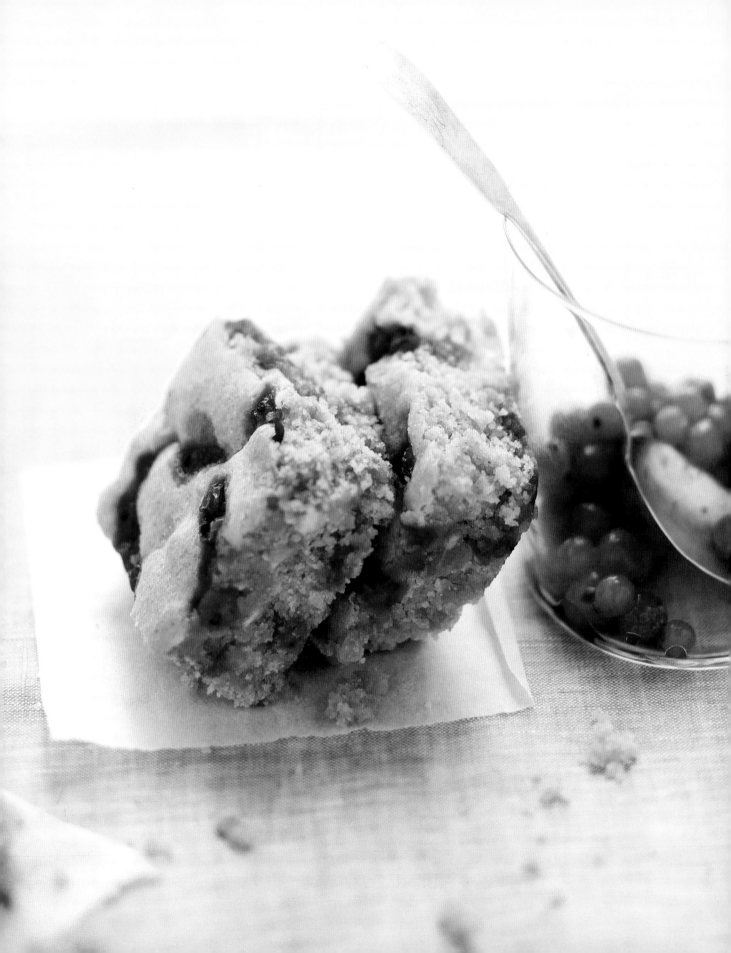

acknowledgments

Thank you to Jon and Miren for being the reason I wake up every day, for putting a smile on my face, and for allowing me to be open and vulnerable. To Chad, who has given me what I treasure most in life, our children, thank you for encouraging me to reach goals that I didn't even know I had.

Thank you to my mom—*eskerrik asko, amatxu*—for always having a pot of food on the stove and for showing me beauty in the subtle details in life. And to my dad (*aitatxu*) for instilling in me a love for the arts and nature. Through both of you I have learned empathy and self-discipline.

Thanks to my family and friends in the Basque Country, who have remained close in spite of the distance between us; to Jokin and Jon, who are my pivot points; to Bego for the best $850 I ever spent; and to Kuadrilla for bringing out the child in me. *Eskerrik asko.*

A special thank-you to Jill and the Bryant family for putting up with me for a whole year and opening my eyes to a new way of being and experiencing life. To my friend Nadia Dole, warm thanks for generosity, patience, and opening your home to me while I worked on this book.

I am grateful to Hilda Smagorinsky for all the hours spent on babysitting duty while we walked the streets of New York City.

To my editor, Michael Sand, thank you for such a smooth collaborative process. Thanks to everyone at Little, Brown and Company for helping create this beautiful book.

A big thank-you to my agent, Judy Linden, for pushing me out of my comfort zone and allowing me to see what I am capable of, and to Amy Atlas for introducing me to the Stonesong family. They have all been very supportive.

Thanks to my recipe testers: Regan Burns-Cafiso, Lauren Jones, Jenny Howard, Kate Ramos, and Vanessa Seder.

Most important, thank you to all the *Cannelle et Vanille* readers who have supported my work throughout the years. This book would not have happened if it weren't for you.

resources

ALTER ECO
Fair-trade grains and other products. My favorite brand of quinoa.
www.altereco-usa.com

ANDEAN DREAM
Quinoa pasta that has great texture.
www.andeandream.com

ANTHROPOLOGIE
Some of my favorite housewares.
www.anthropologie.com

ARROWHEAD MILLS
Great source for gluten-free flours.
www.arrowheadmills.com

AUTHENTIC FOODS
My favorite superfine brown rice flour and other gluten-free flours and baking mixes.
www.authenticfoods.com

BOB'S RED MILL
Another great source for gluten-free flours, whole grains, and baking mixes.
www.bobsredmill.com

CAROLINE SWIFT
British ceramist with delicate bone china spoons and bowls.
www.carolineswift.com

FANCY FLOURS
Great source for baking papers and cake-decorating supplies.
www.fancyflours.com

FRONTIER
Organic, fair-trade vanilla beans that I buy in bulk.
www.frontiercoop.com

INDIAN TREE
Great source for specialty sugars, salts, and spices. This is where I get superfine (caster) and muscovado sugars.
www.indiantree.com

JB PRINCE
Specialty kitchen products like silicone molds, bakeware, knives, and tart molds.
www.jbprince.com

LA TIENDA
Online shop featuring specialty products from Spain, including meats, cheeses, canned goods, and olive oils.
www.tienda.com

MOLLY HATCH
Unique ceramics with signature floral patterns.
www.mollyhatch.com

MUD AUSTRALIA
Modern dinnerware with clean lines.
www.mudaustralia.com

RANCHO GORDO
My favorite brand of heirloom dried beans.
www.ranchogordo.com

SABRE
Colorful and fun flatware from France.
www.sabre.fr

SAMANTHA ROBINSON
Australian ceramist with beautiful floral patterns and one-of-a-kind pieces.
www.samantharobinson.com.au

SHILOH FARMS
Another great source for gluten-free flours and whole grains.
www.shilohfarms.com

SHOP HORNE
Great source for modern housewares and dinnerware.
www.shophorne.com

STARWEST BOTANICALS
Organic bulk herbs and spices.
www.starwest-botanicals.com

SUITE ONE STUDIO
Ceramics by Lindsay Emery with clean lines and beautiful colors.
www.etsy.com/shop/suiteonestudio

SUR LA TABLE
Specialty kitchen shop for bakeware and utensils in general.
www.surlatable.com

WILLIAMS-SONOMA
Another great kitchen shop for bakeware, specialty ingredients, and cookbooks.
www.williams-sonoma.com

index

Page numbers in *italic* refer to illustrations.

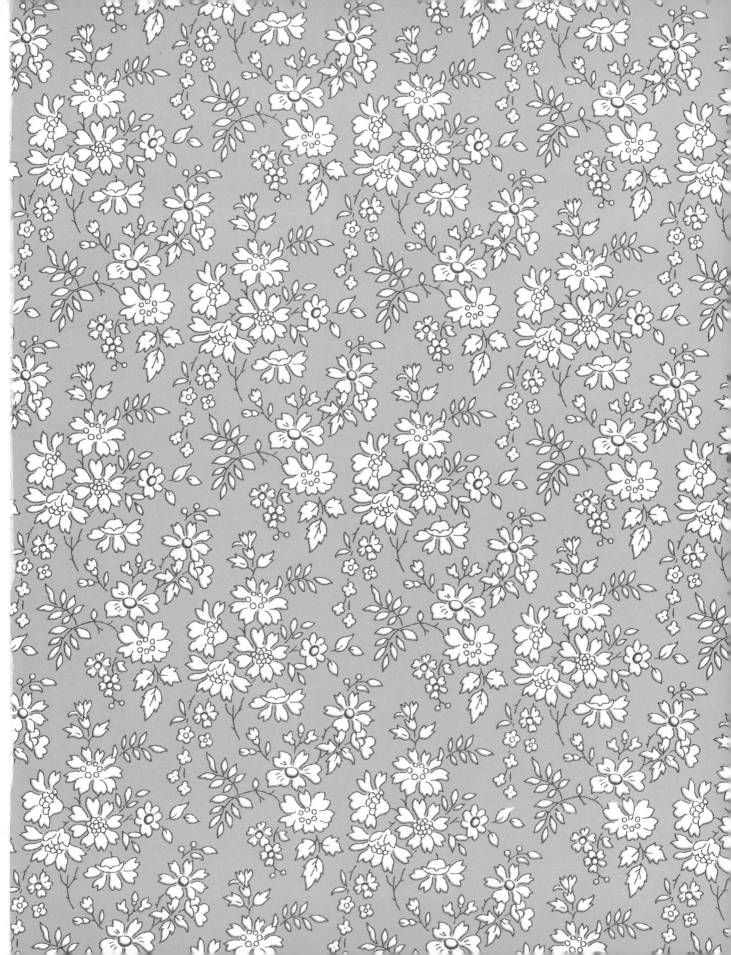

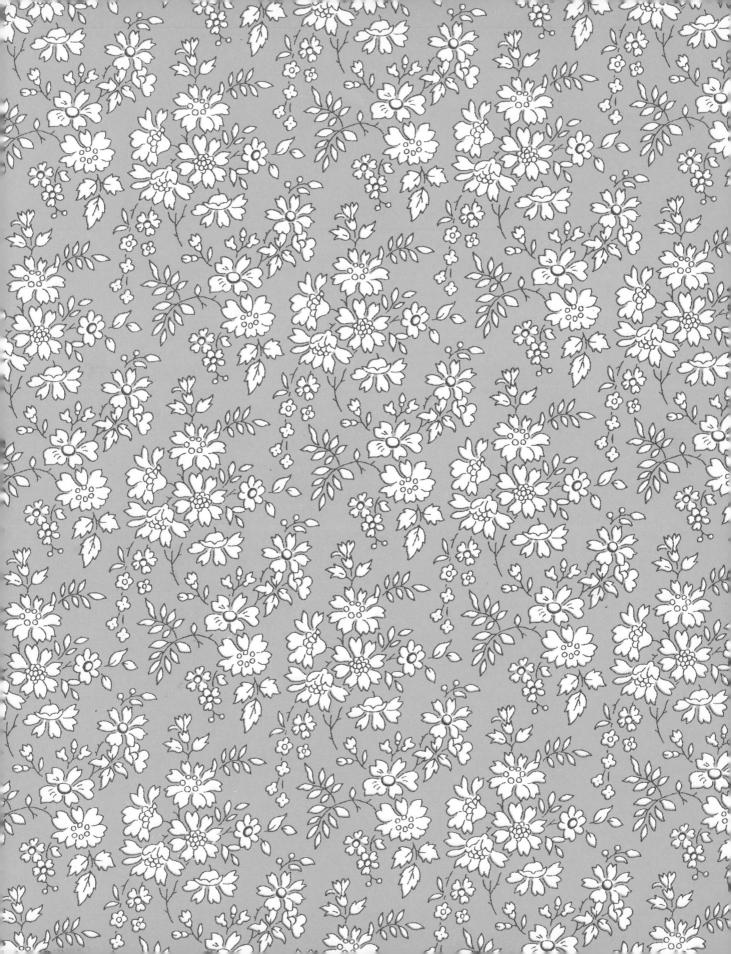